The Way Forward for Chinese Medicine

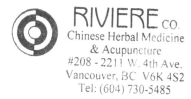

The Way Forward for Chinese Medicine

Edited by

Kelvin Chan

*Institute for the Advancement of
Chinese Medicine
School of Chinese Medicine Hong Kong
Baptist University Hong Kong SAR,
Peoples Republic of China*

and

Henry Lee

*School of Biological, Environmental
and Health Sciences
Middlesex University London, UK*

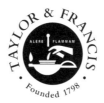

London and New York

First published 2002
by Taylor & Francis
11 New Fetter Lane, London EC4P 4EE

Simultaneously published in the USA and Canada
by Taylor & Francis Inc,
29 West 35th Street, New York, NY 10001

Taylor & Francis is an imprint of the Taylor & Francis Group

Typeset by EXPO Holdings, Malaysia
Printed and bound in Malta by Gutenberg Press Ltd.

Every effort has been made to ensure that the advice and information
in this book is true and accurate at the time of going to press.
However, neither the publisher nor the authors can accept any legal
responsibility or liability for any errors or omissions that may be
made. In the case of drug administration, any medical procedure or
the use of technical equipment mentioned within this book, you are
strongly advised to consult the manufacturer's guidelines.

British Library Cataloguing in Publication Data
A catalogue record for this book is available from the British Library

Library of Congress Cataloging in Publication Data
A catalogue record has been requested

ISBN: 0-415-27720-5

Contents

List of Illustrations

List of Tables

Foreword

I was made aware of this book project when several of the internationally well-known scientists and practitioners gathered together in a vigorous discussion on Chinese Medicine in the coffee shop of a hotel (opposite the famous Confucius Temple; Fu-Zi Miao) in Nanjing, China in the evening of 11th July 1998. We were attending the International Symposium on the Modernisation of Traditional Chinese Medicine (10 to 12 July 1999) there.

Describing to various colleagues in the group (Professors Ke-ji Chen, Pei-gen Xiao and Hin-wing Yeung, Dr Rance Ye and others), Professor Kelvin Chan, a renowned biomedical scientist in the fields of biopharmaceutical and botanical medicines, reported his co-ordination of work on Chinese medicine as described in the book. He explained to us briefly that he was editing a book entitled *The Way Forward For Chinese Medicine*. This project aimed to find out how Chinese medicine is being practised, researched and how its practitioners are being trained in several developed and developing countries and regions all over the world. It will certainly have an impact on the appropriate promotion of Chinese medicine. Professor Chan also wanted to secure some up-to-date applied and clinical research papers for the title. The discussion touched upon several aspects of progress and modernisation of Chinese medicine as supported by the Chinese government.

Chinese medicine is an integral part of the Chinese culture. Over the centuries, various activities and aspects of practising Chinese medicine have made tremendous contributions to the prosperity of the Chinese nation. Its great vitality is demonstrated by the fact that, when compared with other traditional medicine, it's use has never declined over the past several thousand years. During the past fifty years, the Chinese government has advocated "To integrate Chinese and orthodox medicine in the healthcare system", "To inherit and develop Chinese medicine", and "To encourage orthodox medical physicians to study Chinese medicine". In 1996, the Chinese government put forth a further policy, which advocated "To put equal stress on Chinese and orthodox medicines", "To modernise Chinese medicine" and "To promote the integration of the Chinese and orthodox medicines". The above three key points in the policy are complementary. Since the New Drugs Regulation of China was published in 1985, the Ministry of

Health has approved around 1,000 proprietary drugs originated from Chinese medicine at a higher level in order to meet the scientific standard. I believe Chinese medicine shall make a contribution to all human beings throughout the world in the near future.

Professor Chan has made notable contributions in the research of Chinese medicine, apart from his work in pharmacological and pharmacokinetic research in orthodox medicine. In the past years, I have met him several times in scientific and professional conferences. I was deeply impressed by his enthusiasm for the scientific approaches and promotion of Chinese herbal medicines.

The twenty chapters, which are set out in four sections, are very interesting, appropriate and practical because the clinical and theoretical data quoted is comprehensive and up-to-date. The contributors to this book are all experts in their fields within different countries.

In my opinion, the book presents scientifically and professionally proven evidence-based medicine supported with solid data or proven medicine. To promote Chinese medicine, we need to advocate critical and objective assessment by applying recognised principles of scientific investigations and rigorous standards. These approaches are particularly important for the scientific evaluation of effectiveness, safety and quality of any herbal remedies. To offer the highest quality Chinese medicine to the public around the whole world requires vigorous commitment from all professions involved in the healthcare team. I firmly believe that this book can be of help to those who are working in these fields to reach this lofty ideal.

Professor Ke-ji Chen
Academician. Chinese Academy of Sciences
Advisory Panel Member on Traditional Medicine, World Health Organisation
President. Chinese Association of the Integration of Traditional and Western Medicine
President, Chinese Gerontological Society

Preface

Since the early 1990s the increasing interest in Chinese medicine outside of China has stimulated several headlines and investigations on the issues of safety, efficacy and quality of the practice and use of Chinese medicine (CM) in the West. In response to an urgent need, one of us (Professor Kelvin Chan) has attempted to take on the task of bridging the gap between knowledge in the East and West on various areas in the practice of CM and related therapies in mid 1990s. The Winston Churchill Memorial Trust gave Professor Chan a Churchill Travelling Fellowship that allowed him to make a "critical assessment of traditional chinese medicine" in the Far East during the period of February 1995 to April 1996. On 2nd November 1996 he joined force with colleagues from Middlesex University to organise the "Second Annual Conference on Complementary Therapies—Traditional Chinese Medicine: The Way Forward". The signing of an agreement between Beijing University of Traditional Chinese Medicine and Middlesex University to launch the first ever 5-year Degree Course in Chinese Medicine to be taught in an English medium in Europe followed this very significant symposium. Over the past few years, enormous effort has been spent on inviting colleagues from other developed countries for their contribution to this book project. The present book is a consequence of all these happenings.

This book is intended to draw the attention of both orthodox medicine (OM) and Chinese medicine (CM) practitioners and other health-care professionals as to how Chinese medicine has been progressing in the East and other developed countries where it is practiced. It stresses, through various chapters, the importance of open-mindedness and understanding by healthcare professionals of both the concepts of CM and OM in order to benefit complementary medicine, or the integration of both practices. It also points out that modernisation of traditional areas of Chinese medicine is urgently required to cope with the development of technology in the biomedical science fields. An education and training model to cope with both disciplines is needed. The regulatory aspects for both quality of the treatment products and professionalism of practitioners should be worked on with a view to harmonisation.

Professor Kelvin Chan
Dr Henry Lee

Contributors

David J. Atherton
Consultant Practitioner
Department of Dermatology
Great Ormond Street Hospital for Children
London
United Kingdom

Paul Pui-Hay But
Lecturer
Department of Biology
The Chinese University of Hong Kong
Hong Kong SAR
People's Republic of China

Kelvin Chan
Director
Institute for the Advancement of Chinese Medicine
School of Chinese Medicine
Hong Kong Baptist University
Hong Kong SAR
People's Republic of China

Chieh Fu Chen
Director
National Research Institute of Chinese Medicine
Taipei
Taiwan

Lily Cheung
Director/Practitioner
Chung San Acupuncture School
Porchester Garden
London
United Kingdom

Yi Dang
Lecturer
Beijing University of Traditional Chinese Medicine
Beijing
People's Republic of China

Colin C. Duke
Lecturer
Herbal Medicines Research and Education Centre
The University of Sydney
Sydney
Australia

Stefan Hager
Practitioner
TCM-Klinik Kötzting
Kötzting
Germany

Ming Tsuen Hsieh
Director
Institute of Chinese Pharmaceutical Sciences
China Medical College
Taichung
Taiwan

Ka Kit Hui
Director/Practitioner
Centre for East-West Medicine
School of Medicine
University of California
Los Angeles
United States of America

Christoph Kundel
Practitioner
Zentrum Fur Traditionelle Chinesische Medizin
Fulda
Germany

Henry Lee
Director
TCM Course Development
School of Biological, Environmental and Health Sciences
Middlesex University
London
United Kingdom

Qian Li
Lecturer
Herbal Medicines Research and Education Centre
The University of Sydney
Sydney
Australia

Jia-Zhen Liao
Consultant/Practitioner
Dongzhimen Hospital affiliated to Beijing University of TCM
Beijing
People's Republic of China

Xin-Ming-Liu
Researcher
Institute of Medicinal Plant Development
Xi Bei Wang
Beijing
People's Republic of China

Zhan-Wen Liu
Lecturer
Beijing University of Traditional Chinese Medicine and Pharmacy
Beijing
People's Republic of China

Jan Nauta
Practitioner
Department of Neurophysiology, Faculty of Medicine and
Hwa To Centre for Traditional Chinese Medicine
University of Groningen
Groningen
The Netherlands

Fai-Ngor Ngan
Researcher
Chinese Medicinal Material Research Centre
The Chinese University of Hong Kong
Hone Kong SAR
People's Republic of China

Yong Peng
Researcher
Institute of Medicinal Plant Development
Beijing
People's Republic of China

Basil D. Roufogalis
Researcher
Herbal Medicines Research and Education Centre
The University of Sydney
Sydney
Australia

Pang-Chui Shaw
Lecturer
Department of Biochemistry
The Chinese University of Hong Kong
Hong Kong SAR
People's Republic of China

Yau Chik Shum
Researcher
Institute and Department of Pharmacology
National Yang Ming University
Taipei
Taiwan

Anton Staudinger
Director
TCM-Klinik Kötzting
Kötzting
Germany

Pierre Sterchx
Practititioner
St Lievens, Houtern
Belgium

Katsutoshi Terasawa
Director
Department of Japanese Oriental (Kampo) Medicine
Faculty of Medicine
Toyama Medical and Pharmaceutical University
Toyama
Japan

John Tindall
Director
Yuan Clinic and College Clapham
London
United Kingdom

Jennifer M. F. Wan
Lecturer/Researcher
Nutrition/Disease Laboratory
Zoology Department
University of Hong Kong
Hong Kong SAR
People's Republic of China

Jun Wang
Lecturer
Department of Biochemistry
The Chinese University of Hong Kong
Hong Kong SAR
People's Republic of China

Pei-Gen Xiao
Fellow
Chinese Academy of Medical Sciences
Institute of Medicinal Plant Development
Beijing
People's Republic of China

Wei-Yi Yang
Founding Professor
School of Chinese Medicine
Hong Kong Baptist University
Hong Kong SAR
People's Republic of China

Hin-Wing Yeung
Immediately Past Director
Institute for the Advancement of Chinese Medicine
Hong Kong Baptist University
Hong Kong SAR
People's Republic of China

Jun Liang Yu
Lecturer
Centre for East-West Medicine
School of Medicine
University of California
Los Angeles
United States of America

You-Ping Thu
Practitioner/Lecturer
Hwa To Centre for Traditional Chinese Medicine
University of Groningen
Groningen
The Netherlands

Jian-Xiang Zou
Project Director
Project on Modernisation of Chinese Medicine for the State
Administration of Traditional Chinese Medicine
Ministry of Science and Technology
Beijing
People's Republic of China

Lidia Zylowska
Practitioner/Lecturer
Centre for East-West Medicine
School of Medicine
University of California
Los Angeles
United States of America

Acknowledgement

This book project was initiated in response to the increasing interest and concern over the use and practice of Chinese medicine world wide during the mid 1990s. Quite a lot of preliminary groundwork was involved, for the preparation of this text.

We are grateful to the Winston Churchill Memorial Trust for providing the Fellowship to one of us. Professor Kelvin Chan, for the collection of information and building up of connections in the Far East. We thank those colleagues from various universities, organisations and institutes whom Professor Chan met in China Japan, Hong Kong and Taiwan during his Churchill Fellowship in 1995/1996 (See Appendix 1 Chapter 18, for listing). They have A C provided valuable materials in different aspects of TCM, including, teaching, research and development, practice, and regulations on the use and manufacture of Chinese herbal medicinal products. Some of this information has been incorporated and updated in appropriate sections of this text. We express our special thanks to all Contributors who provided valuable texts for various Chapters. We also thank Mr Philip Aston and Mr Edward Hsu for proof reading some of the chapters.

One of us, KC, would like to acknowledge that he has spent a lot of spare time on preparing and editing this book. This should have been spent with his wife, Gail, and children, Debra and Andrew.

SECTION ONE
SOME KEY ISSUES IN CHINESE MEDICINE

1 THE HISTORICAL EVOLUTION OF CHINESE MEDICINE AND ORTHODOX MEDICINE IN CHINA

Kelvin Chan

Introduction

THE EMERGENCE OF COMPLEMENTARY MEDICINE IN ORTHODOX PRACTICE

About 70 to 80% of the world's population, particularly in the developing countries, rely on non-conventional medicine in their primary healthcare as surveyed by the World Health Organisation (WHO, 1991). The rest of the population, in the better-developed countries, have been fortunate receivers of orthodox medicine (OM) or conventional medicine since the early 19th century. Yet in the present era of rapid advances in biomedical science and technology it is astonishing that the public in rich developed countries spends an enormous amount of their earnings on over the counter (OTC) herbal products and related non-conventional therapies. Over the past decade we have witnessed two apparently unrelated trends in the biomedical and biotechnological development of medicinal products (Chan, 1997). There is the rapid development of recombinant DNA technology and related procedure to provide biomedical proteins and related biological products for use as therapeutic drugs, prophylactic vaccines and diagnostic agents. The growth in popularity of OTC health foods (nutraceuticals) and medicinal products from plants or other natural sources have taken a very large share of the healthcare market (*Which?* 1995, Johnson, 1997). Both observations indicate changes in people's perceptions of OM treatment using synthetic drugs or conventional therapies.

In most developed countries where OM assumes full responsibility in national healthcare, most forms of traditionally practised medicine and therapies are considered as complementary or alternative medicine (CAM). Some experts consider that OM is allopathic treatment while many of the CAM involve a holistic approach; the practitioners of OM attempt to intervene in order to block certain body processes while practitioners of CAM focus on supporting and working with the body's innate powers of self-regeneration. The WHO has defined CAM as all forms of healthcare provision which "usually lie outside the official health sector" (Eisenberg, 1993). This definition by WHO embraces formalised traditional systems of medicine (Ayurvedic, Chinese, Hindoo and Unani systems etc.), traditional healers and medicine men, feedback, chiropractic, naturopathy, osteopathy, homeopathy etc. Very little is known of the reasons for the increase in the popularity of CAM in developed countries. Untested assumptions include the side-effects of synthetic drugs, general dissatisfaction of orthodox treatment, diseases that cannot be cured by OM, and patients with chronic illnesses demanding more attention from OM practitioners. Research is urgently needed in these areas to improve healthcare planning (Chan, 1996). CAM treatments are recommended for chronic pain affecting spine, joints or muscles, for the control of nausea, eczema, and other skin complaints, asthma, cancer and migraine etc. (Lewith, Kenyon & Lewis, 1996). There are over 100 different therapies available as CAM treatments, but the five discrete clinical disciplines (acupuncture, chiropractic, herbal medicine homeopathy and osteopathy) are distinguished by having established foundations of training and professional standards (British Medical Association, 1993). However it has been pointed out that not all natural therapies or products related to CAM are free from adverse effects. (Abbot, White & Ernst, 1996; Barnes, 1997).

The acceptance of CAM into orthodox medical practice depends on the proof of good quality of practitioners and treatments with demonstrable efficacy and safety. The practice of OM has been based on a well-established profession that is accepted worldwide. Most of the CAM practitioners receive training that is not widely accepted according to the OM practice in the developed countries. This is because OM has been developed along accepted scientific paths and practised with recognised success in most cases even though the origin of OM comes from traditional practice based on the evolution of the ancient Greek-Roman-Arabic experience.

A BRIEF REVIEW OF THE HISTORICAL EVOLUTION OF ORTHODOX MEDICINE AND ITS INTRODUCTION TO CHINA

The rapid development of modern or western orthodox medicine (OM), mainly in developed countries during the Industrial Revolution period, has a very short history compared with some of the CAM mentioned above.

The evolution of some of the disciplines in OM has been based on ancient traditional medical practices of various ethnic groups that laid down public health laws for the population thousands of years ago. The medical history of the ancient civilisations from various parts of the world differs in their philosophical adaptations to the environments where these civilisations evolved and their practice of fighting diseases developed. Some of these practices have been preserved, survived and modified according to the progress of life on earth. From written records in tablets of clay, on stone steles, on papyrus and on vellum of these civilisations one could find evidence of anatomical and pathological diseases, parasitic infections, bacterial diseases, bone-setting surgery and the use of medicinal plants, animal parts, minerals and other means etc. to treat these ailments. On the other hand the development of the presently accepted practice of orthodox medicine has a comparatively short history. The remarkable medical evolution, or revolution rather, that brought the art of medieval practices into a science-based discipline only took place about 100 years into the 20th century. This tremendously fast rate of success depends on the advance of physical sciences and technology over the past centuries. It will be interested to note some of the noticeable periods that influence the development of modern OM.

As early as 3000BC, the Babylonian, Chinese, and Egyptian cultures had records of medical practice. The Eburs papyrus contains a list of remedies including castor oil seeds. The Edwin Smith papyrus details Egyptian surgery. The earliest records of Chinese herbal medicine (around 2800BC) were found in the *Shen Nong Ben Cao Jing* (The Herbal Classic of Divine Plowman). The Greek inheritance of medicine at around 500BC was derived from the Babylonian and Egyptian medicine with possible influence from practice in the East (Chinese medicine, and Indian Ayurvedic medicine and Hindu surgery which existed around the second millennium). Tuberculosis, smallpox, and leprosy were described. Emetics, purgatives, enemas, sneezing-powders, leeching, cupping and bleeding were practised. Greek physicians handed down this medical knowledge to the Roman. A period of magic and supernatural beliefs along side medicine dominated the healing scene for some time until Greek philosophers such as Pythagoras and Empedocles introduced good sciences to separate medicine from magic. During the time of Hippocrates (460 to 375 BC) medical opinion had largely discarded the concepts of magic and religion. Hippocrates' teaching and writings, including the stress on diagnosis, knowledge of the course of observed diseases and prognosis, has made so much impact for the modern medicine that his legacy

Table 1.1 The evolution of conventional (orthodox) medicine

Origin:	Based on ancient traditional medical practices of various ethics groups.
3000 BC	• Babylonian, Egyptian and Chinese culture & medical records gave initial contribution.
500 BC	• In Europe and surrounding regions, Greek inheritance of Babylonian & Egyptian medicine with influence from the East (Ayurvedic, Chinese, & Hindoo medicines) led the progress.
510 BC to 476 AD	• The Roman Empire brought prosperity, law, Latin language, Christianity to Europe and Mediterranean region, but adopted medical work from the Greek physicians.
476 AD to 14th Century	• Moslem influence on translation and compilation of Greek medical works into Arabic. This formed the source of knowledge for orthodox medicine from the Dark Age, surviving through the Middle Age (4 to 8th century) to modern times.
14th to 17th Century	• Influence of Renaissance, started in Italy to France, increasing knowledge of anatomy and physiology of human body; • Translation of Arabic medical literature to Latin. • Influence of evolution of physical sciences—due to Galileo Galilei (1564–1642), Isaac Newton (1642–1727).
Late 18th Century to 19th Century	• Influence of Industrial Revolution, in Britain (1830) then France & Belgium (after 1870) and Russia (after 1900). • Modernisation of industry, social and economic issues. • Development of natural sciences, such as chemistry, mathematics and physics, laid down the groundwork for medical developments. • A profound influence of this development that helped progress of modern medicine from medieval (religious & superstitious belief) practices into 20th century science based discipline in only 100 years. • Isolation and identification of active ingredients from medicinal plants that were used over centuries and discovery of endogenous compounds with medicinal uses from animal sources. Leading to the first therapeutic revolution of the 20th century.

Table 1.1 The evolution of conventional (orthodox) medicine (*continued*)

Growth:	Period of rapid medical advances. Some key points are listed
Late 19th to 20th century	• Development of public health legislation & education. • Development of immunisation and vaccination for preventative measures. • Development of anaesthetics and anaesthesia (William Morton, 1864) helping surgical progress. • Development of microscope helping bacteriology and sterile techniques that helped indirectly progress of medical surgery (Robert Koch, Louis Pasteur, and Joseph Lister). • Discoveries of chemotherapeutic agents stimulated development of rational therapeutics—emerging pharmaceutical industry.
1905 Early 1990s	• Salvarsan's selective toxicity against syphilis (1905) led the introduction of sulphonamides. • Prontosil's control of streptococcal infections led to the launch of most effective less toxic sulphapyridine in 1938, other antimicrobials included penicillin (1928), streptomycin (1943) chloramphenicol (1949). • Development of rational therapeutics continued under the influence of bioassays and receptor assays using isolated tissues for endogenous neurotransmitters, hormones etc. • Discovery of autonomic functions (due to discovery of pharmacological actions of acetylcholine by Henry Dale in 1940) led to introduction of muscle relaxants, cardiovascular drugs. • Discovery of insulin (action in 1921 by Banting and Best; structure clarified in 1955) standardised by blood sugar concentrations in mice and isolated rat diaphragm. • Discovery of neuroleptics for treatment of schizophrenia (chlorpromazine in 1950). • Discovery of tricyclic antidepressants for treatment of depression (Imipramine 1952) • Introduction of benzodiazepine as tranquillisers and hypnotics (1960's), many other modern synthetic analogues for almost all diagnosed diseases.

Table 1.1 The Evolution of Conventional (Orthodox) Medicine (*continued*)

Growth:	Period of rapid medical advances. Some key points are listed
1961	• The incidence of thalidomide induced malformation of new-borns nearly halted all new drug development due to teratogenic effects. Better quality assurance was demanded for testing toxicity, mutagenicity, carcinogenicity and teratogenicity.
1970s	• Various government interventions on standards and quality assurances in laboratory testing and practice had a great influence on all industries. Good laboratory practice (GLP) guidelines were set to promote and co-ordinate experiments for the purpose of bringing about safety and quality control.
1970 to 1990's	• Setting up legislation by various governments of developed countries to implement GLP, Good Manufacturing Practice (GMP) and Good Clinical Trial Practice (GCTP) for R & D of new drugs and biotechnological products with medicinal uses.
20th Century—Future	• Further development of biotechnology in gene therapy, diagnosis and biotechnological pharmaceuticals. • Development of vaccines against parasites of medical concern. • Preventive medicine, reducing cost of primary healthcare. • Improvement of quality of life. • Acceptance of quality-assured complementary medicines in orthodox medical practice.

has been seen as the code of practice for over 2000 years and continues presently. The extent of the Roman Empire at the height of the power encircled the Mediterranean, reached north to the Rhine, the Danube, and central Scotland and spread into Armenia and Mesopotamia. Interestingly the Empire adopted much medical works from the Greek physicians. Among them, Galen (130–201 AD) was the authority on anatomy and experimental physiology that identified the connection of blood heart and arteries. This medical knowledge had been spread afar throughout Europe and North Africa under the influence of the Roman Empire.

During the period of Middle Ages (after the fall of the Roman Empire from 476 AD to the late 15th century), Greek medical manuscripts were preserved and translated into Arabic. The Moslem influence from 622 AD, spreading from Persia to North Africa and Spain in the west and Afghanistan, India, Indonesia, Malaysia, Pakistan, Turkey, and some of the Balkans, produced many great physicians. Al-Razi recorded his findings for distinguishing smallpox from measles in the 9th century AD. Avicenna (980–1037) wrote the Canon of Medicine, a text in use in France until the 17 century. Abu al-Qasim, (936–1013) of Cordola advanced the status of surgery by his careful illustrated text. These Moslem physicians of that era added to the preserved Greek medicine their own experience and discoveries. The result was a compiled version of Greek and Arabic medicine that became the source of knowledge for Western medicine throughout the Middle Ages right up to early modern times.

During similar period the Benedictines collated and translated the books of Hippocrates and Galen, with the formation of the first secular medical school in Europe at Salerno in Southern Italy. Subsequently other medical schools were set up at Montpellier, Bologna and Padua. Many of the Greek medical works were translated from Arabic into Latin. Thus modern medicine has its origin from this period onward when physical science and later biological sciences began to develop rapidly from the Industrial Revolution at the 18th century (Table 1.1).

While such progress was going on in the West, China had always relied on her own medical practice until the 18th century when the country was open to foreign invasions. Thus the then modern medical concepts from the west were introduced together with all other trades and exchanges. From the early 1900s through the 2nd World till the end of civil war in 1949 between the Communists and the Nationalists orthodox medicine dominated the healthcare scene. After 1950s the practice of Chinese medicine was re-introduced.

THE OBJECTIVE OF THE BOOK

Using Chinese medicine (CM) as an example of a complementary medical therapy, the practice of acupuncture (part of CM practice) is gaining acceptance in the developed countries while the other equally important part of CM practice, Chinese herbal medicine (CHM) is not widely accepted. Both disciplines are receiving world wide attention. Since the early 1990s the popularity of CHM products has been increased in the West due mainly to the successful treatment of atopic eczema in a double blind controlled clinical trial using the decoction of 10 Chinese herbs (Sheenan & Atherton, 1992). CM had been practised in China since 3000BC. Part of this longest practised healthcare system, acupuncture, was introduced to the West in the early 16th century when the West became interested in the Far East. In the early 18th century because of the influence of the West in China, OM was introduced to China and the population was exposed to two healthcare systems while acupuncture was getting more popular in the other parts of the world. Thus it will be useful and interesting to review the historical evolution of CM and compare it with that of OM that has been presently integrated into the healthcare system in China.

The main purposes of the present book have been:

- To examine the progress and development of various aspects of CM practice in different countries,
- To establish the trend for training and education of these traditional disciplines,
- To identify the difficulties and solutions needed for progress to a practice that should give treatment and prevention of illnesses with quality, safety and efficacy,
- To see if it would be possible that the public in the other developed countries can enjoy the integrated discipline of OM and CM as those in China or other regions in the Far East, and
- To discuss various aspects for the modernisation of Chinese medicine that are being carried.

The Evolution of Chinese Medicine

THE EARLY HISTORICAL DEVELOPMENT SINCE 2800 BC

China, a large and developing country, possesses an ancient culture with a very long recorded history of traditional medical practice which has been officially integrated into the health system with orthodox medicine since the 1950s. Orthodox medicine, introduced in the early 1900s to China when she was exposed to western influence, has made a very important impact for treatment of diseases in China, while Chinese medicine (CM) has been the mainstream for healthcare since 2800BC. CM is a complex and holistic system of medicines with its own philosophy, diagnosis systems and pharmacology. It considers the human body in relation to its own natural, physical and social environment. The practice of CM involves physical therapy (non-medication) using acupuncture, moxibustion and related disciplines such as massage and Qi Gong and chemical (medication) therapy using materials of animal, mineral and plant origin in the form of decoctions of combined CM natural products. As most of them are from plants, medical books on CM materia medica through the ages have conveniently referred them as "Ben Cao" (Herbalism). Several authors and editors have written or translated some historic accounts and bibliographies of Chinese medicine and philosophy into the English language (Chan, 1963; Chan, 1995; Deng, 1985; Fung 1953; Kapchuk, 1983; Needham, 1956 and Quinn, 1973). Most of the works described were based on texts written in Chinese and supplemented with references in Chinese. Table 1.2 summarises the periods of the historical evolution of CM.

The practice of acupuncture can be traced back to as early as the Neolithic Age, when the use of a piece of sharp stone, "Bianshi", to treat illnesses marked the beginning of acupuncture. Moxibustion (the burning of an herb, moxa the mugwort or *Artemisia vularis*, at the exposed end of a needle pointing at the meridian point) could be traced back to the days when fire was discovered. With the development of society and civilisation, needling and moxibustion instruments have been constantly improved, providing conditions for further refinement, enhancing curative effects and promoting academic development of acupuncture. During the Shen Nong Period (ca. 2800 BC, a period of agriculture development), the use of herbs was probably started by the folk-lore hero Shen Nong (Divine Plowman) when he identified some medicinal plants and other natural materials which could be beneficial for the treatment of illnesses. In 2697 BC, China's first emperor, Huang Di (Yellow Emperor) and his cabinet members developed techniques in diagnosis and treatments using acupuncture and herbal materials which were later written as the *Huang Di Nei Jing* (The Inner Canon of the Yellow Emperor, recorded in about 100 BC).

The origin of CM herbalism shared similar historical development to acupuncture & moxibustion but more is widely known to be associ-

Table 1.2 The historical evolution of Chinese medicine in China

Period	Three noticeable legendary and dynastic periods
a) Since 2800 BC	• The Shen Nong Period: development of agriculture and use of plant materials by Shen Nong (A Plowman folklore hero) for treatment of illnesses.
	• The use of "Bian-Shi" as sharp stones and moxa for relief of minor complaints marked the origin of acupuncture and moxabustion.
b) 2697 to 1 BC	• Development of techniques for diagnosis and treatment by the first Huang Di (Chinese emperor) and his cabinet members in about 2697 BC
	• Compilation of **Huang Di Nei Jing** by many physicians and pharmacists under the name of Huang Di in about 100 BC (The Inner Canon of the Yellow Emperor) that consists of 2 main parts recording the *Yin Yang Theory*, *Wu Xing* (Five Elements) *Theory*, and all the related information, in question and answer form, on pathology, signs and symptoms (collectively as syndromes), causes of diseases, humanity and the environment, and other principles of Chinese medicine.
	• Compilation of **Shen Nong Ben Cao Jing** (The Herb Classic of the Divine Plowman is the earliest Materia Medica in China) by various scholars in about 1 BC listing of 365 herbal materials of 252, 67, and 46 plant, animal and mineral sources respectively and recording principles of processing, mixing, and formulating them.

Table 1.2 The historical evolution of Chinese medicine in China (*continued*)

Period	Three Noticeable Legendary and Dynastic Periods
c) 221 BC to 1911 AD	Non-stop development and evolution of Chinese medicine and pharmacy throughout can be summarised by the publication of valuable pharmacopoeia and other medical texts. Each dynasty headed by some enlightening emperors would update and compile these texts with the consequence of including more natural products for use as materia medica; only well known ones (including those translated to other languages) are listed here: • **Shang Han Lun** (Treatise of Cold, Disease and Miscellaneous Disorders written by Zhang Zhong-Jing during 25 to 220 AD), a classical dispensary handbook describing syndrome differentiation, treatment, prescription and use of herbs is the foundation of composite prescription. Together with Huang Di Nei Jing and Shen Nong Ben Cao Jing this text played a vital role in the development of Chinese medicine for later generations. • **Tang Ben Cao** (Tang Xin Xiu Ben Cao; Tang Dynasty Materia Medica, commissioned by the Emperor and written by Su Jing with 23 other medical and pharmacy scholars with rectified information) is considered to be the earliest pharmacopoeia in the world. It consists of 54 chapters, 850 herbal descriptions with 20 imported herbs; influencing development of medicine in Korea and Japan; being 800 and 1100 years earlier than the pharmacopoeia from Italy (1499AD) and Denmark (1772 AD). • **Ben Cao Kong Mu,** (Compendium of Materia Medica, authored by Li Shih Zhen, a medical and pharmaceutical practitioner, around 1518 to 1593 AD), consists of 52 volumes, 1892 natural products (350 from minerals, 1099 from plants, 443 from animals), 11096 Fu Fang (composite prescription formulae). This Compendium was published in 1596 AD and was brought to Europe and Japan, translated initially to Latin then in English, French, German and Russian.

Table 1.2 The historical evolution of Chinese medicine in China (*continued*)

Period	Three noticeable legendary and dynastic periods
	• **Introduction of these literature and practice to other countries:** neighbouring countries such as Korea and Japan adopted Chinese medicine as early as the period in Qin dynasty (221 to 207 BC) and 57 AD respectively. • **Acupuncture** was introduced into Europe in the 16th century when some orthodox physicians picked up the techniques in Japan when trading in the Far East was started via the Dutch East India Company.
Post-dynastic Period 1911 to 1950s	**The Influence of Orthodox Medicine and Decline of Chinese Medicine** • The collapse of Qing Dynasty introduced chaos to the country leading to western influence of nearly all aspects of life including political, social and healthcare. • Formation of the Republic in 1911 and introduction of orthodox medicine practically eliminated the practice of Chinese medicine. • Knowledge of acupuncture was introduced to other parts of the world when trade was started with European countries.
Period of Re-introduction 1950 to 1980s	**The Influence of Poor Economic conditions after 2nd World War and the Civil War** • The PRC government re-emphasised the importance of TCM from 1956 onwards due to economic and technical limitation. • Gradual modernisation and regulation of both orthodox medicine and Chinese medicine interfered in between by the cultural revolution from the 1970s to 1980s in conjunction with the nation-wide economic development. • Setting up of specialised universities in Traditional Chinese medicine in major cities in key parts of China: Beijing (north), Chengdu (west), Nanjing (middle), Shanghai(east) and Guangzhou (south).

Table 1.2 The historical evolution of Chinese medicine in China (*continued*)

Period	Three noticeable legendary and dynastic periods
1990s to 21st Century	• International modernisation of Chinese medicine in all aspects: particularly education and training; basic medical scientific investigation of Fu Fang (composite formulae); basic medical scientific investigation on the biochemical and physiological aspects of acupuncture; quality control and assurance of crude herbs and Chinese herbal medicinal products; development of experimental models to relate CM principles and OM pharmacological actions of CHM products; development of modern dosage forms; efficacy and safety of CHM products; • Improve and promote integration approach for orthodox medicine and Chinese medicine in particular on prevention of diseases. • Other key specific projects such as informatics for CHM materials and CM practices; proper promotion of functional food in CM practice etc.

ated with the legendary testing of many herbs or medicinal plants by the folk hero, Shen Nong, whose experience and work in these areas was eventually recorded in *Shen Nong Ben Cao Jing* (The Herbal Classic of the Divine Plowman). Ancient medical records indicated that China began to keep records of medical and pharmaceutical practice as early as three thousand years ago. It is difficult to identify the actual authors of these early records because of the common practice of attributing works to famous authorities and emperors or heroes.

Huang Di Nei Jing (often referred to as *Nei Jing*) is the oldest medicine classic in China. It was written by many physicians and pharmacists under the name of the Huang Di (translated as Yellow Emperor), and consisted of two parts: Part I entitled "Sue Wen (Plain questions and answers) and Part II Ling Shu (Miraculous Pivot). It has 9 separate volumes consisting of various topics such as human anatomy, and physiology, causes of diseases, pathology, signs and symptoms, disease treatment and prevention, health care, the man and the environment, Yin and Yang Theory, the Five Phases (Wu Xing some texts translate it as Five Elements) Theory in medicine, guidelines and principles in CM. It summarised the theories and principles for syndrome differentiation treatment, and the composition and compatibility of ingredients in a prescription.

Shen Nong Ben Cao Jing, the earliest materia medica, published during the Dynasty of Eastern Han (1st century BC). It classified 365 herbal materials into 3 categories: superior, commonly used, and inferior herbs. This Herbal Classic had collections of herbs and folk recipes used by the Pharmacy and Medicine professions. Among them, 252, 67 and 46 are plant, animal and mineral sources respectively. The main contents in this Herbal include the basic theory of materia medica, (a prescription should include four different types of materia medica referred to as the *Jun, Chen, Zuo and Shi*, translated as the Chief, Adjuvant, Assistant, and Guide components, respectively; thus one major active herb and several supporting ones are used together to smooth adverse effects or synergise the pharmacodynamic actions of the others).

DEVELOPMENT THROUGH DIFFERENT DYNASTIC PERIODS FROM QIN DYNASTY (221 BC) TO QING DYNASTY (1911)

Continuous development and evolution of CM in China can be observed from recorded classical texts written throughout different dynastic periods from early AD 214 in Jing Dynasty to 1911 in Qing Dynasty.

Shang Han Lun (Treatise on Cold and Diseases Miscellaneous Disorders, written by Zhang Zhong-Jing in the Eastern Han period, AD 25–220) is considered as the classical dispensary that brings together syndrome differentiation, treatment, prescription and use of herbs in treating diseases and lays the foundation for the formation and development of the science of CM prescription.

Together with *Huang Di Nei Jing* and *Shen Nong Ben Cao Jing* these publications play a vital role in the development of Chinese herbal medicine and materia medica for later generations.

Tang Ben Cao (Tang Dynasty Materia Medica or Tang Xin Xiu Ben Cao, 659 AD, the Tang's Newly Revised Materia Medica commissioned by the Emperor and written by Su Jing with 23 other medical and pharmaceutical scholars with rectified information consequent on mistakes from previous medical texts) is considered to be the earliest official pharmacopoeia in the world, containing 54 chapters and 850 herbal descriptions which included 20 imported herbs from foreign countries. It had great influence on medical practice in China, Japan and Korea and had been used as mandatory text in traditional medical schools during the periods. Internationally, this text was considered as the earliest known official pharmacopoeia published in the world, being over 800 years and 1100 years earlier than the Italian Florence Pharmacopoeia (1499 AD) and the Denmark Pharmacopoeia (1772 AD) respectively.

During the Ming (1304–1644 AD) and Qing (1644–1911 AD) Dynasties no further advancement in CM development was observed although these two dynasties enjoyed quite a long period in the Chinese history. It could be considered that it was a bad time in medical development during some of this era when witchcraft and witch doctors were again popular and serious epidemic diseases and pestilence occurred from time to time.

However the most important and influential contribution to both China and world pharmacy history also came during this period when Li Shi-Zhen (1518–1593 AD, a TCM practitioner and pharmacologist) made an in depth study of all herbs and recipes available at this time by dedicating 30 years of his life to surveying, collecting, examining, and testing in detail these materia medica. Li Zhi-Zhen compiled these findings, together with rectification of errors in previous medical and pharmaceutical writings, in the *Ben Cao Gang Mu* (Compendium of Materia Medica) with illustrative pictures drawn by his son.

The Ben Cao Gang Mu includes 1892 natural products (1099, 433 and 350 of plant, animal and mineral sources respectively) in 52 volumes of written works. It is considered as the complete and detailed pharmacopoeia with descriptions of the shape, characteristics, taste, source and method of collection, preparation, and pharmacological actions of each herb. An appendix of 11096 Fu-Fang (Prescription Formulae) is included. This pharmacopoeia was printed and published in 1596 AD and was brought to Europe and Japan and translated into Latin by Michael Boyd (1612–1650 AD). Subsequently the work was translated into English, French, German Russian and Japanese.

INFLUENCE OF ORTHODOX MEDICINE ON HEALTHCARE IN CHINA AFTER THE DYNASTIC PERIOD FROM 1911 TO PRESENT

The corruption and incompetence of the subsequent government of the Qing Dynasty in the late 1800s exposed China to foreign invasion. In medical and social aspects China suffered the problem of nearly nation-wide opium addiction that weakened her economical, political and physical power. Under the influence of westernisation the practice of orthodox medicine became more popular besides other social or political aspects. This period marked a significant change in the history of China not only politically but also in medical practice. The Republic of China was born after the 1911 Revolution that was led by an ortho-dox medical practitioner, Dr. Sun Yat-Sen. During such a turbulent period it was not surprising that hardly any medical progress was made. It was pointed out in a review by Croizer that the record of Chinese medical developments prior to 1949 was not impressive and before 1927 was dismal.

Civil wars broke out in China one after the other. No efficient meas-ures were taken to get rid of opium smoking. Under the then Nationalist (Guo-Min Dong) government there were over 20 million opium users in China. The practice of orthodox medicine took over the health care and practice of traditional Chinese medicine was not allowed or curtailed. Most chemical drugs were supplied by foreign drug companies and no regulations on drug use and drug quality control were available to check adulterated drugs and misbranded preparations, manufactured domestically or imported, which flooded the market.

Since the founding of the People's Republic of China (PRC) in 1949, in the development of medical practice the government took effective and decisive measures to eradicate opium smoking in just three years. The PRC government re-emphasised the importance of CM practice by campaigning for the rehabilitation of CM with the intention of breaking China's dependence on the West.

The role of barefoot doctors in healthcare during difficult times (Chan, 2000)

During civil wars and after the Second World War, under the direction of Chairman Mao who led the long march the introduction of barefoot doctors into the villages was the only source of healthcare. Chairman Mao's instruction was to put the stress on the rural areas, to adhere to the principles of preventive care first, to combine Chinese and western medicine, to make full use of acupuncture, CHM products and massage therapy. Great tributes have been paid to those barefoot doctors who were the key players in rural medicine for over 30 years since PRC was formed in 1949. The barefoot doctors' knowledge of clinical medicine was minimal, and the practice involved both orthodox medicine and Chinese medicine. They received mainly training in preventive health activities such as hygiene environment and water sanitation and basic curative care. Their functions in healthcare were:

- Organising local health campaigns
- Promoting disease prevention and maternal and child healthcare activities
- Treating common diseases
- Referring more complicated cases to higher level units
- Health education and promotion
- Advising on family planning
- Collecting and reporting health-related information

In June 1965 during the early part of the Cultural Revolution, Chairman Mao announced a new health policy to tackle the shortage of physicians for China's vast rural poor population. He arranged to implement short medical training to produce barefoot doctors who would be upgraded, certified, and paid wages for their full-time medical work. These practitioners would continue to work as agricultural labourers part-time in addition to serving the elementary healthcare needs of fellow workers.

By 1975 there were about 1.6 million barefoot doctors received who had such education/training. They would continue in agriculture labour part-time in addition to serving the elementary healthcare needs of their fellow workers. The name of "barefoot doctor" was replaced by "village doctors". The practice of barefoot doctors was officially abolished in 1986 when the population of "barefoot doctors" was reduced from 1975. The profile of a typical barefoot doctor can be summarised as follows:

Age: Middle aged
Sex: Mainly male
Education: Secondary school level
Work: Generally part-time practising healthcare apart from main job in the farms.

The subsequent integration of Chinese medicine into orthodox medical practice from 1950s

All medical doctors who had been trained in orthodox (western) medicine (OM) were re-allocated to learn Chinese medicine after 1952 when China became more stable after the world war.

Over 10 CM colleges and institutes were established in the coastal provinces and in Sichuan Province. Orthodox physicians were re-educated with CM principles and practice. This marked the start of an integration of education and practice of both OM and CM. The Cultural Revolution (1966–1976) brought Chinese culture and medical progress to a standstill. Barefoot doctors, some with less than 6 months training and no high school education, were sent to rural areas to replace the qualified western-trained physicians and CM practitioners.

Since 1976 China has returned to "normal". Within a period of 3 to 5 years the Ministry of Public Health was authorised to revise and promulgate up to 24 Regulations and Acts for all uses of medicinal products and related businesses. They are concerned with drug administration enforcement, new drug applications, special control of narcotics, psychological drugs, poisons, pharmaceuticals, hospital pharmacy, criteria for punishing violators of drug regulations, drug importation and exportation, introduction of clinical trials, and new drug applications by foreign companies and those through joint ventures between China and foreign companies. Based on these various regulatory development and implementation the first official Chinese Drug Control Law was adopted in 1984. It is believed that continuing development and progress are being made and adopted to comparable international standards. The revision and updating of Pharmacopoeia (1992, 1995) for pharmaceuticals and herbal products have been indicative of attempts to achieve these goals.

The Present Development of CM in China will be described in detail in subsequent chapters. However, it is important to note how the CM education development since the 1950s has affected the healthcare and pharmaceutical development in China. At present the population in China enjoys both OM and CM treatment for their healthcare. This is one of the very few examples where integrated medicine is practised.

DEVELOPMENT OF ACUPUNCTURE AS A SEPARATE DISCIPLINE FOR MEDICAL TREATMENT IN ORTHODOX MEDICINE

Since the founding of the Peoples' Republic of China, acupuncture & moxibustion (A&M) has been developing very fast. Based on the classical theories of acupuncture, various new techniques have been developed: acupuncture analgesia, electrical acupuncture, water acupuncture, ear acupuncture, head acupuncture, face acupuncture, hand acupuncture, and microwave acupuncture. During recent years both inside and outside China, up to 300 different types of diseases in internal medicine, surgery, obstetrics & gynaecology and paediatrics have been benefited by these treatments.

Development outside China of acupuncture has been significant. The practice of A&M had also been introduced to other countries. Zhen Jiu Jia Yi Jing was used as text book in Korea as early as the 6th century; the Ming Tang Tu (Illustrated Manual of Channels, Collaterals and Acupuncture Points) and Zhen Jiu Jia Yi Jing were brought into Japan by a monk, Zhi Cong during the Three Kingdom Period in AD 562 to Japan. In the 17th century, the practice was introduced to countries in Europe such as Austria, Britain, France, Germany, Italy and Switzerland, and spread to Russia before the 1917 Revolution.

Nowadays there are many privately run clinics and schools giving modified tuition on A&M in some of these countries. More recently in the North America and other parts of the world where there were Chinese communities the practice of A&M has been very popular since the 1970s. These include those in Asia, Africa, Latin America, Australia & Oceania, Eastern Europe. Translation of works of CM medical sciences, A&M, CM hebalism and pharmacology, and their related research works appeared in the English language. From 1975, the World Health Organisation (WHO) entrusted the Chinese Ministry of Public Health with the task of running International Acupuncture Training Centres in Beijing, Shanghai, and Nanjing for overseas doctors visiting China. The International Society of Acupuncture & Moxibustion was formed in 1987 by the WHO in Beijing for research and development of various aspects of A&M.

THE OVERALL PROGRESS OF CHINESE MEDICINE IN RELATION TO ORTHODOX MEDICAL PRACTICE

It can be observed that great interest has been shown in Chinese medicine from the complementary medicine viewpoint in the West. However in China Chinese medicine is included as an integral part of the healthcare for the population. It will be most interesting to have a global view of the progress of Chinese medicine from other parts of the world. Section 1 of the book concentrates on "Some Key Issues on Chinese Medicine", Section 2 deals with "Some Examples of Clinical and Scientific Practice of Chinese Medicine while Section 3 deals with "Geographical Development of Chinese Medicine". Finally Section 4 addresses the "Concluding Issues on the Way Forward for Chinese Medicine."

References

Abbot, N.C., White, A.R. & Ernst, E. (1996) Complementary medicine, Nature, **381**, 361.

Barnes, J. (1997) Reports on complementary health care symposium. Pharmaceutical journal, **258**, 76–77.

British Medical Association (1993) Complementary Medicine: new approaches to good practice. Oxford University Press: Oxford, 1993.

Chan, W.-T. (1963) *A Source Book in Chinese Philosophy*, Princeton Paperbacks, Princeton University Press, Princeton, NJ, 1963

Chan, K. (1995) Progress of traditional Chinese medicine, *Trends in Pharmacological Sciences*, **16**, 182–187.

Chan, K. (1996) The role of complementary medicine in healthcare. Biologist **43**: 50–51.

Chan, K. (1997) Regulations for registration of medicinal products from natural sources. In: Proceedings of the 6th Pacific Rim Biotechnology Conference and BioExpo'98. Hong Kong University of Science & Technology, 3 to 5 June 1998, Page 122.

Chan, P.P.F. (2000) The Barefoot Doctor. QED Technology Ltd., Hong Kong, China. In Press.

Deng Q.S. (1985) Historical View on traditional Chinese medicine, *Trends in Pharmacological Sciences*, **6**, 453–455.

Eisenberg, D.M. *et al.* (1993) Unconventional medicine in the United States: prevalence, costs and pattern of use. *New Eng. J. Med.* **328**: 246–252.

Fung Y.-L. (1973) *A History of Chinese Philosophy 2 volumes*, translated by Derk Bodde, Princeton University Press, Princeton NJ, 1953, 1973.

Johnson, B.A. (1997) "Market Report", *HerbalGram, Volume* 40, 1997, p. 49–50.

Kapchuk, T.J. (1983) *The Web That Has no Weaver: Understanding Chinese Medicine*, Congdon & Weed, Inc. Chicago, 1983.

Lewith, G., Kenyon, J., & Lewis, P. (1996) *Complementary Medicine: an Integrated approach*. Oxford University Press,: Oxford, 1996.

Needham, J. (1956) *Science and Civilization in China, Volume 2*, Cambridge University Press, Cambridge, 1956.

Quinn J.R., Ed. (1973) *Medicine and Public Health in the People's Republic of China*, Washington, DC: John E. Fogarty International Center, US Department of HEW, NIH, 1973.

Serturner, F.W.A. (1816) Uber das Morpium eine neue salzfahige, und die Mekonsaure, als Hauptbestandteile das Opium. Gilbet's *"Annalen der physil"* Bd 55, S56, 1816.

Sheehan, M.P. and Atherton A.D. (1992) A controlled trial of traditional Chinese medicinal plants in widespread non-exudative atopic eczema, *British Journal of Dermatology*, **126**: 179–184.

The Pharmacopoeia Commission of P.R.C. (1992) *Pharmacopoeia of the People's Republic of China*. GuangDong Science and Technology Press, GuangDong, China. English Edition, ISBN: 7-5359-0945-O/R 174.

The Pharmacopoeia Commission of P.R.C. (1995) *Pharmacopoeia of the People's Republic of China*. GuangDong Science and Technology Press, GuangDong, China. Two Volumes, Chinese Edition, ISBN: 7-5359-1540-X. (Vol. 1); ISBN:7-5052-1527-5 (Vol. 2).

Which (1995) *Which*? Complementary Therapies, November issue, 1995.

WHO (1991), World Health Organisation's Programme on Traditional Medicines. Guidelines for the assessment of Herbal Medicines, Geneva, WHO, 1991

2 PHILOSOPHICAL ASPECTS OF CHINESE MEDICINE FROM A CHINESE MEDICINE ACADEMICIAN

Zhan-wen Liu

Introduction

Chinese medicine (CM) has evolved over a period of at least 3,000 years. It consists of a complete theoretical system with unique methods of diagnosis and treatment. Because the development of science can never be divorced from philosophy, the ancient Chinese philosophical thinking had influenced the development and growth of CM. The philosophy of CM is different from that of orthodox medicine (OM). To learn and practise CM some understanding of its philosophical and theoretical underpinning is essential. Otherwise it would be like prescribing antibiotics with no knowledge of physiology and pharmacology of the human body.

A broad philosophical perspective in seven sections is presented in this chapter. Section 1 describes the general concepts embodied in CM such as monism of *Qi* as well as the concept of "*Yin & Yang*" and "*Five Elements*". Section 2 deals with the basic viewpoint of life. CM views life as a natural phenomenon and the inevitable outcome of the evolutionary movement of substances in the universe at a certain stage. Section 3 gives an overall description of the essence and cause of diseases. Section 4 is concerned with the holistic concept of CM, with emphasis on the human body as an organic whole, the unity of man and natural environment, and the unity of man and social environment. Section 5 examines the methodology of CM. Section 6 covers dialectical viewpoint of CM, focusing on treatment based on syndrome differentiation, treating the same disease with different methods and treating different diseases with the same method, and distinguishing root versus branch, urgent versus less urgent. Section 7 is a general introduction to the principles of health preservation in CM, including correspondence between man and the universe and conformity to nature, preserving both physique and vitality, association of motion and rest, and regarding the genuine *Qi* as the foundation of life.

Chinese Medicine's View of the Universe

MONISM OF *QI*

The philosophers of the Spring and Autumn and Warring States periods in ancient China believed that *Qi* was the fundamental substance which constituted the world, and all things in the cosmos were produced by the movement and changes of *Qi*. That is to say, *Qi* and an object were dialectically unified. This was how the ancient philosophers tried to understand the relationship between the universe and man. This primitive understanding was introduced into medical theory to become the basic concept of *Qi* in CM. Accordingly; *Qi* is the basic substance, which makes up the human body. When *Qi* gathers, it forms the organic body, when it disperses, the organic body dies. The Internal Classic (Huang Di Nei Jing) explains that *Qi* which constitutes nature and transforms all things biologically may be classified into two categories, namely *Yang-Qi and Yin-Qi*, the former characterized by being clear, light and active. It rises and is warm, while the latter by being rough, heavy and stationary, sinks and is cold. Hence, the vast heaven is composed of the moving and flying *Yang-Qi*, while the substantial earth consists of the coagulated *Yin-Qi*. Owing to the interaction of *Yin-Qi* and *Yang-Qi* in the universe, non-living matters and living objects or things, including human beings, animals and plants, appeared and existed in the world. Much of the existence of objects or things in the universe are pre-determined by different properties, quantities and integrative modes of *Qi*. For instance, the so called *Evil-Qi*, namely, the substances which can damage health and cause diseases, pertains to the natural-Qi. In the human body there are *nutritive-Qi, defensive-Qi, pectoral-Qi* and many other *Qi*, which help maintain all functions of life. The monism of *Qi* in CM affirms the unity and diversity of the universe, thus laying a simple and scientific epistemological foundation for solving some complicated and abstract problems that CM had been confronted with.

THE NOTION OF CONSTANT MOTION

Qi is vigorously dynamic and is in constant motion. It is believed to be the origin of all matter or things. That is to say, new matter continuously emerges and grows from small to big and from weak to strong. Simultaneously, the old matter gradually declines from big to small and from strong to weak. This basic understanding of CM about the universe in continuous evolution is also known as a dynamic motion.

There are two kinds of changes in the universe. The quantitative change, namely, a gradual or not obvious change involving only quantitative variance. The second type is qualitative change. This is a variance in the quality when the quantitative change of a matter reaches a certain point. In other words, it refers to sudden transformation of a matter from one kind of substance into another. The Internal Classic (Huang Di Nei Jing, referred to in Chapter 1) points out clearly the distinction and connection between the two kinds of changes: "The generation of an object indicates the qualitative change, while its course of change from the beginning to the end means the quantitative change". Nature has its own intricate laws. For example, the evolution and the changes depend on the interaction of *Yin-Qi* and *Yang-Qi*; in other words, the unity of opposites of *Yin-Qi* and *Yang-Qi* gives impetus to the movement and the changes of everything. *Yin-Yang* is therefore the source of changes and the motive force of every matter from birth to decline. Time and space characterize such evolution and the changes. CM too emphasizes the need to take into consideration, when diagnosing and treating ill health, the periodical variations in the four seasons of a year and their effects upon the activities of the human body. These variations include the diversity and particularity of the dynamic changes due to the different geographic orientations and regions.

BASIC CONCEPT OF YIN-YANG AND FIVE ELEMENTS THEORIES

Basic concept of "Yin & Yang"

The root of many of the ideas in CM, and in fact much of the outlook of Chinese traditional culture, lies in the theories of "*Yin-Yang*" and "*Five Elements*" which originated in ancient China. They possess the basic connotations of materialism and dialectics. These theories have been expanded beyond their original meanings respectively. *Yin* and *Yang* are concepts of the fundamental duality in the universe, a duality that is ultimately unified. The original meaning of the concept of *Yin* and *Yang* is very simple. Initially, it referred to whether or not a place was facing the sunlight. The sunny place was called Yang, while the shady side was called Yin. The ancient philosophers gradually observed that there was a dialectical existence in the natural world, such as heaven and earth, sun and moon, day and night, cold and hot, bright and dim, death and life, and male and female. Consequently, the meaning and the use of *Yin* and *Yang* were extended into a concept of opposites. Gradually, it was realized that all matters in nature have two opposite aspects, and that their interactions promote change and development. Subsequently, Yin and Yang have become a pair of philosophical categories instead of a specific thing. The ancient scholars drew a diagram called Tai ji in order to express the primitive meaning relating to the sunlight as well as the deeper signification of tension and transformation, between Yin and Yang (See Figure 2.1).

The black part stands for Yin and white part for Yang. Both exist in an entity as indicated by the big circle. The white point within the black part and black point within the white part denote respectively *Yang* within *Yin* and *Yin* within *Yang*, as well as the inter-dependence and inter-transformation between *Yin* and *Yang*. It also confirms the mutual waxing and waning and dynamic change of yin and yang. As a pair of philosophical categories, *Yin* and *Yang* were specially defined by the quality of their characteristics, phenomena and matters, which cannot be interchanged. For instance, cold and heat are a pair of *Yin-Yang*, however, cold only belongs to *Yin* and heat to *Yang*. The delineation of *Yin* and *Yang* in property is regarded as a regulation that should be complied with when classifying the attributes of matters to *Yin* and *Yang*.

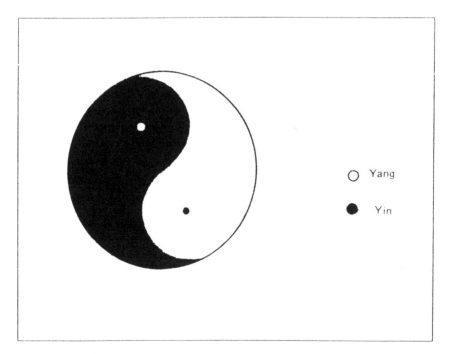

Figure 2.1   Diagram for Tai ji

Because the *Yin-Yang* concept is all-pervasive in Chinese thought, the ancient physicians of Chinese medicine naturally adopted it. Consequently, the Yin-Yang theory underlines the philosophy and practice of CM. That is Yin-Yang is used to explain the human anatomy, physiology and pathology in order to guide clinical diagnosis and treatment.

Basic concept of five elements

The Chinese used another set of concepts in their attempt to understand the phenomena of the physical world. These were the *"Five Elements"*: *Metal, Wood, Water, Fire,* and *Earth*. The original meanings of five elements refer to the five kinds of raw materials, which were vital to the ancient people for their daily living. They had already realized that these five materials had different, but important, functions for livelihood. For example, it is recorded in the Chapter Dazhuan of Shangshu (an ancient texture authority), that *Fire* and *Water* were essential in the production of food, *Metal* and *Wood* for the conditions of work and rest, *Earth* for growth in all living things. Armed with these discoveries, the ancestors further realized that these five kinds of materials are the original source of materials constituting everything in the material world. Since the time of the Warring States, the concept of the *Five Elements* began to evolve further. The ancient scholars emphasised the functional phases and properties that the *Five Elements* stood for. Their meaning was not defined by the simple description of metal, wood, water, fire, and earth. For example, Chapter Hongfan in Shangshu states, "*Water* is characterized by moisturizing downwards, *Fire* by flaming upwards, *Wood* by flex and extension, *Metal* by reforming, and *Earth* by farming". This shows that at that time the five elements referred not just to the five kind of raw materials, but to an abstract philosophic conception representing the properties of five overriding categories of things. For example, water is not only considered as the substantial water, but also stands for the state and property of moisturising downwards as well as other things with the same or similar state and property. Hence, all things are classified into five categories in terms of phases and properties of metal, wood, water, fire, and earth. The intrinsic connections among the five categories and changes were then explored to form the Theory of Five Elements, which identify the features of and the interaction among these five elements (See Figure 2.2).

There are two basic relations of the five elements, i.e., inter-generation and inter-restraint. The abnormal relations after the break down

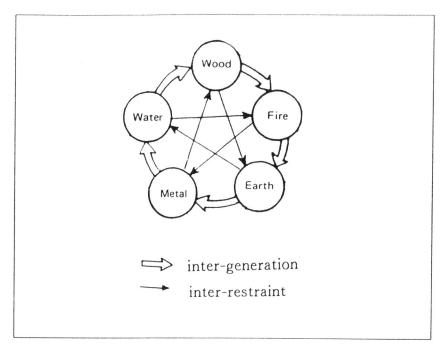

Figure 2.2   Diagram for inter-generation and inter-restraint of the five elements

of the normal inter-generation and inter-restraint, are mainly the inter-over-restraint and inter-counter restraint among them.

Inter-generation implies the relations of generating, benefitting and complementing each other. The order of inter-generation among the five elements is: *Wood* generates *Fire, Fire* generates *Earth, Earth* generates *Metal, Metal* generates *Water,* and *Water* generates *Wood.*

Inter-restraint means mutual restriction, conquering and suppression. The law of inter-restraint among the five elements is: *Wood* restrains *Earth, Earth* restrains *Water, Water* restrains *Fire, Fire* restrains *Metal* and *Metal* restrains *Wood.*

Anyone of the five elements may have a direct connection with the other four elements. The law of keeping natural normality is a consequence of interplay from both inter-generation and inter-restraint of the five elements. They are two indispensable activities, on which matters or things can exist and move normally. In this way, the ecological balance in the universe and the body's physiological stability can be ensured. In CM, the theory of the Five Elements is chiefly applied to generalize the functional properties of viscera and structure, to demonstrate the internal law of mutual relationships among the five *Zang*-viscera systems (which is the anatomical system in CM) and to sum up mutual relationships between man and his environment. It is used to guide clinical analysis and treatment of illnesses due to an imbalance in the body.

The monism of *Qi*, the theories of *Yin-Yang* and *Five Elements* all reflect the way the philosophers and physicians in ancient China perceived the world and the existence of life. They represent a summation of multiple disciplines and are important components of CM. It is therefore important that the ancient philosophy is studied first when studying CM, as its basic characteristics are different from the other disciplines.

The View of Life in CM

ESSENCE AS THE BASIS OF LIFE

Medicine can be defined as the scientific study of normal and abnormal life activities. It is the science of the prevention and cure of disease and of health maintenance. CM does not agree with any use of superstitions but recognises that life is a natural phenomenon as the inevitable outcome of the evolutionary movement of substances in the universe.

Chapter 9 in Plain Questions of the Huang Di Nei Jing (Su Wen, an ancient text of medicine) states: "The heaven supplies man with the *Five Qi* while the earth provides him with the *Five Flavours*". Chapter 25 in the same book says: "Man depends on the combinative *Qi* of the heaven and earth for his birth, and his growth and development depend on the natural law of four seasons". That is to say, only while the *Yin-Qi* and *Yang-Qi* in the universe mutually inter-flow and mix together, can there be life which is based on a combination of the *Essence* and Qi from the heaven and earth. The life activities include the inherited and acquired *Essence* and *Qi*, which are the essential substances to life. Thus Chapter 9 in Spirit Pivot of the Huang Di Nei Jing (Ling Su, an ancient medical text) states: "The original substances of life are called *Essence*, the life-force created by the combination of *Yin* essence and *Yang* essence is named for vitality".

The *Essence* is regarded as the basis of life and has three meanings besides the organic life combination of *Essence Qi* from both *Yin* and *Yang* in nature. First, a new life is formed when the reproductive *essences* of both sexes combine after the sexual union between a man and a woman. Then, the human body, including internal organs, varied tissues, etc. possesses manifold essence which stems from the *congenital essence*. This is then supplemented from the acquired nutrition; finally, a person's life span from birth to senescence as well as health or disease is related directly to the abundance or deficiency and normality or abnormality of the *essence*.

UNIFICATION OF PHYSIQUE AND VITALITY

Physique, the configuration and constitution of a human body, is composed of *zang fu viscera, meridians* and *collateral, essence, Qi, blood, body fluid, five sense organs, nine orifices, limbs as well as tendons, vessels, muscle, skin and bone*. Vitality, can be defined broadly as a general term for the external manifestation of life processes of the human body. These include the various physiological or pathological signs and symptoms that are manifested externally; or internally as spirit, consciousness and thinking, and a series of such psychological activities as emotion, thought and character. The concept of unity of physique and vitality is conceived as the combination of the body and mind or the unity of form and function. This is an important concept in the basic theories of CM as well as one of the theoretical bases of the science of health preservation.

According to CM theory, physique and vitality are closely related to each other. Physique is the material basis of vitality while vitality is the functional manifestation of physique; vitality cannot exist without physique, and without physique there would be no vitality. A strong physique leads to a vigorous vitality, while lethargic physique results in an exhausted vitality. On the other hand, vitality dominates the physique. Chapter 13 in Plain Questions (Su Wen) of the Huang Di Nei Jing states "Patients with vitality will be cured; otherwise, they will die". Chapter 70 in the same book says "The life process ends as soon as vitality dies away". It is thus evident that in the dialectical relationship of interdependence and mutual opposing, there exists also a complementary relationship between the body and mind of the human being. Physique is the place for vitality to lodge while vitality is the functional activities of the physique. This relationship has an important significance for clinical practice to correctly assess the relationship of the unity of the opposites between the body and mind to enable diagnosis, treatment and prevention of disease.

VITAL *QI* CONNECTING WITH THE UNIVERSE

"*Vital Qi* is connected with nature" is a celebrated thesis on the relationship between man and nature in the Huang Di Nei Jing. It means that life activities are linked closely with the universe according to certain categories of relationships. Firstly, the human body relies on the unceasing exchanges of both substance and energy with the natural environment to sustain life functions, e.g., taking food, excretion and breathing. Secondly, the human body has through experience become adaptable to the variations in natural environment. When days are hot, blood moves towards the body surface with profuse sweating to cool the body and passing a smaller amount of urine. During cold days the skin contracts to retain the blood within to keep warm and the body produces hypohidrosis and polyuria. Thirdly, the human body is not completely passive when adapting to changes in the natural environment. Indeed, the human body actively manages natural activities to its advantage to prevent harmful calamities.

CM uses the adaptation of the law of seasonal *Yin-Yang* as the main principle to promise health and treat ill health. CM has always attached great importance to the influences of the environmental variations on the individual. It is therefore important that observations and research on the human life activities should include the environmental influences to enhance the quality of treatment and care.

The Concept of Disease in CM

KNOWLEDGE OF DISEASE

There exist many views regarding the conception, essence and causes of disease in modern or ancient times in China or elsewhere. These views, indeed, influenced people throughout the history of different cultures to adopt different strategies against diseases. Before CM was established, ghosts and gods were believed to be responsible for the diseases that were prevailing in ancient China. Those believers had adopted a passive and fatalistic attitude towards illnesses. They usually turned to the sorcerer or sorceress for help and with devout prayers whenever they were not well.

To counter those superstitious beliefs CM argues that contracting diseases is a natural occurrence but can be avoided. As there are climatic variations in the four seasons of a year, life also alternates between health and ill health. Not all ill health is unavoidable. It can be prevented and cured. For example, Bian Que, a well-known physician in the Warring States, was very critical of the society's belief and practice of sorcery as he considered these practices distorted the effectiveness and efficacy of medicine. According to CM, the signs and symptoms of the diseases help to understand the pathological processes and changes before and after a treatment is instituted. CM also refutes the notion of incurability and considers that if a disease is not cured it is because the physician's knowledge on the disease is not correct or not clear; a definite and effective therapy has not yet been found.

HOLISTIC IMBALANCE

Life activities are accomplished by the cooperative work of all the parts constituting the whole body. Observations and researches on either normal or abnormal life activities should be underpinned by the totality of the human body within the environment with which it interacts.

CM believes that in the healthy state, the relatively balanced and harmonious relationships among the various parts inside the body as well as between the body and its environment are maintained, and once these relations are broken down, disease occurs. The medical scholars of ancient China used to take the theory of *Yin-Yang* literally to mean the unity of the opposites existing in either the whole body or a component part of the body. As a result health was described as a dynamic balance of the body's *Yin* and *Yang* and any imbalance will cause ill health. This, in fact, has become CM's central philosophical and theoretical base to explain health and ill health, diagnosis, treatment and health promotion.

Generally, there is a regulating mechanism in a person to enable him or her to adjust his/her life activities in response to both internal and external changes to maintain health. When a pathogenic agent breaches the body's ability to respond to maintain health disease will occur. CM therapies are based on this principle of holistic dynamic equilibrium and harmony in the body.

STRUGGLE BETWEEN THE *GENUINE-QI* AND THE *EVIL-QI*

According to CM diseases are influenced by the body's relative functional state. When the body has low resistance against diseases, attacks of various *Evil-Qi* will follow. The disease will affect either the body's *Genuine-Qi* and *Evil-Qi*. The *Genuine-Qi* refers to the functional activities of the body and its ability to prevent disease, struggle against diseases, and repair injured tissues. The *Evil-Qi* refers to various harmful factors that lead to diseases, such as the six climatic evils, seven emotions, pestilence, phlegm, fluid retention, stagnant blood, and retention of the food and drink taken into the body. Therefore, in CM ill health is a reflection of the struggle between the *Genuine-Qi* and the *Evil-Qi*. Ill health is a process in which the body's immune system is fighting off the *Evil-Qi*. In this process, the internal unity of the body and the external environment is in continuous interaction and when the body's *Genuine-Qi* becomes too weak to resist the *Evil-Qi* or the *Evil-Qi* is too intense for the *Genuine-Qi*, an illness occurs. This internal struggle between the *Genuine-Qi* and *Evil-Qi* continues even during the therapeutic stage until *Genuine-Qi* is strengthened and has overcome the *Evil-Qi*. The inter-changes in the intensity of the *Genuine-Qi* and the *Evil-Qi* in this process need to be understood in order to understand CM

Concept of Holism in CM

Holism in CM Holism is another important philosophical concept to understand the physiology, pathology, diagnostics, therapeutics, and prevention of diseases. It refers to the unity and integrity of the body, in relation to the universe and the human body. The universe is the macrocosm, while the human body is a smaller microcosm within the larger macrocosm. The holism therefore includes two aspects: Firstly, the body itself is an organic whole. This concept is applied to the study of the physiology and the pathology of the body, and in the diagnosis and treatment of disease. Secondly, both the body and the universe are in harmony.

REGARDING THE HUMAN BODY AS AN ORGANIC WHOLE

In CM, the human body consists of various viscera, tissues and organs with separate functions to form a functioning system that is not related to the orthodox medical concept. The activities of this system determine the body's ability to maintain itself through the coordination and balance of its physiology. Each body component is intimately connected and inter-related thereby capable of producing complicated physiological and pathological reactions. This interrelationship is formed by the *Five Zang Viscera* as the centre, and is brought into existence through the connecting action of the meridian system. These systems are bound together forming the physiological, pathological, diagnostic, therapeutic and other aspects of CM. The *Five Zang Viscera* in CM actually stand for the human body's five big functional systems bringing together all component parts and functional activities of the body. Thus, the theory of visceral manifestation taking the *Five Zang Viscera* as the Centre is seen as a cornerstone around which the concept of holism of CM can be established.

Normal and steady life activities of the whole body depend on all the organs and tissues functioning properly as well as on the integration of the mutual coordination and restraint among them. The functional division and cooperation in the whole body reflect the concept of holism in CM. For instance, each of the *Five Zang Viscera* has its own special functions. The heart holds the leading position because of its functions of governing and coordinating *Five Zang Viscera* and the whole body. The complicated regulatory mechanism between the *Zang Viscera* and other tissues in the body in CM can be expounded in terms of the principles of the unity of the opposing of *Yin* and *Yang*, and the inter-generation and inter-restriction of the *Five Elements*.

CM explores the human life activities from the view of holism, and furthermore sees the whole pathological process from the perspective of the local morbid condition in combination with its entirety. Importance is attached to both the connection of partial pathological changes with the relevant *Zang Viscera* and *meridians* and the influences of the morbid *Zang Viscera* and *meridian* over others, which embodies the concept of holism in the doctrine of pathogenesis. When diagnosis is made, the pathogenesis of an internal organ or even the whole body can be ascertained according to the signs and symptoms accessible by sense organs, tongue, pulse etc. This is regarded as a practical application of the dialectically united relationship between the human body as a whole and its separate parts. For example, the disorders of ear, such as tinitus, deafness and neuralgia, are considered as resulting from the *Kidney* deficiency or *Damp-Heat* in the *Liver* and *Gallbladder* in CM. So the satisfactory effect gained by tonifying the *Kidney* or removing *Damp-Heat* from the *Liver-Gallbladder*. Another example is treating an illness in the head by acupuncture-needling on the foot and treating a sickness in the left side of the body by acupuncture-needling on the right side. Both achieve favourable results because they regulate the entire functions and harmony of the whole body's *Yin* and *Yang*.

THE UNITY OF HUMAN BODY AND THE UNIVERSE

The human body is an organic whole, a small part of the universe. CM believes that in the universe there are prerequisites to sustain life, such as air, water, sunlight, animals and plants, etc. and the body's activities can be directly or indirectly influenced by the external environment. The human body acquires the self-regulating and self-controlling abilities to adapt to the variations of his environment. Of course, if the changes in the universe are beyond the body's adaptability, or the adaptability is too weak to cope with the change, illness will occur.

The effects of season, climate, geography and other natural changes on life are very important considerations in CM. The Internal Classic (Huang Di Nei Jing) points out that during seasonal variations and alternations of day and night, the physiological regulations on the body's visceral functions, the circulation of *Qi* and blood, all influence each other's actions. This is to maintain the dynamic balances between *Yin* and *Yang* inside and outside of the body. For example, the body's Qi and blood flows outward accompanied by a floating and large pulse in spring and summer, but flows inward with a deep and small pulse in autumn and winter. In the daytime the body's *Yang-Qi* circulates mainly in the body surface, and at noon reaches to the most exuberant extent. However, at night it is stored in the inner body in a dormant state. These phenomena correspond to the rhythms of *Yin-Yang* alternation in nature. Different diseases will occur according to the changes in the environment.

To sum up, the human body and its environment are considered as an organic whole according to the CM concept. Today we call this chrono-biology that refers to the physiological activities or pathological changes of the body that manifest themselves in periodic rhythms in order to allow the human body to adapt to natural changes. The changes of *Qi*, blood, *Yin* and *Yang* correspond with the objectively existing waning and waxing, and with the prosperity and decline of *Yin* and *Yang* in the universe.

THE UNITY OF THE HUMAN BODY AND SOCIAL ENVIRONMENT

The human body is not merely a biological entity, but also a psychosocial being that is in constant interaction with the changing environment. Social position, economic status, occupation, ideology, education as well as the relationship with others influence its health. CM has long recognized this influence and applied it in the medical practice.

The Internal Classic (Huang Di Nei Jing) explains that because rich people were accustomed to fatty meat and fine grain, and addicted to extravagant and dissipated life style, they tended to suffer from debilitated internal viscera, frail tendons and bones, and floating, shallow *Qi*-blood; while poor people eat only coarse food, grain and vegetables, and lead to an industrious and plain life, hence tending to have the firm internal viscera, tough tendons and bones, and deeper stable *Qi* and blood.

The influence of social environment over the human body is an important factor in CM etiology. CM believes that violent social changes, a worsening economy, lowering living standard, war, stress, meeting with misfortune etc. can seriously damage mind and body, and can give rise to psychosomatic conditions and other difficult and complicated disorders. They may complicate the disease process. Since different social environments bring about different causes, types, natures and even courses of the diseases, the therapeutic principles adopted should be appropriate and individualised. That's why the Internal Classic (Huang Di Nei Jing) stresses that a doctor should not only understand astronomy and geography, but also social sciences. Orthodox medicine too is gradually shifting from its original medical mode of biomedicine into psycho-social medical mode, emphasizing that man and society are a united whole. Consequently, in CM an overall analysis of patients is underpinned by the natural and social influences on their body and mind. When treating a patient it is essential that his conditions and needs are based on his environmental context including seasonal and local conditions,. For mental disorders caused by social factors CM aims to help the patient to readapt to the societal values.

Methodology of Diagnosis in CM

Three common methods for diagnosis and research are described in this section.

HOLISTIC SYSTEMATIC METHOD

The holistic systematic method refers to a combination of holistic and system approaches

The CM views the health of a human body and its life activities as a whole system interacting with the environment. All the internal organs, *Qi*, blood and body fluid, five sense organs and nine orifices, four limbs and skeleton, as well as the mental activities in the body are closely interrelated and influenced by the environment. Therefore, a local disorder cannot be separated from the whole and should be diagnosed and treated as a partial manifestation of the whole body's disorder. The holistic method of CM emphasizes the whole body and its environment instead of viewing various medical problems individually. The system is an organic whole with particular functions. It consists of a number of component parts that are interacting and interdependent. Each system is seen as a component part of a bigger system to which it belongs. This method is discussed in the theory of the *Five Elements*, which divides the human life activities into the five great functional systems. The theory considers the *Five Zang Viscera* as the core, and different parts of the body and their activities are respectively related to the five systems. This classification is also extended to the matters in the universe and reconnected back to the *Five Zang Viscera* correspondingly. Consequently, the human body is regarded not only as a system characterized by a whole connection, but also as a subsystem of the bigger eco-system.

CM divides the body into layers, such as the exterior and interior, upper and lower, ascending and descending, *Qi* and blood, *Nutrient Qi* and *Defense Qi*, body fluid, vitality, *Yin meridians* and *Yang Meridians*. The two opposing sides of unity make up the organic whole, but the organic whole is not equal to the simple addition of parts. This is one important concept of the system theory in modern methodology. For example, we know that the internal organs and tissues of the body surface are physiologically interrelated and they interact with one another.

METHOD BASED ON ATTRIBUTION OF MATTERS ACCORDING TO ANALOGOUS PHENOMENA

This is an analogy in which some features of the relevant matters are inferred to be similar to each other according to their properties. They are attributed to the same category with further interconnection. The appearances or features are represented as images that can classify and induce the disorderly and unsystematic appearances according to their common features. Some new knowledge may also be deduced.

The method of attributing things according to analogous phenomena is commonly used as a way for recognizing nature and man, as well as the relationship between them. For example, the functional features of the *Five Zang Viscera* bear some analogy to the attributes of the *Five Elements* (*wood, fire, earth, metal* and *water*) in nature. The numerous appearances and objects in both the human body and nature are classified and interconnected in the same way, thereby, offering certain theoretical inference to the functional activities and pathological changes in the body. An analogy could be the blood in the body compared to the water in rivers. Water congeals because of the extreme cold and boils because of extreme heat. Blood has the same analogous features giving a plain and clear exposition for the pathological presentations of cold and heat disorders.

The method of attributing matters according to analogous phenomena is effective in many cases, but it also has some limitations. Firstly, the outcome of an analogy remains a probability instead of a certainty and needs to be verified through practice. Secondly, correct reasoning from the analogy depends upon the extent of interrelation between the analogized objects. Therefore, two matters that have little relation cannot be analogized.

METHOD OF INFERRING THE INTERIOR FROM THE EXTERIOR

This method surmises that internal changes in the human body are reflected in exterior appearances. The ancient scholars thought that the essence of a disease hidden inside could always be reflected outside. Therefore, by observing and analyzing the exterior phenomena we can recognize the essence of interior changes. This process further reinforces the holistic concept.

In CM, this method is chiefly used in the formation of the theories of visceral manifestation and pathogenesis, as well as ascertaining the syndrome through differentiating symptoms and signs. Accordingly, the internal organs are linked closely with the external tissues on the body surface such as the five sense organs, and the nine orifices, etc. mainly through the *Meridians, Qi* and blood. The functional states of the *Zangfu Viscera* can be detected by observing and analyzing the external manifestations. This theory also points out that any changes in locality would reflect, to some extent, the information of the locality and integrity. On this basis, CM formulates its diagnosis and treatment, and creates many unique guidelines for doing so. The "Five facial colour diagnosis", "tongue diagnosis", "pulse diagnosis", "ear diagnosis", etc., are all designed to deduce the internal reaction status based on the external local changes. The internal pathological changes could thus be detected externally.

The human body is a living organism and its physiological functions cannot be observed without modern instruments available in OM, through either autopsy or other experimental means. However, the method of inferring the interior from the exterior in CM need not invalidate the object of study, and need not cut off or break down the body's inherent dynamic connections. The method infers the law of internal activities from external signs. Moreover, the human activities are the most complicated among the living things because of the multi-lateral, multi-channel and multiform systematic links in the body. The inherent connections are inferred to by examining the exterior. This method is better than the straightforward causality obtained by a general local analysis, hence its conclusion maybe more close to the original states of human activities.

Treatment Based on Syndrome Differentiation

The treatment based on syndrome differentiation is a basic principle for recognizing and managing diseases of the body during ill health, and is also a fundamental law of clinical practice in CM. It was formed in the light of the concept of holism. Both syndrome differentiation and holism reflect the features of CM theoretical system. The Chinese character "zheng" points to the symptom, which refers to the clinical manifestation of a disease, such as cough, vomiting, or headaches. Syndrome, or symptom complex, is different from symptom. Syndrome refers to the pathological generalization of a group of closely related symptoms at a given stage during the course of the disease development. A syndrome can demonstrate the specific part, reason, property, and relationship of the evils and the body resistance and essence of pathological change at a given point of the disease's development. It also provides a more multi-faceted view of the development and essence of a disease than a symptom observation.

Syndrome differentiation refers to analyzing and summarizing the relevant information gathered from the four diagnostic methods (inspection, auscultation and olfaction, interrogation, and pulse feeling and palpation). The symptoms and signs are the objects of differentiation and syndrome is the result of differentiation. A syndrome derives the typical status of a reaction process within the body during ill health. Clinically, a CM doctor obtains pathological information directly from his observations of the patient, then analyzes and summarizes the information. Finally, the functional status of the patient is distinguished. This provides the foundation for syndrome differentiation. Thus, a disease is understood in terms of the body reactions to its ill health. It is recognized that the inherent relationship of clinical manifestations is that of analyzing the existing symptoms and signs. The treatment requires the establishment of the proper therapeutic principles and methods based on this analysis. Syndrome differentiation is the premise and basis of treatment, while treatment is the medium and method of curing diseases.

In CM, establishing the therapeutic principles and general rules is of first importance; this is followed by the formulation of prescriptions and therapeutic measures because the latter depends on the former for guidance. On the other hand, the outcome of a treatment will indicate whether or not the diagnosed syndrome and therapy formulated are correct. Among the basic steps of CM clinical practice, the four examination techniques help to confirm the signs and symptoms that, in turn, serve as means to work out the therapy. Finally, the therapy directs the formulation of a specific prescription and selection of herbs. These five steps are interlinked, interconnected and indispensable.

A treatment based on syndrome differentiation is different from the symptomatic treatment that aims at relieving patient's complaints or main symptoms as often done in OM. It demands that the patient's morbid state be ascertained in order to change an individual characteristic. For example, a patient with chronic diarrhea should be treated by the herbs for invigorating the *Spleen* to benefit *Qi* according to the syndrome that the spleen is unable to carry out the transforming and transporting function. In OM this condition is often treated with antidiarrhoea and antispasmodic drugs due to the symptoms of diarrhoea and abdominal pain; or using antiseptic and anti-inflammatory agent due to the bacterial infection of the intestines. So treatment based on syndrome differentiation requires a physician to include clinical manifestations, syndrome, therapeutic principles and prescription during the diagnosing-treating process in full consideration of every patient's specific condition.

TREATING THE SAME DISEASE WITH DIFFERENT METHODS AND TREATING DIFFERENT DISEASES WITH SAME METHOD

A treatment based on syndrome differentiation is the basic principle of disease diagnosis. One disease may exhibit several different syndromes, and conversely, different diseases may exhibit the same syndrome in the course of their development. Thus, CM may treat different diseases with the same therapeutic method, or it may treat the same disease with different methods. Treatment of the same disease with different methods may differ according to the patient's constitution, climatic and seasonal changes, geographical environment, or differences in manifestation or pathogenesis. For example, giving treatment to a patient with a definitely diagnosed common cold is not easy using the CM principles. This is because a common cold is usually divided into two types of syndrome according to differences of the evil factors involved and the patient's individual responses. The common cold could be caused by "*Wind-heat*" invading the exterior and "*Wind-cold*" tightening the exterior. Herbs pungent in flavor and cool in property can relieve the exterior syndrome of the former cause, while herbs pungent in flavour and warm in property can relieve the exterior symptom complex of the latter. Thus the CM doctor must correctly diagnosed the type of syndrome through further differentiation, then formulate a therapeutic scheme to achieve a satisfactory curative result.

Moreover one disease occurring in different individuals or existing in different morbid stages may show different types of syndrome resulting respectively the corresponding syndrome. For example, among the patients with peptic ulcer, according to differentiation of the symptoms and signs, one may belong to the syndrome of *cold deficiency of the Spleen*, one may belong to that of hyperactive *Liver-Qi* attacking the *Stomach*, and another to that of retention of *Damp-Heat* in the *Stomach*. In this situation different therapeutic principles as well as the relevant prescriptions and herbs should be adopted to suit the individual patient.

It is possible to treat different diseases that exhibit a syndrome with the same characteristics using the same therapeutic principle. For instance, chronic dysentery and prolapse of the rectum and uterus, are different diseases, but exhibit the same syndrome of sinking *Middle-Qi* at a certain pathologic stage of ill health development. Thus, both can be treated with the prescription of nourishing and elevating *Middle-Qi*. According to syndrome differentiation, patients who have contracted lumbago, oedema, diarrhea and enuresis, may be cured with the identical therapeutic principle, warming and recuperating *Yang* of both the *Spleen* and *Kidney*, provided they are all diagnosed as suffering from the syndrome of insufficiency of both the Spleen-*Yang* and *Kidney-Yang*,.

Thus, the syndrome apart from the diagnosis chiefly decides the treatment of diseases in CM. The appearances of a disease, its symptoms and signs, should be considered in accordance with the syndrome. The same disease can be cured with different principle because of different types of syndrome caused by different pathogenesis of the disease; and different diseases can be cured with the same principle because identical types of syndrome are caused by identical pathogenesis of different diseases. The dialectical principle that the contradictions with different properties are solved by different methods offer the advantage of treatment based on syndrome differentiation display.

This principle of treatment not only pays attention to the similarities and differences of diseases, but also places an emphasis on the similarities and differences between syndromes. The principle also adopts different problem-solving methods in response to different qualities of contradictions in the course of disease development.

It is worth mentioning that combination of information obtained from differentiating syndrome and progress of the disease will encourage reflection and improve the curative rate. For example, a patient with bacilliary dysentery is treated, in addition to treatment based on syndrome differentiation, with inclusion of specific Chinese herbs (antimicrobial and anti-inflammatory) to enhance their curative effect. For this reason, the diagnosing-treating model according to differentiation of pathogenesis combined with differentiation of disease has been considered of paramount importance.

DISTINGUISHING ROOT VERSUS BRANCH, URGENT VERSUS LESS URGENT

In treating a disease, CM stresses the unity of the human body and its environment. CM therapeutics dictates that treatment of diseases should vary in accordance with different geographical environment, seasons and individuality in order to achieve the goal of eliminating the causes and curing the disease. This is what is known as treating the root of disease. This basic principle of the treatment is based on syndrome differentiation.

The "Root" is opposite to the "Branch". In the process of the occurrence and development of a disease, there are always primary and secondary contradictions to good (balanced) health. The primary contradiction or the primary aspect of a contradiction is the root, while the secondary contradiction or the secondary aspect of a contradiction is, comparatively speaking, the branch. The root has a dominating effect on the branch; while the branch is subordinate to the root. These are comparative concepts; they have a variety of meanings and can be used to indicate the relations between primary and secondary contradictions, or the primary and secondary aspect of a contradiction in any pathogenic process. The occurrence and development of a disease can be manifested by its symptoms, which are only the appearance of the disease rather than its "root". Only with detailed assessment and complete understanding with comprehensive analysis of the clinical material can one see through the appearance to the essence, to find the underlying causes and to adopt suitable therapeutic methods. In clinical practice, treating the root of the disease can be achieved in three stages: treating the branch first in emergency cases; treating the root in less urgent cases; and treating both root and branch simultaneously.

Treating Branch First in Emergency Cases: The primary contradiction to good health or the primary aspect of a contradiction is root, not branch. Usually treating the root of a disease is the cardinal principle. But in some complicated and variable cases, the primary (root) and the secondary (branch) may transform into either one. Some conditions may have to be treated first or immediately, while some conditions can be dealt with afterwards. For example, in massive haemorrhage, emergency measures must be taken to stop the bleeding first regardless of the cause. Only when the bleeding is stopped and the patient's condition relieved, can one tackle the root or the cause.

Treating the Root in Less Urgent Cases: This principle means that in general conditions, doctors must identify the cause, administer treatment against the root cause of the disease, and resolve the basic contradiction to good health. For instance, pulmonary tuberculosis is, according to the theories, a syndrome with symptoms such as cough, low fever, dry mouth and throat, hot sensation in the five centers, red cheek and night sweat. *Yin deficiency, endogenous Heat* and deficiency-*Fire* injuring the *Lung* induce these symptoms. The symptoms are branch, while *Yin deficiency, endogenous Heat*, and the *Lung* injury caused by deficiency *Fire* are the root cause. So for this syndrome, the treatment is to nourish *Yin* and moisten the *Lung*, to resolve the contradiction of *Yin deficiency*, rather than attempting to remove phlegm and relieve the cough. Only by improving the body's resistance to disease, can this syndrome be cured.

Treating Branch and Root Simultaneously: This principle is also commonly used in clinical practice in CM when both branch and root conditions are serious and urgent. One should treat both simultaneously. For example, dysentery usually has symptoms such as abdominal pain, mucous bloody stool, tenesmus, yellow greasy coating of the tongue, and a rapid slippery pulse. The cause of this disease, the root, is *Damp-Heat*. So the method of clearing *Damp-Heat* is to treat the root; but at the same time treatment must include a therapy of soothing the intestines and regulating Qi to relieve the abdominal pain and tenesmus, as these symptoms are usually severe.

The practitioner must be very alert and should not approach the condition mechanically. Sometimes, the root of a disease must also be treated in emergency cases, for instance, when dealing with exhaustion of Qi which occurs after massive hemorrhage, the method of replenishing Qi is to stop bleeding, and this is also treatment of root. On the other hand, in less urgent cases, it is wise to treat the branch because of its effect on the root. The basic principle is to treat what is urgent regardless of branch and root. In clinical practice, it is very important to treat the disease from the root if the transformation of the branch and the primary contradiction or the primary aspects of a contradiction are diagnosed.

View of Health Preservation in CM

Health preservation, is one of CM's preoccupations to achieve longevity through disease prevention. As early as 2,000 years ago, the discipline of health preservation in CM was already well established with rich experiences and theoretical knowledge. Those theories and principles of health-preserving are still effective and valid in guiding modern CM practices.

CORRESPONDENCE BETWEEN THE HUMAN BODY AND NATURE AND CONFORMING WITH NATURE

Chinese medicine holds that the human body, living in the natural world, is closely related with the changes in the natural environment. The cycle of the four seasons in a year, the changes from daylight to night and from dawn to dusk in a day, the differences of geographical surroundings and so on, all exert important influences on the physiological functions and pathological changes of the human body. Thus, the Spirit Pivot states: "Man is related with heaven and earth, and corresponds with the sun and moon".

This explains why CM believes that the human body can achieve good health and prevent ill health once it understands and knows well the changing patterns of the four seasons, the six kinds of climate, as well as the features of the various different natural environments. It conforms to the changes in the natural world, and keeps its body in harmony with the environment. Chapter 2 in Plain Questions (Su Wen) states: "The changes of *Yin, Yang* and the four seasons signify the beginning and end of the growth of all things and constitute the fundamentals of man's life and death". It added: "The change patterns of *Yin, Yang* and the four seasons are fundamental to the growth of all things on the earth. Therefore, the wise man preserves *Yang* in spring and summer and nourishes *Yin* in autumn and winter to conform to the fundamental".

Consequently, CM stresses that all the life activities of the human body must comply with the objective law of the relative waning and waxing and transformation of *Yin* and *Yang* throughout the four seasons. Otherwise, diseases will occur, which may even endanger the human body; as indicated in Chapter 8 in Spirit Pivot that: "The wise man will surely conform to the changes of the four seasons, adapt himself to the cold of winter and the heat of summer, neutralize joy and anger and live a regular life". Thus people must attempt to balance mental activities with their physical work. For instance, spring and summer are of *Yang* nature while autumn and winter are of *Yin* nature with sprouting in spring, growing in summer, harvesting in autumn and storing in winter. People should, accordingly, nurture *Yang-Qi* (with the vital energy for sprouting and growing) in spring and summer and nurture *Yin-Qi*, (to harvest and store the vital essence) in autumn and winter, CM believes that man's relationship with nature is not passive. Man can not only understand the change patterns of the natural world and actively adapt himself to nature, but gradually can also modify nature to be in good health and to prevent diseases.

Today, the general ethos is to promote health and prevent ill health, confirming the general expectation of CM philosophy.

PRESERVING BOTH PHYSIQUE AND VITALITY

The unity of physique and vitality is a very important concept based on the principle of preserving both the physique and the vitality. Preserving the physique means protection and nourishment of the *Zang-fu Viscera*, the *Essence, Qi* and blood, the limbs, the five sense organs and the seven orifices and so on. As physique is a mindset to explain the normal spiritual activities Zhang Jingyue, a physician of the Ming Dynasty, in his book on the Treatise on Preserving Physique, repeatedly stressed the significance of taking good care of the physique: "For a man who is good at keeping himself in good health, how can he not start with preserving the physique to provide a healthy residence for the mind? For a person who is good at curing diseases, how can he not begin treating physique troubles to furnish a sound base for the recovery and prosperity of the body?" he asked. The five *Zang-fu Viscera* constitute the centre of the functional activities of the physique. It is of paramount importance in protecting the physique, to nurture the vital essence and coordinate the functions of the *Zang-fu Viscera*, in particular, the *Heart* that is the master of the five *Zang Viscera*, the six *Fu-Viscera* and the house of the mind. This explains why in health preservation, care must be taken to keep the twelve *Zang-fu viscera* in peak condition and to harmonize and coordinate their functions.

A good physique is achieved through diet and a proper balance between work and rest, a regular life, and avoiding cold and heat, and physical training. Chinese *Qi Gong* and other activities are also appropriate.

Preserving vitality means achieving a balanced emotional state. According to CM theories, the changes in man's spirit and emotions are an important component part of the physiological activities. And it is normal to react to them. Their emotional changes are expressions of normal psychological activities in life process and also help to maintain health, resist disease and prolong life. If the spiritual stimuli are acute or protracted for any length of time they can impair the five *Zang Viscera* or affect the functional activities of *Qi*, resulting in various diseases. This, confirms the importance of maintaining spirit and emotional health. The theory of health preservation in CM emphasizes preserving the vitality, demanding that man should keep the mind calm, refrain from activities that over excite the mental state to avoid damage to vitality and *genuine-Qi*. Physique forms part of vitality and vice versa. Hence preserving vitality can ensure a perfect physique while safeguarding a perfect physique can achieve vitality. They complement each other and neither can exist alone.

ASSOCIATION OF MOTION AND REST

The theory of health preservation in CM maintains that *Qi* and blood need motion while the vitality needs calm, only by associating activity with rest can the goal of preserving health and preventing diseases be achieved.

Motion includes work and exercise. The classic book *Lüshi's Spring and Autumn* points out that running water is never stale and a door-hinge never gets worm-eaten, because they are always in motion. This is analogous to the physique and energy of the human body. If the physique does not move, the *genuine-Qi* does not flow; the functional activities of *Qi* become stagnate. Over the long process of evolution, many effective physical fitness exercises with distinctive motion features have been created, for examples, the five mimic animal boxing, the muscle bone strengthening exercise, etc. According to the theory, these fitness exercises can ensure normal functional activities of *Qi*, promote the flow of *Qi* and the circulation of blood, relieve the rigidity of muscles and joints and increase the resistance against diseases. Modern medical science has also proved that constant motion can promote metabolism of the body, invigorate various organs and defer their senility.

Rest, which is opposite to motion, includes avoiding mental stress in the relative quietness of the physique. It plays an important place in the studies on health preservation. The Internal Classic (Huang Di Nei Jing) points out that serenity and quietness lead to the striae being hermetic and the internal organs being strong so that even violent pathogenic factors cannot impair them. Physicians of later generations also emphasize the importance of keeping a clear and quiet mind and abstaining from improper desires, to achieve a state of serenity. The internal exercise of Chinese *Qi Gong* usually does not involve any movement of the limbs and the trunk. The human body carries out the internal self-training and self-regulation by specific postures, specific breathing techniques and specific mental activities in order to achieve the goal of regulating, repairing, constructing organisms.

The Chinese medicine argues that both motion and rest must be active to a moderate degree; any excess or deficiency will bring about harmful effect on one's health, resulting in diseases. Chapter 23 in Plain Questions (Su Wen) suggests that "Protracted use of eyes impairs blood; protracted lying damages *Qi*; protracted sitting injures the muscles; protracted standing injures the bone; protracted walking injures the tendons". Therefore, it is necessary to undertake regular physical training, and use the brain frequently. But care must be taken not to overtax it. Thus motion will not cause extreme fatigue and rest will not result in excessive ease and pleasure.

In short, motion and rest are both opposite and complementary to each other. The *Genuine-Qi* refers, in general, to the normal physiological functions of the human body and its capacity to resist diseases and to rehabilitate. Health preservation aims at strengthening and protecting the *Genuine-Qi* to keep a person in good health.

In pathogenesis, CM pays special attention to the *Genuine-Qi* of the human body, and believes it to be the decisive factor in the occurrence, development and change of, as well as the recovery from, a disease. Generally, the human body has sufficient *Genuine-Qi* to ward off the *Evil-Qi* and the invasion of diseases. Therefore, chapter 72 in Plain Questions (Su Wen) states: "When the *Genuine-Qi* keeps itself inside the body, the *Evil-Qi* will be unable to attack". Only when the *Genuine-Qi* is weak, the superficial defensive system will be weakened to the resistance against the attacks by *Evil-Qi*. Thus, Chapter 33 in Plain Questions (Su Wen) says: "When the *Evil-Qi* gets a chance to attack the body, there must be a deficiency of *Genuine-Qi*". However, CM does not rule out the beneficial action of the *Evil-Qi*. Under certain circumstances, it may play the leading role in causing a disease; it advocates that certain effective measures be taken to avoid the attack of *Poison-Qi*, which, too, is thought to be an important aspect of preserving health and preventing diseases.

In the course of CM rehabilitation, strengthening the *Genuine-Qi* to consolidate the constitution has been considered an important principle. This means enhancing the ability of body to resist diseases and to recover health, to assist in removing the *Evil-Qi*. Consolidating the constitution is to reinforce the *Primordial-Qi* so as to promote the rehabilitation of the body from diseases. Thus, strengthening the *Genuine-Qi* is a very important part of health promotion.

In the light of this theory, health preservation aims to preserve the *Genuine-Qi* by such practices as doing more physical exercises, resorting to proper diet and invigorating daily life and mental activities.

This chapter attempts to give a broad perspective on CM philosophy to promote a good foundation from which to CM and related subjects. When studying CM, one should emphasize the dialectical materialism and historical materialism in practice. Together, they make up the general principle, which enables students, along with much clinical practice, to fully understand the basic theories of Chinese medicine.

Because orthodox medical theory vastly differs from that of Chinese medicine, students studying CM must focus on mastering the unique characteristics and philosophies of CM. They must attempt to remain unbiased in their distinction between the two medical systems, and refrain from mechanically copying orthodox medicine's basic disregard of symptoms in favour of a disease specific label.

References

Liu, Zhanwen (1998), Basic Theories of Traditional Chinese Medicine, Academy Press, Beijing, China.

Zhang, Liutong and Chang, Zaozhi (1996), The Basic Theories of Traditional Chinese Medicine, Wuhan University Press, 1996.

Zhang, Enqin (1990), Health Preservation and Rehabilitation in A Practical English Chinese Library of Traditional Chinese Medicine, Publishing House of Shanghai College of Traditional Chinese Medicine.

O'Connor J. and Bensky, D. (1981), Acupuncture, A Comprehensive Text, Eastland Press.

3 THE THEORY AND APPLICATION OF FUNCTIONAL FOOD IN CHINESE MEDICINE

Yi Dang

Introduction

"Health for all by the year 2000" was the global strategic goal put forward by the World Health Organisation. Application of functional food is one of the most important aspects to realize this goal. What is the concept of functional food? What is the difference between common food and functional food?

Functional food has different names in different countries: For examples, "Functional Food" is used in Japan, Korea, the U.S.A. and Europe and "The Foods for Maintaining Health" in China. It refers to those group of foods that carry out not only functions in nourishment and perceptibility for human sensory that any food should have, but also those functions in adjusting human physiology which are not common to food in general. These functional foods may have not enjoyed so much attention. Nowadays, the cure and prevention of some diseases and maintaining health by means of functional food have become a general focus. Many medical researchers in China are exploring and researching on the functional food in traditional Chinese Medicine.

History of Functional Food in Traditional Chinese Medicine

Functional foods in Traditional Chinese Medicine have more than 3000 years' history in China. When primitive people gathered wild fruits, they could not tell what was food and what was medicine. To satisfy their hunger, they often ate poisonous plants, which would lead to vomiting, loose bowels and giddiness. So gradually people came to identify some plants or food from natural sources of medicinal values.

The invention of fire brought light and warmth, and people learned to cook their food. Cooked food was much more digestible and the result was better mental and physical development.

During the pre-Qin Dynasty period (Before 207 BC), food therapy began to take shape. Many history books recorded that the people in Yin Dynasty drank wine. During that time, the wine offered in the sacrifices to the Gods was "Chang", a fragrant herbal wine made by more than a hundred kinds of herbal grasses. In the book *Shuo Wen Jie Zi*, the Chinese character "醫" (i.e. treatment) was explained by "wine", showing wine was used to cure diseases. From the inscriptions on oracle bones and turtle shells found in the Yin ruins, we can see that fish had been used to cure stomach diseases, showing Yin people already knew how to use certain food to cure illnesses. During the time of the Shang Tang period (1500–1000B.C.), an officer, named Yi Yin wrote *Tang Ye Jing*, the earliest book on food therapy, thus becoming the father of food therapy.

As early as the Western-Zhou Dynasty (1000–771 BC), there already were food doctors (nutritionists). According to the recording in the book of *Zhou Li. Tian Guan*, there were four kinds of doctors at that time: namely "food doctor", "physician", "surgeon" and "veterinary surgeon". The food doctors were given the leading position, for they were considered as the most important. The functional food designed by the nutritionists at that time were probably the earliest ones in the world.

In the *Huang Di Nei Jing* (Emperor's Canon of Medicine), herbal wine was recorded to be able to cure prolonged illnesses and serious illnesses, and encouraged patients to cooperate during the rehabilitation period by eating as much cereal, meat, fruit and vegetable as possible. That is, restoring the vital energy by means of eating and drinking. It was recorded in *Huainanzi* of West Han Dynasty (206 B.C–24 AD) that the ancient emperor Shen Nong (the father of agriculture) tasted wild plants and came across seventy varieties of poison in one day. Primitive people got to know about animal medicine from their hunting activities. They learnt that gall bladder could loosen the bowels and that liver was good for the eyes.

There were 14 kinds of classical medical books of the Western-Han Dynasty (206 B.C–24 AD), unearthed from Han Tomb at Chang Sha Ma Wang Dui, recording about the medicated porridge for treatment. In the East Han Dynasty (25 A.D.–220 AD), the practitioner, Zhang Zhongjing, was able to cure chronic diseases through the use of herbal medicine combined with functional food. He used red bean and angelica powder to cure Huhuo illness, he cured consumptive illnesses and "coldness" using Chinese Yam pill, he cured poor appetite using lilly egg soup. He also used thin porridge to strengthen the effect of the herbal medicine used.

Shen Nong Ben Cao Jing (Shen Nong's Materia Medica) is the earliest book about Chinese medicinal materials used in China. There were 365 kind of herbs listed in this book. At least half of them can be used as medicine as well as food.

Sun Simiao, a famous doctor in the Tang dynasty, wrote a book named "One Thousand Precious Prescriptions" with a chapter entitled "Food Therapy" which mentioned the functions of 154 kind of foods in the four classification including fruits, vegetables, grains, birds, beasts, worms and fish. In this book, Dr. Sun Simiao pointed out: "Doctors should first understand the pathogenesis of the disease, and then treat it with food. Drug should only be used if food therapy fails." He said that animal liver would cure night blindness. That vitamin A would cure night-blindness was discovered only in recent years. For goitre patients, Sun prescribed lamb cheeks or deer cheeks. For oedema patients, Sun prescribed grain husks that contained a lot of vitamin B. His research in this field made possible the prevention of illness due to malnutrition. The Tang dynasty saw the first publication of the food therapy book written by Meng Xian.

During the Yuan Dynasty (1271 AD–1368 AD), the doctor Wu Rui wrote Materia Medica for Daily Use. Soon after it was published, the imperial court's food doctor Hu sihui wrote the book Essentials of Food and Drink. These two books have their own benefits, and each was based on different principles and approaches to the concept of food therapy. They both included the concept of "food fortifying" in healthy persons. This formed the basis for Chinese clinical medicine's nutritional work. In addition, the "Essentials of Food and Drink" furthered the development of studying the medicinal aspects of regular foodstuffs.

Li Shizhen, a famous doctor in the Ming Dynasty (1368 A.D.–1644 AD), collected more than 500 kind of herbs for food therapy in his book named *Ben Cao Gang Mu* (Compendium of Materia Medica).

In the Qing Dynasty (1644 A.D.–1911 AD), functional food in traditional Chinese medicine developed very quickly. A lot of books about food therapy were published.

Chinese medical doctors in modern times have promoted the development of functional food. Along with China's reform and opening to the outside world, it has found itself in thousands upon thousands of homes well since the early 1980's when people in most areas began to progressively extricate themselves from difficulties of food and clothing. The domestic broad market serves as the main force behind the development of the functional food. The functional food factories amounted less than one hundred on 1980, but exceeded three thousand by 1992, producing over three thousand varieties of such food, with an annual output value at twenty billion RMB Yuan ($), about ten percent of the entire food industry. The total sales that year were well over four hundred and fifty million Yuan ($) in Beijing area alone.

Entering the 1990's, it has seen a new aspect of leaping forward in the functional food industry, where a multi-assortment and multi-functional framework is taking shape. As the functional food production forges ahead toward industrialization, modernization and a commercial scale of operation, large quantities of brands and highly competitive products have been introduced. Moreover a number of large and middle-sized new enterprises and group of companies with a yearly output value from one hundred million to even one billion yuan have been established with so many nation-wide, well-known enterprises coming to the fore.

In recent years, researches on functional food were brisk and were paid great attention at home and abroad. The many research results of functional food by the experts and scholars showed improved strength and health was directly related to the effects from taking the functional food.

The Current Status and Prospect of Functional Food in Chinese Medicine

Article 22 of Food Hygiene Law, which was enacted by the Standing Committee of the National People's Congress of Peoples' Republic of China (PRC) on 30 October, 1995, stipulates that any food product or its specification claiming functions for health must be submitted to the Ministry of Public Health under the State Council for examination. The Ministry of Public Health will examine the hygienic standard as well as the production, marketing, and management of the food products. The Measures of Functional Food Administration (MEASURES) have been enforced since 1 June, 1996 to regulate the use, examination, production, marketing and sales, labeling, specification, advertising, and monitoring of functional food in China.

Table 3.1 77 种已批准的既是食品又是药品的名单

Drug Latin name	Chinese name	English name	Latin name
Agkistrodon	蝮蛇，Fushe	Pallas Pit Viper	*Agkistrodon balys*
Arillus Longan	龙眼肉，Longyanrou	Longan Aril	*Dimocarpus longan*
Bulbus Allii Macrostemi	薤白，Xiebai	Longstamen Onion Bulb	*Allium macrostemon*
Bulbus Lilii	百合，Baihe	Lily Bulb	*Lilium lancifolium; L. brownii var. viridulum; L. pumilum*
Concha Ostreae	牡蛎，Muli	Oyster Shell	*Ostrea gigas; O. talienwhanensis; O. rivularis*
Cortex Cinnamomi	肉桂，Rougui	Cassia Bark	*Cinnamomum cassia*
Endothelium Corneum Gigeriae Galli	鸡内金，Jineijin	Chicken's Gizzard-skin	*Gallus gallus domesticus*
Exocarpium Citri Rubrum	橘红，Juhong	Red Tangerine Peel	*Citrus reticulata*
Flos Carthami	红花，Honghua	Safflower	*Carthamus tinctorius*
Flos Caryophylli	丁香，Dingxiang	Clove	*Eugenia caryophylata*
Flos Chrysanthemi	菊花，Juhua	Chrysanthemun Flower	*Chrysanthemum morifolium*
Folium Mori	桑叶，Sangye	Mulberry Leaf	*Morus alba*
Folium Nelumbinis	荷叶，Heye	Lotus Leaf	*Nelumbo nucifera*
Folium Perillae	紫苏叶，Zisuye	Perilla Leaf	*Perilla frutescens*
Fructus Amomi	砂仁，Sharen	Villous Amomum Fruit	*Amomum villosum; A. villosum var. Xanthioides; A. longiligulare*
Fructus Anisi Stellati	八角茴香，Bajiaohuixiang	Chinese Star Anise	*Illcium verum*
Fructus Aurantii	代代花，Daidaihua	Orange Fruit	*Citrus aurantium "Daidai"*

Table 3.1 77 种已批准的既是食品又是药品的名单 (continued)

Drug Latin name	Chinese name	English name	Latin name
Fructus Canarii	青果，Qingguo	Chinese White Olive	Canarium album
Fructus Cannabis	火麻仁，Huomaren	Hemp Seed	Cannabis sativa
Fructus Chaenomelis	木瓜，Mugua	Common Floweringqince Fruit	Chaenomeles speciosa
Fructus Citri	香缘，Xiangyuan	Citron Fruit	Citrus medica; C. wilsonii
Fructus Citri Sarcodactylis	佛手，Foshou	Finger Citron	Citrus medica var. sarcodactylis
Fructus Crataegi	山楂，Shanzha	Hawthorn Fruit	Crataegus pinnatifida var. major; C. pinnatifida
Fructus Foeniculi	小茴香，Xiaohuixiang	Fennel	Foeniculum vulgare
Fructus Gardeniae	栀子，Zhizi	Cape Jasmine Fruit	Gardenia jasminoides
Fructus Hippophae	沙棘，Shaji	Seabuckthorn Fruit	Hippophae rhamnoides
Fructus Hordei Germinatus	麦芽，Maiya	Germinated Barley	Hordeum vulgare
Fructus Jujubae	大枣，Dazao	Chinese Date	Ziziphus jujuba
Fructus Lycii	枸杞子，Gouqizi	Barbary Wolfberry Fruit	Lycium barbarum
Fructus Momordicae	罗汉果，Luohanguo	Grosvenor Momordica Fruit	Momordica grosvenori
Fructus Mori	桑椹，Sangshen	Mulberry Fruit	Morus alba
Fructus Mume	乌梅，Wumei	Smoked Plum	Prunus mume
Fructus Piperis	胡椒，Hujiao	Pepper Fruit	Piper nigrum
Herba Cichorii	菊苣，Juju	Chicory Herb	Cichorium glandulosum; C. intybus
Herba Moslae	香薷，Xiangru	Haichow Elsholtzia Herb	Mosla chinensis
Herba Menthae	薄荷，Bohe	Peppermint	Mentha haplocalyx

Table 3.1 77 种已批准的既是食品又是药品的名单 (*continued*)

Drug Latin name	Chinese name	English name	Latin name
Herba Pogostemonis	广藿香，Guanghuoxiang	Cablin Patchouli Herb	*Pogostemon cablin*
Herba Portulacae	马齿苋，Machixian	Purslane Herb	*Portulaca oleracea*
Mel	蜂蜜，Fengmi	Honey	*Apis cerana; A. mellifera*
Pericappium Citri Reticulatae	陈皮，Chenpi	Dried Tangerine Peel	*Citrus reticulata*
Pericarpium Zanthoxyli	花椒，Huajiao	Pricklyash Peel	*Zanthoxylum schinifolium; Z. bungeanum*
Poria	茯苓，Fuling	Indian Bread	*Poria cocos*
Radix Angelicae Dahuricae	白芷，Baizhi	Dahurian Angelica Root	*Angelica dahurica; A. var. formosana*
Radix Glycyrrhizae	甘草，Gancao	Liquorice Root	*Glycyrrhiza uralensis; G. inflata; G. glabra*
Rhizoma Apiniae Officinarum	高良姜，Gaoliangjiang	Lesser Galangal Rhizome	*Alpinia officinarum*
Rhizoma Dioscoreae	山药，Shanyao	Common Yam Rhizome	*Dioscorea opposita*
Rhizoma Imperatae	白茅根，Baimaogen	Lalang Grass Rhizome	*Imperata cylindrica var. major*
Rhizoma Phragmitis	芦根，Lugen	Reed Rhizome	*Phragmites communis*
Rhizoma Zingiberis Recens	生姜，Shengjiang	Fresh Ginger	*Zingiber officinale*
Semen Armeniacae Amarum	杏仁，Xingren	Apricot Seed	*Prunus armeniaca var. ansu; P. sibirica; P. mandshurica; P. armeniaca*
Semen Canavaliae	刀豆，Daodou	Jack Bean	*Canavalia gladiata*
Semen Cassiae	决明子，Juemingzi	Cassia Seed	*Cassia obtusifolia; C. tora*

Table 3.1   77 种已批准的既是食品又是药品的名单 (*continued*)

Drug Latin Name	Chinese Name	English Name	Latin Name
Semen Coicis	薏苡仁，Yiyiren	Coix Seed	*Coix lacrymajobi var. Ma-yuen*
Semen Euryales	芡实，Qianshi	Gordon Euryale Seed	*Euryale ferox*
Semen Ginkgo	白果，Baiguo	Ginkgo Seed	*Ginkgo biloba*
Semen Lablab Album	白扁豆，Baibiandou	White Hyacinth Bean	*Dolichos lablab*
Semen Myristicae	肉豆蔻，Roudoukou	Nutmeg	*Myristica fragrans*
Semen Nelumbinis	莲子，Lianzi	Lotus Seed	*Nelumbo nucifera*
Semen Persicae	桃仁，Taoren	Peach Seed	*Prunus persica; P. davidiana*
Semen Phaseoli	赤小豆，Chixiaodou	Rice Bean	*Phaseolus calcaratus; P. angularis*
Semen Pruni	郁李仁，Yuliren	Chinese Dwarf Cherry Seed	*Prunus humilis; Prunus japonica; P. pedunculata*
Semen Raphani	莱菔子，Laifuzi	Radish Seed	*Raphanus sativus*
Semen Sesami Nigrum	黑芝麻，Heizhima	Black Sesame	*Sesamum indicum*
Semen Brassicae Junceae	黄芥子，Huangjiezi	Yellow Mustard Seed	*Brassica juncea*
Semen Sojae Preparatum	淡豆豉，Dandouchi	Fermented Soybean	*Glycine max;*
Semen Torreyae	榧子，Feizi	Grand Torreya Seed	*Torreya grandis*
Semen Ziziphi Spinosae	酸枣仁，Suanzaoren	Spine Date Seed	*Ziziphus jujuba var. spinosa*
Thallus Laminariae	昆布，Kunbu	Kelp or Tangle	*Laminaria japonica*
Zaocys	乌梢蛇，Wushaoshe	Black Snake	*Zaocys dhumnades*
Fructus Phyllanthi	余甘子，Yuganzi	Emblic Leafflower Fruit	*Phyllanthus emblica L.*
Flos Lonicerae	金银花，Jinyinhua	Honeysuckle Flower	*Lonicera japonica Thunb.; Lonicera hypoglauca Miq.; Lonicera confusa DC.; Lonicera dasystyla Rebd.*
Herba Houttuyniae	鱼腥草，Yuxingcao	Heartleaf Houttuynia Herb	*Houttuynia cordata Thunb.*

Table 3.1 77 种已批准的既是食品又是药品的名单 (*continued*)

Drug Latin name	Chinese name	English name	Latin name
Fructus Alpiniae Oxyphyllae	益智，Yizhi	Sharpleaf Glangal Fruit	*Alpinia oxyphylla Miq.*
Semen Sterculiae Lychnophorae	胖大海，Pangdahai	Boat-fruited Sterculia Seed	*Sterculia lychnophora Hance*
Herba Lophatheri	淡竹叶，Danzhuye	Lophatherum He	*Lophatherum gracile Brongn.*
Radix Puerariae	葛根，Gegen	Kudzuvine Root	*Pueraria lobata (Willd.) Ohwi.; Pueraria thomsonii Benth.*
Herba Taraxaci	蒲公英，Pugongying	Dandelion	*Taraxacum mongolicum Hand.-Mazz.; Taraxacum sinicum Kitag.*

THE CONCEPT AND DEFINITION OF FUNCTIONAL FOOD

The concept and definition of functional food are very difficult to determine. They are still to be settled after being debated for decades. The definitions of functional food are different from country to country. The term "functional food" was first used in Japan and is now widely used in Europe and America [Verschuren, 1996; Analysis, 19962]. The earliest definition by Japanese Public Health Ministry in 1962, is as follows: "Functional food is the food which comprises a kind of functional factor relating to biological protection, biological rhythmic regulation, disease prevention and health restoration, has been processed, and has a significant effect on the regulation of body functions." [Jin, 1995]

Basically, functional food is (1) made from raw materials or ingredients of daily food; (2) taken as diets by usual ways; and (3) labeled to specify its function in biological regulation [Jin, 1995]. Functional food is commonly understood in Korea as "therapeutic food", as appreciated in IUFOST'96 Regional Symposium on Non-nutritive Health Factors for Future Foods [Proceeding, 1996], which was sponsored by South Korea's Food Science Technology Society. "Health food" and "Pharm food" [Etkin & John, 1996] are also common terms for functional food in the U.S.A. The term "improvement food" is commonly used in Germany.

According to the World Food Research Institute, there are two categories of health food, i.e., natural health food and prescribed health food.

Natural health food comprises:

(1) The food for good health (narrow scope), which helps maintain and improve health;
(2) Natural food, which is free of food additives; and
(3) Nutritional supplement food, which is nutrition supplements and modifiers.

Prescribed functional food may be also used for therapeutic and corrective purposes. In China, it is called medicated food [Wong, 1982], medicated diet [Zhang, 1990], therapeutic food, food for health care, food for maintaining health [Dang, 1995], and diet for nutrition, food for nutrition and health care, etc. Old terms such as imperial diet [Dang, 1996], rare diet [Hu, 1987], food recipe for therapy, etc. are also widely used [Cheng, 1986; Sun, 1995, Zhao, 1962].

In spite of the great difference in nomenclature and classification of functional food in different countries, a consensus is to focus on the function for health care, so-called the third function of food. The MEASURES provides such a unified concept of Chinese functional food. As stipulated in Article 2 of Chapter 1 of the MEASURES, functional food is the food with specific function for health care. Functional food is suitable for use by specific group of people to improve their body functions but it is not aimed at treating disease [The Ministry of Public Health, 1996a].

In a word, a good definition for functional foods is this: they are foods which can be part of our everyday diet but which have properties that provide an additional health benefit.

THE REQUIREMENT FOR EXAMINATION OF FUNCTIONAL FOOD

To implement the MEASURES for scientific examination and standardization, the Ministry of Public Health established the Committee of Food Hygiene Examination and promulgated some regulations (RULES), including Rules of Technology in Functional Food Examination, Functional Evaluation and Examination Methods for Functional Food, Rules of Functional Food Labeling, and General Requirements of Functional Food Hygiene. Responsible governments in different municipalities, provinces and autonomous regions authorized some institutes to conduct testing of functional food. Without the formal approval by the Ministry of Public Health or application submitted to the Health Administration under the State Council, any production, marketing, or sales under the name of functional food is illegal and will be prosecuted according to the Law of Food Hygiene. As yet, about 2000 Chinese functional food items have been approved by the Ministry of Public Health and entitled to have a Label of Functional Food on their packages.

THE EVALUATION AND TESTING OF FUNCTIONAL FOOD

Before promulgation of the RULES, it was difficult to have standard methods for functional food testing. Common Standards for Functional Food (STANDARDS) were published by the National Technology Supervision Bureau on 28 February 1997 and have been enforced since 1 May 1997. At present, the authorized institutes for testing functional food need to perform the following 30 tests on functional food products:

Immune regulation; Postponement of senility; Memory improvement; Promotion of growth and development; Anti-fatigue; Body weight reduction; Oxygen deficit tolerance; Radiation protection; Antimutation; Blood lipid regulation; Blood glucose regulation; Gastrointestinal function improvement; Sleep improvement; Improvement of nutritional anemia; Protection of liver from chemical damages; Lactation improvement; Vision improvement; Promotion of lead removal; Removal of "*intense heat*" from the throat and moistening of the throat; Blood pressure regulation; Enhancement of bone calcification.

抗氧化　antioxidant
祛痤瘡　reducing acne
祛黃褐斑　removing chloasma
改善皮膚水分，油分　improving skin moisture or oil
調節腸道菌群　regulating intestinal bacterial growth
改善消化　improving digestion function
潤腸通便　moistening the bowels to relieve constipation
對胃粘膜有輔助保護作用　protecting stomach mucous membrane
減輕放化療毒副作用　relieving the side-effects of radiotherapy or chemotherapy

The published STANDARDS avoid arbitrary descriptions of the functions of functional food. For examining any functional food, which has not yet been classified by STANDARDS, functional food manufacturers could propose some testing and evaluation methods. The proposed methods will be verified by the experts assigned by the Ministry of Public Health before acceptance and listing of the methods in the STANDARDS [The Ministry of Public Health, 1996b]. Regarding the appearance and other sensory characteristics, the STANDARDS stipulate that functional food must have defined shape, color, smell, taste, and quality. Any annoying smell or taste is not allowed.

THE EXTENSION OF FUNCTIONAL FOOD TO CHINESE MEDICINE PRESCRIPTIONS

Which material qualities as functional food but not Chinese medicine, or vice versa is still a debate. It has been long believed that food and medicine share a common origin in Chinese tradition. To resolve this problem, the Ministry of Public Health [Department of Hygiene Supervision, 1997] has formally recognized 77 items as both food and

Chinese medicine (Table 17.1). It is difficult to distinguish these listed 77 items of dietary Chinese medicine for use as functional food or traditional Chinese medicine.

The number of items in the list will increase with further research and development of dietary Chinese medicine products, which must be safe, reliable, and with defined functions for health care.

The items which are not listed as dietary Chinese medicine require Safety and Toxicology Evaluation, as stipulated in the Evaluation Methods and Testing Measures of Food Safety and Toxicology, before application for inclusion in the functional food listing.

THE STEADY DEVELOPMENT OF FUNCTIONAL FOOD PRODUCTS

As seen from the 2000 kinds of food which had passed the functional food evaluation, the current research and development of Chinese functional food is performed very well in formulation design, development of product categories, functions for health care, practical use, etc.

Formulation Design

Most of the approved functional food items were developed by using modern technology in accordance with modern nutritional science, and traditional Chinese nutrition knowledge in Chinese medicine. Novel formulation and processes were found in the production of many functional food items. For example, the Tiao Zhi Ling (a golden remedy for regulating fat) comprises fermentation liquid of hypha of Lingchih (*Ganoderma sp.*), honey, and fruits of Chinese Wolfberry (*Lycium barbarum*).

Product Categories

The China markets for functional food has great potential. There are a variety of functional food products in the China market. Effective functional food has been specially developed and produced for use in specific groups of people (e.g., specific races) in a specific environment (e.g., geographical regions, climate, body conditions, etc.). The popular categories of functional food take the forms of health-care wine, health-care tea, health-care drinks, health-care vinegar, health-care cake, health-care powder, health-care rice, health-care flour, nutritional liquid, health-care chewing gum. In addition to local functional food product, foreign products such as shark's cartilage, melatonin, fish oil, spirulina have also entered into China's functional food market.

Health-care Functions
The vague terms such as "suitable for both the old and young", which is commonly used in the past, are not allowable. More definite terms such as "postponement of senility" and "immune regulation" are used instead. According to our preliminary statistics, some foods that are grouped as the most common health-care function categories are as follows:

Immune regulation
American ginseng (Panax quinquefolius)
Ginseng (Panax ginseng)
Acanthopanax (Acanthopanax senticosus)
Barbary Wolfberry Fruit (Lycium barbarum)
Astragalus (Astragalus membranaceus; A. Membranaceus var. Mongholicus)
Chinese Caterpillar fungus (Cordyceps sinensis)
Gingko leaf (Ginkgo biloba)
Walnut (Juglans regia)
Chinese Date (Ziziphus jujuba)
Royal Jelly,
Chinese Angelica (Angelica sinensis)
Glossy Ganoderma (Ganoderma applanatum)
Mulberry Fruit (Morus alba)

Postponement of senility
Roxburgh Rose (Rosa roxburghii)
green tea (Camellia sinensis)
Fleeceflower root (Polygonum multiflorum)
Black Sesame (Sesamum indicum)
honey
Mulberry Fruit (Morus alba)
Barbary Wolfberry Fruit (Lycium barbarum)

Blood lipid regulation
Hawthorn fruit (Crataegus pinnatifida)
Soybean (Glycine max)
Peach Seed (Prunus persica)
Chrysanthemum Flower (Chrysanthemum morifolium)
supper vinegar
Spine Date Seed (Ziziphus jujuba var. spinosa)
fish oil,
corn oil (Zea mays)

extract of Flax seed (Linum usitatissimum)
Safflower seed (Carthamus tinctorius)
Liquorice Root (Glycyrrhiza uralensis; G. inflata; G. glabra)
Dried Tangerine Peel (Citrus reticulata)
Barbary Wolfberry Fruit (Lycium barbarum)

Blood and urine glucose reduction
Five leaf Gynosttemma (Gynostemma pentaphyllum)
Hawthorn fruit (Crataegus pinnatifida)
Chinese Yam (Dioscorea opposita)
Buckweat Poria (Fagopyrum esculentum)
Cocos Poria (Poria cocos),
extract of Pumpkin (Cucurbita moschata)
extract of pig pancreas
powder of Spirulina (Spirulina princeps)
Germinated Barley (Hordeum vulgare)
Barbary Wolfberry Fruit (Lycium barbarum)
Mulberry Fruit (Morus alba)

Oxygen deficit tolerance
Safflower seed (Carthamus tinctorius)
Chrysanthemum Flower (Chrysanthemum morifolium)
Glossy Ganoderma (Ganoderma applanatum)

Improvement of nutritional anemia
Chinese Date (Ziziphus jujuba)
Barbary Wolfberry Fruit (Lycium barbarum)

Radiation protection
Cassia Bark (Cinnamomum cassia)
Glossy Ganoderma (Ganoderma applanatum)

Other common function categories include anti-fatigue, body weight reduction.

Practical application
It is appreciated that the legislation in China did not narrow the scope of functional food application. The approved functional food products include those suitable for the aged, children, men, and women in pregnancy and puerpera.

Concluding Remarks

Long history and rich experience of traditional Chinese medicine in food therapy provides us with a number of traditional functional foods e.g., *Herba Houttuyniae Houttuynia cordata Thunb.*, and Vaccinium bracteatum (*Vaccinium fragile Franch.*). With the development of advanced technology, a new generation of Chinese functional food is emerging. In addition to the human and animal testing for the effects of functional food on the body regulation, the structure and quantity of active ingredients of some functional food are also determined. The new generation functional food will have higher quality and popularity in international markets.

The Theory and Use of Functional Food in Traditional Chinese Medicine

According to traditional Chinese Medicine, food has 4 properties: cold, cool, warm and hot, and five tastes: sour, bitter, sweet, pungent and salty just like medicinal herbs. Besides, food also has other properties, such as the lifting, lowering, floating and sinking actions, meridian's tropism, and compatibility and so on just like medicinal herbs.

Foods with cold or cool properties have the function of clearing away heat, purging fire-evil and removing toxic material. They can be used to treat carbuncle, diarrhea, and cough due to lung-heat. Such foods include crab, bitter melon, mung bean, pear, etc..

Foods with warm and hot properties have the function of warming, clearing away coldness. They can be used to treat asthenia-cold of the spleen and stomach, lassitude in the loins and legs, etc.. Such foods include mutton, walnut, peppers, etc.

Foods with mild properties can be used by ordinary people. These foods are carrot, an edible fungus, eggs, grapes, etc.

The five tastes refer to as sour, bitter, sweet, pungent and salty. Foods with different tastes have different functions.

Foods with sour taste have the function of contraction. If a patient suffers from abdominal pain and loose stool due to dyspepsia, what can we do?

> "Chinese hawthorn, a fruit with sour taste can cure this disease. Fry Chinese hawthorn into coke and grind them into fine powder. Take 9 grams, and add some brown sugar. Pour in boiling water, and mix. Take it all when it is warm."

Foods with bitter taste can dry the wetness-evil, and clear away heat.

Foods with sweet taste have the functions of nourishing blood and *Qi* and relieving convulsive disease. For example, a patient who suffers from weakness, anemia and neurasthenia can take mulberry syrup, which has a sweet taste.

> "Take 10–15 grams each time, 2–3 times a day. Take it together with warm water or yellow wine together."

Foods with pungent taste have the function of dispersing exopathogens from superficies of the body and regulating Qi (vital energy) and relieving pain.

Foods with salty taste have the function of dissipating a mass, nourishing *Yin* and suppressing *Yang*.

> "The theory of Yin and Yang is an ancient philosophical concept used in Traditional Chinese Medicine. It means the two fundamental principles or forces in the universe, ever opposing and supplementing each other. Traditional Chinese holds that 'functional movement' belongs to Yang, 'nourishing substance' to Yin."

Different tastes can go into different meridian. According to the theory of traditional Chinese medicine, it is easy for sour taste to go into the liver and gall bladder. It is easy for bitter taste to go into the heart and small intestine. It is easy for sweet taste to go into the spleen and stomach. It is easy for pungent taste to go into the lung and large intestine, and it is easy for salty taste to go into the kidney and urinary bladder.

After getting into the body, the functions of foods can go upward or downward in direction based on the different properties. Most foods which are thin and light in taste have the actions of lifting and floating and pungent, sweet tastes and warm or hot properties. In contrast, most of the thick in taste and heavy foods with the actions of lowering and sinking have bitter, sour, salty tastes and cold or cool properties.

The lifting, lowering, floating and sinking actions can also be altered through the processing and joint use of foods. Using eating the crab as an example, the property of crab is cold and the taste is salty. So it is not good for the patient with weakness and cold constitution. However, if they insist to eat crab they can do so by eating some food with the actions of lifting and floating and the properties of warm or hot together, such as ginger, Chinese onion, vinegar, wine, etc.. In this way, the cold property of crab can be changed or suppressed.

To change the warm or hot property of peppers, one can add some food with cold or cool property when cooking peppers, such as bitter melon. In this way, the hot property of pepper can be changed.

To get good effect with food therapy in the clinic one can apply knowledge of the different properties of food, meridian's tropism, and the properties of lifting, lowering, sinking and compatibility. Traditional Chinese medicine holds that medicine and food share a common origin. Some foods can be used to prevent and treat diseases just like medicine. This can be illustrated by using garlic and radish, common vegetable food, for example:

"Apart from such nutrients as protein, carbohydrates, vitamin, calcium, phosphorus, etc., garlic contains a volatile ingredient such as allicin (Suan La Su) which has good antibacterial effects against some micro-organisms. The presence of garlic juice in culture medium prevents growth of staphylococcal dysentery, escherichia coli, and hemophilus pertussis. Even aflatoxin, which can produce a very strong substance to cause cancer, was eliminated by garlic juice. Thus garlic is not only a food of rich nutrition but also a medicine with many functions to disinfect bacteria"

"Radish, a common vegetable, can be cooked into very delicious dishes, but can also be used as medicine. Radish can relieve some syndromes like retention of food due to over-eating, indigestion, abdominal distention and so on. This is because radish contains a kind of oil with pungent and hot taste named mustard oil (Jie Zi oil) in white radish, which can promote the movement of stomach and small intestine, promote digestion, improve appetite and regulate Qi. In addition, fried shredded radish with beef has the functions of reinforcing spleen and stomach, strengthening tendon and bone, promoting the circulation of blood and eliminating sputum, etc."

"The mixture of sliced radish and garlic paste has the functions of invigorating stomach, relieving dyspepsia, and eliminating phlegm. So it can be used to treat indigestion and high blood pressure."

"Xin Li Mei, a kind of sweet radish with green peel and red insides, is treasured as ideal vegetable during such dry seasons as winter and spring. An old saying in China, 'If you eat more reddish in winter and more ginger in summer, you needn't see the doctor.' indicates the reasons behind the usefulness of eating medicinal food.

Foods rich in fiber can prevent and treat the troubles in stomach and intestinal, especially for the cancer of colon and rectum. Eating more fruits and vegetables with green, red and yellow color, one can replenish a lot of carotene, vitamin C, therefore, some diseases caused by lack of vitamins can be cured. Many people have known this.

Corn is rich in nutrients. The fat contained in corn is 4–5 times than that in rice and flour, and the fat in corn is rich in unsaturated fatty acid, especially for linoleic acid which is 6 times higher than pig fat and 25% higher than peanut oil. So it can reduce serum cholesterol and prevent high blood pressure and myocardial infarction. The recent years' research has proved that corn has the function of anti-cancer. The fiber in corn can promote the movement of stomach and small intestine. It can clear away the poison and prevents the cancer of intestine. Corn also contains a factor called glutathione. It can catch or hold the substance that causes cancer just like handcuffs and then excrete them out through the digestive tract.

The most important application principle of functional food is that different patients need different functional food. For some serious diseases, the patient should also take some medicine to supplement the effects of functional food. With the development of Chinese hygiene and health care courses, functional food is attracting more and more attention from the doctors and the broad masses of the people. We believe that the functional food will have a bright future.

References

Analysis and Perspective. (1996) Eastern and Western Scientists share perspectives on functional foods at International Conference. World Food Regulation Review, Jan. 1996, 17–19.

Cheng, Zhi (1986) the Song Dynasty, A New Book for Longevity and Health of the Aged (Reprinted in 1986 by China Bookstore, Beijing).

Dang, Yi (1995) Science of Nutrition Dietary Therapy of Traditional Chinese Medicine, Beijing, Science Publishing House.

Dang, Yi (1996) Medicated Diet Textual Research on the Term "Medicated Food", Collection of Research Document of TCM, Beijing, TCM Classic Publishing House.

Department of Hygiene Supervision of the Ministry of Public Health (1997) Collection of Administration Laws of the Functional Food, Jilin Science and Technology Publishing House.

Etkin and John (1996) Medicated Food and Nutritious Agent: Transformation of Biological Therapy Model, a speech at International Symposium on Food Applied in Food and Medicine, London.

Hu, Sihui (1987) the Yuan Dynasty, Principles of Correct Diet (Reprinted in 1987 by the Peoples' Medical Publishing House, Beijing).

Jin, Zonglian (1995) Evaluating Principles and Methods of Functional Food, Beijing, Peking University Publishing House.

Proceedings of IUFOSI (1996) Regional Symposium on Non-Nutritive Health Factors for Future Foods.

Sun, Simiao (1995) the Tang Dynasty, Prescription Worth a Thousand Gold for Emergencies (Reprinted in 1955 by the People's Medical Publishing House, Beijing).

The Ministry of Public Health of the People's Republic of China (1996a), Measures of Functional Food Administration.

The Ministry of Public Health of the People's Republic of China (1996b) The Functional Evaluating Process and Testing Measures of the Functional Food.

Verschuren, Paulus M. (1996) Functional Food Science in Europe, Proceedings of IUFOSI '96 Regional Symposium on Non-Nutritive Health Factors for Future Foods.

Wong, Weijian (1982) A Collection of Choice Specimens of Medicated Diet Recipes, Beijing, The People's Medical Publishing House.

Wong, Weijian (1992) Nutriology of Traditional Chinese Medicine Diet, Shanghai, Shanghai Science Publishing House.

Zhang, Wengao (1990) Chinese Medicated Diet, Shanghai, Publishing House of Shanghai College of Traditional Chinese Medicine.

Zhao, Jie (1962) The Song Dynasty, Imperial Encyclopedia of Medicine (Reprinted in 1962 by the People's Medical Publishing House, Beijing).

4 UNDERSTANDING THE TOXICITY OF CHINESE HERBAL MEDICINAL PRODUCTS

Kelvin Chan

Introduction

Chinese medicine (CM) is a complex and holistic system of medicine with its own philosophy, diagnosis systems and treatments. It considers the human body in relation to its own natural, physical and social environments. The practice of CM involves physical therapy using acupuncture, moxibustion and related disciplines such as medical massage and Qi Gong, and chemical therapy using CM natural products. Thus Chinese herbal medicine (CHM) is an integral part of the Chinese medicine which has several thousand years of history in China, and is playing an important role in the medical care of Chinese people even nowadays, in parallel and often integrated with orthodox medical practice. It is the generalisation and summation of the experiences of CM practitioners' and scholars' long-term struggle against diseases. Its development has evolved into, based on the culture and philosophy of balancing body functions, a medical system through repeated tests and verification in clinical practice. The theories involved may not be easily interpreted in terms of those understood in orthodox medicine (Refer to Chapter 2 for detail).

Through centuries of using various types of CHM materials, possibly initiated by the folklore hero Shen Nong (translated as Divine Plowman) at around 2800 BC, records of cumulative experience had been kept. During these early periods, two important works appeared. The Shen Nong Ben Cao Jing (the earliest recorded materia medica of Shen Nong's herbal experience, translated as The Herbal Classic of the Divine Plowman) recorded 365 herbal materials. The Huang Di Nei Jing (the Inner Canon of the Yellow Emperor, in 100 BC) contained records of diagnosis and treatments using acupuncture and CHM materials. Later, a major updating of herbal experience and medical treatment was carried out by Li Shi Zhen who complied a comprehensive Pharmacopoeia, Ben Cao Gang Mu (Compendium of Materia Medica), in AD 1590, during the Ming Dynasty period. It consisted of 52 volumes, which took the author 30 years for its completion. It lists a total of 1,892 medical substances with more than 1,000 illustrations and about 11,000 composite prescriptions or formulae (Fu Fang) with detailed description of the appearance, properties, methods of collection, processing procedures and use of each herbal substance. These texts were first translated into Latin and then other languages during the 17th century. In recent years, more herbs have come into use through development, experience and research. These have been incorporated in successive editions of the Chinese Pharmacopoeia. There are now about 4,000 herbs, but generally some 500 are in common use. They are grouped under 18 classes according to their effects for treatment (See Chinese Pharmacopoeia 1992). The natural products, CHM materials, used in Chinese medicine consist of a combination of animal, mineral and plant origins in the form of mostly aqueous decoctions. As most of them are from plants, medical books on CM materia medica throughout the long history of development have conveniently referred them as "Ben Cao" (herbalism). The parts of plants used as crude herbs are processed roots, rhizomes, fruits, seeds, flowers, leaves, woods, barks, vine stems and sometimes, the whole plants. Most of these CHM natural materials are incorporated as composite prescriptions (formulae) that contain 3 to as many as 30 herbs. The herbal mixture is prepared as aqueous decoction by boiling all the herbal ingredients in a fixed amount of water. After simmering down to about one-third of the original volume the warm decoction is consumed orally immediately.

Apart from the commonly used decoctions other types of preparations are also administered. These CM medications are often known as "Zhong Cheng Yao" (ready-made CHM products). These are Powder (*San-ji*), Pill (*Wan-ji*), Extract (*Gao-ji*), Ointment (*Ruan-gao*) Plaster (*Ying-gao*), Liquor (*Jiu-ji* an alcoholic solution), Medicated tea (*Cha-ji*), and Tablet (*Pian-ji*). Some of the well-known prescriptions have been manufactured into ready-made CHM products in dosage forms, similar to those of orthodox medicinal products that are convenient for patient use. Noticeable problems are those involved with quality control of these products.

Some of these materials are poisonous and some with confusing species according to the classification in the Ben Cao Gang Mu (the Compendium of CM Materia Medica, published in 1596AD). The most recent listings have been published in successive pharmacopoeia (English version, one volume published in 1992; the Chinese version has 2 volumes published in 1995). They will cause intoxication, side effects or even death if they are not identified or used properly. Yet when processed, formulated and used properly they are useful parts of the composite prescriptions or ready made CHM products (Zhong Cheng Yao). Therefore it is not correct to consider that all herbal materials are safe. Clearly the concepts conceived in the principles of CM do utilise natural materials which are considered poisonous. From orthodox medical viewpoints these poisonous plants are not accepted for medical uses. It will be more helpful to understand the background and reasons behind the use of poisonous medicinal natural materials in Chinese medicine. However we must be open-minded and cautious when utilising medicinal herbs. Chapter 3 has illustrated that some of those well-used and non-toxic medicinal plants are used as functional food.

Recent Problems Concerning Toxicity of Chinese Medicinal Herbs

EXPERIENCE IN HONG KONG

During the late 1980s and the early 1990s the public in Hong Kong had experienced several severe cases of poisoning due to Chinese medicinal (CM) herbal materials, mainly crude herbs and ready-made herbal products, purchased from the local herbal shops for their own use. Some government bodies and academic institutes investigated some of these cases. The major reasons behind these unfortunate incidents have been due to lack of legal control on the use of CM crude herbs and ready-made products, mistakes of supplying the wrong herbs that should not be available freely to the public, and the lack of expertise in identifying commonly available potent and poisonous crude herbs.

In 1989, two persons in Hong Kong suffered serious neuropathy and encephalopathy after consuming the roots of Guijiu (*Podophyllum hexandrum*). This toxic herb was supplied as Longdancao (*Gentiana rigescen*) by a supplier in China (Ng *et al.* 1991). The same herb was also found as a substitute in the samples of *Clematis* species (Weilingxian) leading to 14 cases of neuropathy in Asian countries in 1995–96 (But *et al.* 1996). But (1994) reported 4 cases of drowsiness attributed to erroneous dispensing of Yangjihua (flower of *Datura metel*) instead of Lingxiaohua (flower of *Campsis grandiflora*).

Subsequently, over the past decade the Hong Kong's governmental Ministry of Health, who has set up working parties, together with the help of academic institutes has made tremendous and continuing effort to update databases and take action for all aspects of Chinese medicine. These include legal control on supply of CM materials, CM practitioners' and professionals' qualifications, education and training, and promotion of research & development in herbal manufacturing, and quality assurance measures on CM herbal products.

The selection of CM materials was from those available, after surveying, in the market at the time of the project in the early 1990s (i.e. before the implementation of regulations being started at present in Hong Kong). The 48 specimens obtained from commercial sources were also recorded in the Pharmacopoeia of the People's Republic of China (described here as the Chinese Pharmacopoeia, CP, 1992 English Edition), as potent and poisonous materia medica and also in similar literature in Taiwan; all of the 48 items were considered as poisonous and potent CM materials. They are recorded as poisonous in the CP. Therefore, the choice was considered appropriate. The project was a practically oriented investigation and documentation. It was not just a literature search; except some of the information on clinical symptoms due to poisoning and for treatment were derived from literature available in journals written in Chinese language. The results on authentication, identification and determination of LD-50 were experimentally obtained. The Chinese version of the Compendium was the result of these investigations. The two co-editors of the Chinese version directed the completion of the project and publication of the Chinese version of the Compendium by Commercial Press (Hong Kong) Ltd. in August 1994 (Xu & Chan, 1994).

The text is divided into four main sections. The Preface highlights how this Compendium was conceived. The Introduction gives a brief concept of guide for the use of each of the main monographs. The Main section consists of 48 monographs. Each monograph follows a pattern that is organised for easy access to information concerning the poisonous material under 10 headings such as Alternative names, Source, History, Locality of growth or production, Identification of crude herb, Chemical composition, Main functions & indications, Toxicity, Clinical toxicity, and Rescuing treatment. At the end of each monograph a list of specific references is given for further information. The Appendices section has 3 sub-divisions. Appendix 1 is newly added into the English version. It deals with the processing of CM materia medica from freshly collected materials. These materials should be processed, according strict procedures, before used as "crude" herbs. Such procedures are specified in the CP to ensure the usability of the crude materials. During the processing stages the toxic ingredients of the poisonous herbs will be removed. Appendix 2 gives a general description of the toxicology procedures used to determine the LD_{50} of each poisonous CM material. Appendix 3 summarises the list of general references. Table 4.1 gives the pin yin names and Latin names of these 48 poisonous natural CM materials included in the Compendium.

This Compendium will be of interest to teachers and students in Schools of Pharmacy and other university departments running Chinese medicine courses, and courses on toxicology and plant chemistry, scientists in Regulatory Authorities and Poisoning Units with particular interest in natural products. The information from the Compendium can be utilised in several ways in order to prevent and treat accidental poisoning due to these substances. It also helps regulatory bodies to consider regulatory aspects of products containing these items.

PROBLEMS OF TOXICITY FROM CHINESE HERBAL MEDICINAL SUBSTANCES REPORTED IN DEVELOPED COUNTRIES

Over the past few years, the popularity of CM herbs and herbal products has grown in a very rapid way and caught the attention of the public in western developed countries (Jin *et al.* 1995) in both sides of the Atlantic. This has been due to the well known double-blind clinical trial on the successful use of a decoction of 10 CM crude herbs to relief atopic eczema that was resistant to orthodox medical treatment. At the same time the public, medical communities, herbal suppliers and manufacturers and academic professionals in these developed communities also express their fear and uncertainty over the safety, efficacy and quality of CM herbs and products available in the markets (Chan, 1996). Adulteration was responsible for an epidemic of severe kidney damage (de Smet 1992) in Belgium where the herb Fangji (*Stephania tetrandra*) was substituted by the nephrotoxic Guangfangji (*Aristolochia fangchi*).

Lack of understanding of how to use CHM substances
One of the major problems has been the lack of understanding how CHM materials should be used properly. When used according to guidelines in CM practice, often as Fu-Fang (composite formulae), even poisonous herbs can be beneficial to certain treatments. For example, Bai Xia (*Rhizoma pinelliae*, monograph 7 in the Compendium) is considered as poisonous according to the CP. But it is included, in properly

Table 4.1 Potent or toxic medicinal materials included in the pictorial compendium of poisonous Chinese medicinal herbs available in Hong Kong (Edited by Xu & Chan, 1994)

Common Pin Yin names	Latin names
Radixes and rhizomata	
1. Chuan Wu	(*Radix Aconiti*)
2. Da Ji	(Hong Da Ji; *Radix Knoxiae*)
3. Shan Dou Gen	(Guang Dou Gen; *Radix Sophorae tonkinensis*)
4. Tian Ma	(*Rhizoma Gastrodiae*)
5. Tian Nan Xing	(Hu Zhang Nan Xing; *Rhizoma Pinelliae pedatisectae*)
6. Shui Ban Xia	(*Rhizoma Typhonii flagelliformis*)
7. Ban Xia	(*Rhizoma Pinelliae*)
8. Gan Shui	(*Radix Kansui*)
9. Fu Zi	(*Radix Aconiti lateralis preparata*)
10. Cao Wu	(*Radix Aconiti*)
11. Chong Lou	(*Rhizoma Paridis*)
12. Tao Er Qi	(*Radix et Rhizoma Sinopodophylli*)
13. Lang Du	(Guangdong Lang Du; *Rhizoma Alocasiae*)
14. Chang Shan	(*Radix Dichroae*)
Cortices	
15. Ku Lian Pi	(*Cortex Meliae)*
16. Xiang Jia Pi	(*Cortex Periplocae*)
Flowers	
17. Yuan Hua	(*Flos Genkwa)*
18. Nao Yang Hua	(Yang Jin Hua; *Flos Daturae*)
Fruits and seeds	
19. Tian Xian Zi	(*Semen Hyoscyami*)
20. Mu Bie Zi	(*Semen Momordicae*)
21. Ba Dou	(*Fructus Crotonis*)
22. Zao Jia	(*Fructus Gleditsiae*)
23. Ku Xing Ren	(*Fructus Armeniacae amarum*)
24. Wu Zhu Yu	(*Fructus Evodiae*)
25. Ma Qian Zi	(*Fructus Strychni*)
26. Ji Xing Zi	(*Fructus Impatientis*)
27. Tao Ren	(*Fructus Persicae*)
28. She Chuang Zi	(*Fructus cnidii*)
29. Qian Niu Zi	(*Fructus Pharbitdis*)
30. Bi Ma Zi	(*Fructus Ricini*)
31. Ya Dan Zi	(*Fructus Bruceae*)

Table 4.1 Potent or toxic medicinal materials included in the pictorial compendium of poisonous Chinese medicinal herbs available in Hong Kong (Edited by Xu & Chan, 1994) (*continued*)

Common Pin Yin names	Latin names
The whole plant	
32. Xi Xin	(*Herba asari*)
Resin	
33. Gan Qi	(*Resina Toxicodendri*)
Animals used as medicine	
34. Tu Bie Chong	(Jin Bian Tu Bie, *Opisthosplatia*)
35. Shui Zhi	(*Hirudo*)
36. Quan Xie	(*Scorpio*)
37. Meng Chong	(*Tabanus*)
38. Hong Niang Zi	(*Huechys*)
39. Ban Mao	(*Mylabris*)
40. Wu Gong	(*Scolopendra*)
41. Qi She	(*Agkistrodon*)
42. Chan Su	(*Venenum Bufonis*)
Minerals used as medicine	
43. Mang Xiao	(*Natrii sulfas*)
44. Zhu Sha	(*Cinnabaria*)
45. Liu Huang	(*Sulphur*)
46. Xiong Huang	(*Realgar*)
47. Qing Fen	(*Calomelos*)
48. Fan Dan	(*Chalcanthitum*)

processed form, as one of the 6 ingredients in the famous Fu-Fang, Liu Jun Zi Tong (Decoction of Six Noble Ingredients, available also as ready-made product as Liu Jun Zi Wan). The six ingredients are Dang Shen (*Radix Codonopsis pilosilae*), Fu Ling (*Poria*), Bai Shu (*Rhizoma Atractylodis macrocephalae*), Gan Cao (*Radix Glycyrrhizae*), Chen Pi (*Pericarpium citri reticulatae*), and Ban Xia (*Rhizoma pinelliae*). This Fu Fang is used to regulate gastrointestinal disorders and immune system and has anti-gastric ulcer action. The CM description for its use is "It benefits *Qi and Spleen* aids deficiency of *Spleen and Stomach Qi*, relieves abdominal distension and rectifies loose stools". However, Ban Xia alone is poisonous. Many other examples are available for inclusion of potent and poisonous CM materia medica in composite formulae. The CP under the sections on "Zhong Cheng Yao" or

"Ready-made Preparations" include these potent and toxic natural materials as ingredients in the formulae for Fu-Fang (composite prescriptions) that are approved by the Authority.

Some heavy metals have been included as ingredients in the ready-made formulae products. For examples, Liu Shen Wan, a popular readymade product, contains toad toxin (*Venenum Bufonis*), Realgar as one of the potent and poisonous ingredients. At the dose used according to the Pharmacopoeia it is safe to take. Unfortunately the quality control of the OTC products is variable as we observed (Hong *et al.* 1995), thus potential accidental poisoning will happen when the public acquire poor QC products of these sort.

Supply of fake or substituted CHM substances

The other concern has been the authenticity of CM materials available in the market. We over the years identified fake or substituted CHM crude substances in the UK market (Yu *et al.*, 1995). Recognition and identification of CM materials requires expertise. These expert professionals are not plentiful in the west. It has been therefore the intention of this English version of the Compendium (Chan & Xu 2001), to bridge the gap, for the time being, as reference information. Professionals in CM practice, those engaged in toxicology and poison centres, suppliers of CM materials, and scientists in academic and research institutes may benefit from the text. Recent episodes of liver or kidney toxicity consequential to the use of slimming CM product in Belgium were not straightforward kidney "poisoning" cases (Vanherweghem 1995). The herbal example for weight reduction involving "Fang-Ji" (*Radix Stephaniae tetrandrae*) was a good one illustrating the use of wrong herbs. Guang Fang-Ji was included in the mixture recipe (containing orthodox amphetamine analogue and diuretics together with two CM herbal items), of which Guang Fang-Ji, instead of Fang-Ji was one identified. Guang Fang-Ji, contains aristocholic acid that caused renal failure which the proper Fang-Ji should have no such chemical ingredients. Nevertheless Fang-Ji is not considered as a poisonous herb in the CP.

Inclusion of orthodox drugs into CHM products

Some imported CHM products contain orthodox drugs such as anti-biotics, anti-inflammatory drugs (both non-steroids and steroids) and pain-relieving agents (Karunanithy & Sumita, 1991). The toxicity, and efficacy claimed of the CHM products may be manly to those of the orthodox drugs included. Such inclusion in ready made CHM products was not considered as a positive attribute of CM in the west

(Chan, 2000), although some ready made CHM products containing orthodox drugs appear in the Chinese Pharmacopoeia. The licensing authority in China has approved these products.

Pricinples for Using Poisonous Herbs in Composite Prescriptions (Fu-Fang)

PRINCIPLES OF ACTIONS OF CM HERBS AND THEIR COMBINATIONS

From an orthodox medical viewpoint, some CHM natural herbs listed in the Official Chinese Pharmacopoeia (CP) are considered poisonous or toxic due to the presence of poisonous or toxic chemical constituents in the herbs. Of these there are about 50 of animal, plant and mineral natural materials in total included in the CP. In CM they are seldom prescribed or used alone. Each CM herb has its own specific characteristics and functions. CM herbs are generally classified into different categories.

- *Category a): Four Energies* (cold, hot, warm and cool, or neutral in terms of their energetic actions) **and** *Five Tastes* (sour, bitter, sweet, pungent-spicy and salty or tasteless) as defined by their actions to promote, disperse, harmonise, or tonify.
- *Category b): Ascending, Descending, Floating or Sinking*: Herbs that ascend and float move *Qi* (inner essence) upward and outward as they promote sweating and raise *Yang*, and causing vomiting and opening the orifices. Herbs that descend and sink promote urination and defaecation subduing *Yang* and calming the mind. In general, the functional tendency of an herb is related to its taste, property, quality, and processing. Herbs with features of ascending and floating must be pungent-spicy or sweet in taste and warm and hot in property, while herbs with characteristics of descending and sinking must be bitter, sour or salty in taste and cool or cold in property.
- *Category c): Herbs Entering Specific Meridians*. An herb may selectively act on a particular part of the body to relieve pathological change in specific meridians and organs. For example, *Ephedra* root (Mahuang) is indicated for fever, chills and absence of sweating due to invasion by *exogenous pathogenic wind and cold*, dysuria and oedema

by promoting sweating, soothing asthma and benefiting urination via the entrance to the lung and urinary bladder meridians.

- *Category d). Herbs with Toxicity and Non-toxicity*: The words "toxic, non-toxic, very toxic or slightly toxic" are often used in Chinese Materia Medica. Non-toxic herbs, sometimes referred to as "Superior Class", are moderate in nature and, generally speaking, do not possess any side effects. Examples are Jujube (Dazao) and Poria (Fuling). Toxic herbs, sometimes referred as "Low Grade" herbs and used for specific purposes in a TCM prescription, can cause symptomatic reactions and adverse effects. No overdose of these should be given. Examples are processed aconite root (Fuzi) and *Nuxvomica* seed (Maqianzi).

CM herbs are often prescribed in *Fu-Fang* (composite formulae) according to CM principles of diagnosis and treatment. This approach of combination of processed poisonous or toxic herbs with other non-toxic herbs may also neutralise or reduce toxicity of the poisonous herbs. The different characteristics of herbs in the prescription, consumed orally as an aqueous decoction, rectify the hyper-activity or hypo-activity of *Yin* and *Yang* in the unwell body, consequently curing the diseases that have caused the imbalance of *Yin* and *Yang*, and restoring health. Different combinations of herbs can cause variation in therapeutic effects. Traditionally the results of combining herbs can be classified as *Mutual reinforcement; Mutual assistance; Mutual restraint or Mutual counteraction; Mutual suppression; and Mutual antagonism*. The present text is not involved with the detail of the pharmacology, treatment use or principles of *Fu-Fang-Xue* (Studies of Herbal Combination) of CM herbs. It is hoped that this brief description helps to explain why poisonous herbs have been used in CM. Based on the CM principles of *Fu-Fang-Xue*, the poisonous herbs present the formulae have been included in some well-used prescriptions over a long period according to recorded experience. The poisonous herbs that are included in Fu-Fang should be processed according to laid down procedures listed in the Pharmacopoeia or other CM guidebooks.

COMPOSITION OF A CHINESE HERBAL MEDICINAL (CHM) PRESCRIPTION

During the development of prescriptions, an early CHM prescription contained only one herb or might be two or more. Some prescriptions gradually became established for specific diseases that were later modified in clinical practice according to differentiation of syndromes. Different herbs have different properties, flavours and tastes, and each has its own specific functions and deficiencies. Thus the purposes of having a combination of herbs in a prescription are:

1) To select herbs according to the differentiation of syndromes of the whole diseased body for curing complicated cases;
2) To enhance the therapeutic effects of individual herbs by promoting their synergism; and
3) To inhibit the adverse effects of other potent herbs or to counteract the toxicity of poisonous ones in the prescriptions.

In the selection of proper herbs for a prescription, it is necessary to distinguish between the principal herbs and the secondary ones, making sure that they complement and antagonise in the right ways of one another in order to produce the most effective results in the treatment of diseases. The principles for the composition of prescriptions, as first described in the Huang Di Nei Jing (The Inner Canon of the Yellow Emperor), stipulate that a prescription should include four different herbs. They are the *Chief or Principal (Jun)*, the *Adjuvant (Chen)*, the *Assistant (Zuo)* and the *Guide (Shi)* according to the different roles they play in the prescription.

The Chief Herb or Principal Herb (Jun), being essential in a prescription, aims to produce the leading effect in treating the cause of the main symptom of a disease. It plays the principal curative role.

The Adjuvant Herb (Chen) helps to strengthen the curative actions of the Chief Herb or treat less important symptoms by its own.

The Assistant Herb (Zuo) aims at producing the leading effect in treating the accompanying diseases or symptoms, helps to strengthen the effect of the principal herb by playing a significant role in treatment, and counteracts the potent effects or toxicity of the Chief and Adjuvant Herbs.

The Guiding Herb (Shi) leads the effects of other herbs to the diseased parts of the body and to balance the actions of the other herbs in the prescriptions.

As a rule, the *Chief Herb* should be used as the dominating one in a prescription, with the *Adjuvant, Assistant* and the *Guiding Herbs* subordinate to it. The four herbs supplementing one another play the curative role together. However, not every prescription is composed of the four kinds of herbs together. It may be composed of the principal herb with any one of the other three kinds depending on the conditions of the diseases, characteristics of the herbs and therapeutic needs. In some prescriptions the *Chief Herb* or the *Adjuvant Herb* itself possesses the action of the *Assistant* or *Guide Herb*.

METHODS OF PROCESSING CHINESE MATERIA MEDICA CMM

The procedure of preparing each of the CMM substance described in text books or Pharmacopoeia is the cumulative experience of users of poisonous or toxic herbs recorded in Pharmacopoeia such as the Shen Nong Ben Cao Jing in the past. The use of unprocessed herbs or herbs that are not prepared properly should be avoided.

The preliminary processing procedures remove foreign matters, soak and soften or cut medicinal herbs into small pieces ready for decoction. Common methods of processing include:

a) *Stir-baking (Chao)* refers to baking the herbs in a pan with constant stirring. The methods of stirring for different herbs vary in terms of time and temperature. The herb can be baked until yellow, brown or complete carbonised. For example, *Rhizoma Atractyodis Macrocephlae, when* baked until yellow, has the ability to strengthen the spleen.

b) *Stir-baking with adjuvants (Zhi)* refers to baking the herbs with liquid adjuvants such as honey, vinegar, wine, ginger juice and salt water. The adjuvant is soaked or attached into the herb during the baking period. The adjuvant may itself possess therapeutic effects and the processed herb with the adjuvant has its own therapeutic effects enhanced. For example, Radix Astragali seu Hedysari stir-baked with honey produces an improved effect in strengthening the middle *Jiao* and replenishing *Qi*

c) *High temperature stir-baking (Pao)* is, basically, similar as the procedure mentioned above, but is done rapidly over high temperature making the herb loose and cracked. Some herbs such as Radix Aconiti lateralis Preparata and Semen Strychni, are heated in hot charcoal ashes until brown and cracking but not yet carbonised. After such processing treatment the poisonous contents are reduced or removed.

d) *Calcining (Duan)* refers to the processing by burning an herb directly or indirectly over fire to make the herb light, crispy and easily crushable so as to bring out all its effects. Those mineral or shell-fish materials are usually calcined directly until they turn red.

e) *Wet-coated baking or roasting (Wei)* refers to baking or roasting the herbs coated with wet paper or wet dough in an oven until the coating turns black. This process reduces the fat contents and moderates the action of the herbs. *Rhizoma Zingiberis Rececs Preparata* and *Semen Myristicae Preparata* are prepared according to this procedure.

f) *Steaming (Zheng)* refers to steaming the herbs with other adjuvants over a slow fire until they are cooked. Raw *Radix Rehmanniae* has a cold nature and acts to purge heat, cool the blood, replenish yin and promote the generation of fluids. *Raw Radix Rehmanniae*, has a cold nature and acts to purge heat. After steaming with rice wine its cool nature is changed into a warm one and makes it effective in replenishing yin and blood.

Boiling (Zhu) refers to the processing by boiling the herbs in water or with other adjuvant. For examples, Radix Aconiti is boiled with bean-curd in order to reduce contents of poisonous ingredients.

Grinding in water (Shui Fei) refers to the process of crushing the insoluble minerals and shell-fish.

It is through these various procedures that the toxic components in the herbs can either be removed or reduced. However the dosage of each poisonous substance included in any prescription depends on the presence of other herbs in the prescription that is used for treating the conditions of the patient. The herbs described in the Phemacopoeia are seldom prescribed singly. It is probable that the inclusion of other herbs according to the TCM formulary often takes into account of the interacting actions to reduce toxicity.

GENERAL DISCUSSION ON HOW CHM PRODUCTS PRODUCE TOXIC EFFECTS WHEN NOT USED PROPERLY

Similar to using orthodox medicines it is understood that all drugs are toxic at high doses. Although the 48 Chinese medicinal materials described in the Pictorial Compendium (Xu & Chan 1994) are recorded in Pharmacopoeia as poisonous herbs they are used in herbal combinations with other non-toxic herbs according to CM diagnosis and treatment. With practice, experience and good knowledge of CM herbs the practitioners seldom come across any problems. Among many factors, possible reasons for occurrence of adverse effects and toxicity in using CM can be discussed as follows:

Authenticity or Poor Quality of CM Herbs: Popularity and scarcity of certain CM herbs may encourage traders to provide poor quality. Misuse and confusion of names of certain CM herbs enhances difficulty in identifying the right herbs in the market. Some traders supply fake herbs that are poisonous.

Substitution or adulteration with more toxic herbs may occur erroneously, when the herb is incorrectly identified, or deliberately for economic reasons when a cheaper herb is supplied to replace a safer, more expensive one. The most widely publicised reports were the cluster of cases of rapidly progressive interstitial nephritis in Belgium. It turned out that, after some investigation, this problem was attributed to the substitution of *Aristolochia fangchi* instead of the CM herb *Stephania tetrandra* in a combined slimming regimen that included some orthodox medications. Aristolochic acid from *Aristolochia fangchi* is a known nephrotoxin, and the other orthodox drugs present such as acetazolamide in the slimming medication could have potentiated this toxic effect. Most of the cases involved were young women, and some developed irreversible end-stage renal failure or carcinoma in the urinary tract.

The Consequence of Processing of CM Crude Herbs: All CM herbs are processed or prepared from fresh after collection with appropriate procedures before use. The processing, apart from cleaning and preserving purposes, has removed or reduced the toxic components in the unprocessed crude herbs which when taken alone will cause fatal effects. Certain processing changes the effects of some herbs. For example, raw *Radix Rehmanniae* is mainly used to purge heat, or cool the blood and promote the generation of body fluids. But *Radix Rehmanniae Preparata* has a warm property and becomes especially effective for enriching blood. After processing the therapeutic effects of some herbs will be enhanced. For example, *Rhizoma Corydalis* processed with vinegar has greater analgesic effect. If the supplied herbs in the market of developed countries have not been processed properly toxicity will be possible, especially so when used without composite prescriptions.

The Quantity of CM Herbs Prescribed: This refers to the dosage of each herb used in the composite prescriptions (Fu Fang) and depends on how well trained and experienced the practitioner who prescribes. General guidelines are listed in each of the monographs of CM herbs and composites formulae as reference for use. Thus overdosing should be avoided. This is also related to the quality of herbs supplied. Potent or poisonous herbs, if not properly processed and checked, will produce adverse effects even when used as components in composite formulae.

The likelihood of drug-CHM products interactions

Available in the literature, reports have reviewed potential interactions between herbal medicines and drugs. These have focused mainly on the herbs used in the west but have covered ginseng and ginkgo biloba, which are widely used in Asian countries. Ginseng has been reported to interact with phenelzine and other monoamine inhibitors causing a CNS stimulant effect (Jones and Runikis, 1987). The anticoagulant effect of warfarin was decreased when ginseng was also taken simultaneously (Janetzky and Morreale 1995). Digoxin levels became elevated when a patient took a preparation labeled as Siberian ginseng, *Eleutherococcus senticosus*, (McRae 1999), but there were no signs of toxic effects. We supported some clinical observations on interactions between popular CHM herbs with warfarin and confirmed our findings by some animal study data. *Danshen (Salvia miltiorrhiza)* had effects on both the pharmacodynamics and pharmacokinetics of warfarin in rats (Chan *et al.*, 2000), whereas *danggui (Angelica sinensis)* affected the pharmacodynamics but not the pharmacokinetics of warfarin in rabbits (Lo *et al.*, 1992).

However, not many literatures in the English language report interactions between CHM substances and orthodox drugs. We have recently compiled some comprehensive information on these (Chan and Cheung, 2000). We also observed that not all interactions between CHM products and orthodox drugs were harmful; some were beneficial when both CHM products and OM drugs are combined. All commonly used CHM crude herbs and readymade CHM products have been listed against orthodox drugs for warning of likely and clinically important herb-drug interactions.

The presence of heavy metals in CHM products

Contamination or adulteration of CHM products with heavy metals such as lead, mercury, cadmium, arsenic, or thallium has been a problem. A number of case reports have been published, and the problem was reviewed in previous articles. However some CHM products do contain heavy metals as essential ingredients. The poor quality control of these products causes health hazard as some products may present unusually high concentrations of potent and poisonous ingredients that will be fatal.

The conditions of the patients' well-being and disease state

Many patients are very ill by the time they consult the CM practitioners. Some would consider CM treatment as their last hope for recovery

(See Chapter 5). The incidents of adverse effects would be higher in this group of patients. Because of the aging processes many elderly patients would have their body functions compromised; in particular, the cardio-vascular system, liver function, and renal function. Moreover many of these patients have been put on poly-pharmacy scheme of drug treatment. Therefore the likelihood of getting drug-CHM products interactions is high.

Suggestions on Control of Poisonous Chinese Herbal Medicinal Substances

PROPER USE OF POTENT CHM PRODUCTS BY TRAINED CM PRACTITIONERS & PROFESSIONALS

Potent or poisonous CHM substances should only be used or prescribed by experienced CM prescribers who should be trained adequately. Such training has to be addressed in a different context (training and education, professionalism; see Chapter 19). Perhaps strict regulatory control on the availability and educational exposure to the general public will reduce the number of accidental poisoning cases. Nevertheless the present text has identified some of the problems involving the use and mis-use of potent and poisonous CHM products.

BASIC RESEARCH APPROACH

Basic research programmes on CHM substances should be encouraged to focus on the toxicity and efficacy relationship according to the doses applied similar to orthodox drug approach.

Due to the out-cry of toxicity, poor quality and adulteration of ready made herbal medicinal products in the market the priority of research on products-related treatment, in particular herbal product, is to ensure quality, efficacy, and safety of the end products used by patients. In majority of the cases, the biologically active chemical compounds of these products are unknown even other known chemical entities are isolated. It has also been shown that single compounds isolated from organic solvents are either too toxic or with no activities. Most traditional medicinal herbs are used as aqueous decoction. Therefore research projects should centred on development of analytical and biological procedures for use to give the quality assurance and control, and clinical assessment of efficacy and safety of these products. I have been involved with institutes in China to develop procedures linking analytical and bio-activity patterns or finger-printings together and interpreted with fuzzy logic computing techniques on Chinese medicinal herbs and herbal prescriptions (official Fu Fang-mixtures of several herbs together, administered as decoction). After a series of "training set" inputs of the authenticated aqueous herbal extracts, single herbs or mixtures of herbs, a "standard" pattern is used as the reference guide for subsequent assessment. This type of approach will generate patterns as reference and for prediction and recognition purposes for further research for pure active single chemical entities.

REGULATORY ASPECTS

All CHM products when supplied, as medications should be regulated for safety, quality and for *appropriate* evidence of efficacy. It advocates the establishment of a new category of licensed herbal medicines, prepared in accordance with current Good Manufacturing Procedures (cGMP), which meet standards for safety and quality, and which are regulated by the Medicines Control Agency in the UK.

The licensing requirements in this new category may not be as demanding as those that currently apply to licensed medicines. Specifically, the "level of proof" of activity may not need to be as high as for allopathic medicines. Efficacy may be accepted on the basis of documentation of traditional use over a long period.

Safety may deem to have been demonstrated by virtue of traditional use. However, these products ought to be required to substantiate a history of safe use, preferably in the EU for the dosage and indications to be approved, and the license should clearly indicate the inappropriate conditions of use (contra-indications). It would be dangerous to agree product safety as the basic, default position. In addition, the "test of time" criterion detects common acute adverse events, but not rare adverse events or those with a long latency. Also, today's users of herbal remedies may differ from those in earlier eras.

The governmental departments in China, such as State Drug Administration, authorise for the issue of regulations and registration guidelines and procedures for Chinese herbal medicinal (CHM) products for Traditional Chinese Medicine. State Drug Administration. Consultation with these guidelines will help to set up regulation in the UK or other developed countries on CHM products. Consultation of the Commission E structure from Germany will also help to formulate Regulatory Guidelines for herbal products as medicines.

There is a need for regulation on the quality assurance of both practitioners and products-related treatment involving herbal products for medicinal uses. In the case of Chinese herbal medicinal products in the UK nearly all of them are imported. Some are "manufactured" by small herbal firms from imported dried granules. They are crude herbs and ready-made products of well-used prescription products. Quality assurance and control of these have been loose and unsatisfactory. They reach the UK market probably as food or nutritional category. There is a lack of expertise in the professional aspects of checking the identity of them. Language problem is another aspect as herbal ingredients are supplied with similarly named substitutes that could be toxic. Appropriate regulations may help to sort out problems on the quality assurance and control side.

One way of giving guidelines for regulation is to spell out monographic control of herbs and herbal products imported. For some herbs used in the EU there are monographs issued for all of them in common use. The Commission E in Germany has produced standard monographs for controlling herbal medicines. ESCOP has commissioned the writing of standards for 50 European herbs. With quality of herbal medicinal products assured the efficacy of them can be assessed by RCT before licenses can be issued. The consequence of such procedures will certainly single out "cow-boy" practice, but also discourage manufacturers to register their products as medicines due to the high cost for getting the licences. A suitable approach should be needed without compromising the issue on quality, efficacy and safety of these products.

References

But, P.P.H. (1994) Herbal poisoning caused by adulterants or erroneous substitutes. *Journal of Tropical Medicine & Hygiene*, **97**, 371–374.

But, P.P.H, Tomlinson, B., Cheung, K.O., Yong, S.P., Szeto, M.L., Lee, C.K. (1996) Adulterants of herbal products can cause poisoning. *British Medical Journal*, **313**, 117.

Chan, K. (1996). The role of complementary medicine in health care. *Biologist*, **43**, 50–51.

Chan, K. (2000) Chapter 8 In: *Interactions between Chinese herbal medicinal products and orthodox drugs* (Chan, K. & Cheung, L, Ed), Harwood Academic Publishers, The Gordon & Breach Publishing Group, 2000.

Chan, K., Lo, A.C.T., Yeung, J.H.K. & Woo, K.S. (1995) The effects of Danshen (*Salvia miltiorrhiza*) on warfarin pharmacodynamics and pharmacokinetics of warfarin enantiomers in rats. *Journal of Pharmacy & Pharmacology*, **47**, 402–406.

Chan, K. & Xu, G.-J. (2001) *Pictorial Compendium of Poisonous Chinese Herbal Materials (English edition)*, Harwood Academic Publishers, The Gordon & Breach Publishing Group, in printer's.

De Smet, P.A.G. (1992) *Aristolochia* species. In P.A.G. De Smet, K. Keller, R. Hansel, and R.F. Chandler, (eds.), *Adverse Effects of Herbal Drugs*. Volume 1, Springer-Verlag, Berlin, pp. 79.

Hong, Z., *Chan, K.*, Yeung, H.W. (1992) Simultaneous determination of bufadienolides in the traditional Chinese medicine preparation. Liu-Shen-Wan, by liquid chromatography. *Journal of Pharmacy & Pharmacology* **44**, 1023–1026.

Janetzky K. & Morreale A.P. (1997) Probable interaction between warfarin and ginseng. *American Journal of Health-System Pharmacy*, **54**, 692–693.

Jin, Y., Berry, M., & Chan, K. (1995) Chinese herbal medicine in the U.K. In: Abstract of Pharmacy Practice Research, *Pharmaceutical Journal*, **255**, **Suppl.**, R37.

Jones B.D. and Runikis A.M. (1987) Interaction of ginseng with phenelzine (letter). *Journal of Clinical Psychopharmacology* 7, 201–202.

Karunanityh, R. and Sumita, K.R. (1991) Undeclared drugs in traditional Chinese anti-rheumatoid medicines. *International Journal of Pharmacy Practice*. **1**, 117–119.

Lo, A.C.T., *Chan, K.*, Yeung, J.H.K. & Woo, K.S. (1992) The effects of Danshen (*Salvia miltiorrhiza*) on pharmacokinetics and pharmacodynamics of warfarin in rats. *European Journal of Drug Metabolism & Pharmacokinetics*, **17**, 257–262.

Lo, A.C.T., Chan, K., Yeung, J.H.K. & Woo, K.S. (1995) Danggui (*Angelica sinesis*) affects the pharmacodynamics not the pharmacokinetics of warfarin in rabbits. *European Journal of Drug Metabolism & Pharmacokinetics*, **20**, 55–60.

McRae, S. (1999) Elevated serum digoxin levels in a patient taking digoxin and Siberian ginseng. *Canadian Medical Association Journa*, **155**, 293–295.

Ng, T.H, Chan, Y.W, Yu, Y.L, Chang, C.M, Ho, H.C, Leung, S.Y, But, P.P.H. (1991) Encephalopathy and neuropathy following ingestion of a Chinese herbal broth containing podophyllin. *Journal of Neurological Sciences*, **101**, 107–13.

Vanherweghem JL, Deplerreux M, Tielemans C, Abramowicz, D, *et al.* (1993) Rapidly progressive interstitial renal fibrosis in young women : association with slimming regime including Chinese herbal medicines *Lancet* **341**, 387–391.

Xu, G-J & Chan, K. (1994) *A Pictorial Compendium of Poisonous Traditional Chinese Medicinal Herbs Available in Hong Kong.* Commercial Press Ltd., Hong Kong, August 1994.

Yu, H., Zhong, S., Chan, K., & Berry, M. (1995) Pharmacognostical investigation on traditional Chinese medicinal herbs: Identification of four herbs from the U.K. market. *Journal of Pharmacy & Pharmacology,* **47, Suppl.,** 1129.

Yu, H., Berry, M., Zhong, S., & Chan, K. (1997) Pharmacognostical investigations on traditional Chinese medicinal herbs: Identification of six herbs from the UK market. *Journal of Pharmacy & Pharmacology,* **49 (Suppl. 4),** 212.

SECTION TWO
SPECIAL ASPECTS OF CLINICAL AND SCHEMATIC PRACTICE IN CHINESE MEDICINE

5 THE PRACTICE OF CHINESE MEDICINE IN TCM-KLINIK KÖTZTING IN GERMANY

Jia-zhen Liao
Stefan Hager
Anton Staudinger

Introduction

The establishment of the TCM (Traditional Chinese Medicine) Klinik Kötzting near Munich in Germany was approved by the Bavarian government. In March 1991 it was set up by the cooperation between Beijing University of TCM and German entrepreneur Mr. Anton Staudinger. It is the first hospital for TCM in Germany. In this 76-bed hospital, there are ten Chinese physicians from Beijing University of TCM. The Beijing staff consists of 3 internists, 3 Tuina-Massage doctors, 2 acupuncture doctors, 1 Qi-Gong doctor and 1 statistical doctor, who collaborate with six German physicians, and 2 professional translators who facilitate communication. Patients can be referred to the hospital directly by their family general practitioner (GPs) who are qualified orthodox medical (OM) doctors. Public health insurance companies in Germany have agreed to pay the medical expenses for the inpatients who have joined their insurance scheme. The patients who want to be treated in the hospital have to make an appointment for admission and usually wait for about one and a half years.

Mission and Tasks

TCM-Klinik Kötzting carries out the following three major missions and tasks education, scientific research and medical service.

EDUCATION

A Medical School for Training in traditional Chinese Medicine (CM) was founded at the hospital in 1992. Its main purpose was to train orthodox medical practitioners in the practice of CM, teaching them the basic theories of CM which include *Yin-Yang Theory*, the *Five Elements Concepts*, the structure and functions of the human body (*Zang-Fu*), etiology and pathogenesis, differential diagnosis in accordance with the Eight Principal Syndromes and differential diagnosis and treatment according to the pathological changes of viscera (*Zang-Fu*). The participants all are western medical doctors. The period of training extends over 2 years. It is divided into 8 courses; each course consists of a 3 day period (a total of 24 hours).

During the first 3 courses the participants learn the basic theories of CM, in the remaining 5 courses the differential diagnosis and treatment for 50 kinds of common diseases are taught. In each course there is a clinical practical work for a half day, five patients are selected as the typical teaching cases. The teaching materials are written mainly by the in-house Chinese professors of CM. The classroom teaching is done by Chinese professors and German chief doctors. Since 1992 there were 8 training classes for western doctors to learn CM. Such arrangements had been utilized throughout and more than 200 doctors had finished the training. When they passed the examination the students would get the certification that is admitted by German government. Now many of them can apply Chinese medicine and acupuncture to treat the patients in their clinics. As Professor Liao has abundant clinical and educational experiences, his lectures were integration of theory with practice and also of traditional with western medicine. These approaches of training for CM resulted in very good effects and outcomes, and were much appreciated by the trainees.

Another CM treatment procedure, the Chinese Tuina-Massage, has shown good effects for treatment of lumbar syndromes, cervical syndromes and soft tissue strain etc. This was of great interest to the patients and the German OM doctors. Since 1996, 4 training classes for German massage practitioners to learn the Chinese Tuina-Massage have been conducted and more than 50 trainees had finished the training. Because of the fact that Chinese Herbal medicines (CHM) have been increasingly used in Germany, a training course for German pharmacists to learn the common sense of CHM, such as taste, nature, *Channels*-entered and effects etc. of the imported Chinese herbal medicines had also been stored at the hospital.

Scientific Research

Since 1993 two subjects of scientific research have been carried out at the TCM-Klinik Kötzting.

THE EFFECT OF ACUPUNCTURE ON RELIEVING ACUTE MIGRAINE ATTACK

The main objective was to observe the effect of acupuncture on relieving acute migraine attack. A total of 180 inpatients with typical migraine were divided into 3 groups at random. Group A (60 cases) was treated by acupuncture, group B with "Sumatriptan" 100 mg by intramuscular injection, group C with intramuscular placebo injection. This clinical investigation was finished in the end of March 1999. The results showed that the effective rate of relieving acute migraine attack was 62.07% and 58.38% in group B and group A respectively, but only 29.51% in group C. There is no difference between the group A and group B. This research project received the financial support of the German government.

ANALYSIS OF CRUDE CHINESE HERBAL MEDICINAL (CHM) MATERIALS USED IN THE HOSPITAL

The objective of this study was to analyse 100 crude CHM materials used locally in the hospital with modern scientific methods.

The studies in each herb included the following headings: pharmacopoeia origin (first cited in), official herbal ingredients, substitute herbs, description of the official herbs, falsification and indications according to traditional Chinese medicine principles, main constituents, pharmacology, toxicology, Thin Layer Chromatograph (TLC), High Liquid Chromatograph (HPLC) fingerprint analysis and evaluation as well as discussion.

Illustration using the monograph of Radix. Astragalus as an example:
The evaluation of experimental data for Radix Astragalus indicated that the TLC fingerprint analysis of the *Astragalus* herb samples 1–5 exhibited a relatively homogeneous flavonoid profile varying mainly in the concentration of isomucornulatol glycoside/aglycone and 9-methoxy-nissolin

glycoside/aglycone. Some additional differences could be determined in the astragaloside pattern. Together with the consideration of the observation of the pharmacological and therapeutic effects of the *Astragalus* herb it is important to note the synergism of saponins and flavonoids in the herb. Thus, the TLC and the HPLC fingerprint analysis of both classes of compounds is necessary for an unambigious identification and standardization of the *Astragalus* root.

The HPLC-fingerprint spectra of the ether-acetone-precipitated n-BuOH-phases of several *Astragalus* roots exhibit different (valuable) astragaluside patterns depending on their provenance, harvest and storage time.

The publication of monographs of CM herbs:
Thus far we have finished the studies of 12 crude Chinese herbs. Among these, 8 monographs were published by Verlag für Ganzheitliche Medizin Dr. Erich Wühr GmbH, Kötzting/Bayer. Wald, Germany. The study has been led by Professor Dr. rer. nat. Hildebert Wagner and sponsored by Mr. Anton Staudinger. The results showed that these data are of significant value for determining the quality of crude CM herbs imported for use in the hospital.

Medical Services

THE POLICY OF DIAGNOSIS FOR PATIENTS ADMITTED TO THE HOSPITAL

Medical service is the principal work of the TCM-Klinik Kötzting. There is an accepted procedure for diagnosis of all patients admitted to the hospital as a general policy. For each patient, on the day of admission, a German OM physician, a CM physician from China and a translator acting together will obtain the patient's illness history and make the examination. Both the CM and OM doctors will record their diagnostic findings separately. At the end of the admission procedure, the two physicians decide together on the following issues: diagnosis according to CM principles (differentiation of the symptoms and signs according to the theories of TCM), principle of treatment and prescriptions, frequency and dosage of CM therapy.

The experience of running of the hospital services and the outcome of treatment for patients admitted to the hospital can be summarised under the following headings:

Medical Statistics Obtained from Patients Admitted to the Hospital

(1) CLINICAL DEMOGRAPHICAL DATA

- *Number*   A total of 7585 inpatients were treated from 18th March 1991 to 31st December 1998.
- *Sex*:   male 27.8%, female 72.2%
- *Age*:   An average age of 52.6 +/– 14 years
- *Duration of diseases*: An average of 12.1 +/– 10.9 years. In 64.5% cases it was over 5 years.
- *Number of previous treatments* (within one year before admission the patients were treated by other doctors): It was a mean of 4.4 +/– 2.3 times.
- *Duration of hospitalisation*: The patients stayed at the hospital on average for 27 +/– 5.3 days.
- The diseases or syndromes treated in the hospital were classified as follows:

    Primary disease: It was the main diseases or syndromes that the patients were admitted to the hospital for treatment.
    Secondary diseases: Apart from the primary diseases, the patients suffered with other diseases or syndromes at the same time that were classified as the secondary diseases.

During the hospitalisation the principal treatments were used for the primary diseases but the secondary diseases were also treated properly.
    The statistics of the efficacy of the primary and secondary diseases were calculated respectively and will be given in the following sections.

(2) METHODS OF TREATMENTS

Treatments with CM
According to different diseases or syndromes the patients were treated with combination therapy by various Chinese therapeutic methods:

- Decoction: 95.1% of cases were treated with decoction.
- Acupuncture: 98.4% of cases were treated with acupuncture. Moxibustion was not used in the hospital.
- Tuina-Massage: 60.9% of cases were treated with Tuina-Massage
- Qi-Gong: 15.8% of cases were treated with Qi-Gong.

Treatments with OM

- When the patients were admitted to the hospital, 46.8% of cases had been treated with various orthodox medicines. After treatment with CM the following changes appeared.
- In 67.88% of the patients the dosage of orthodox medicines was reduced or stopped.
- In 31.22% of the cases the orthodox medicines were used as before.
- In 0.9% of the patients the dosage of orthodox medicines was added or increased.

(3) THE EFFICACY OF TREATMENT AS MEASURED BY A SET STANDARD

The efficacy of treatment over the period specified has been assessed according to the following criteria:

- Effective: The symptoms and signs were improved by 20–40%.
- Markedly effective: The symptoms and signs were improved by equal or over 50%.
- Remission: The symptoms and signs were relieved completely.
- Ineffective: The symptoms and signs were not improved or less than 20%.
- Aggravation: The symptoms and signs were aggravated.

The changes of intensity of diseases were evaluated by the physicians and the patients respectively on a scale ranging from 1 (no complaints) to 10 (intolerable).

(4) RESULTS OF TREATMENT OVER THE PERIOD FROM 1991 TO 1998

Results of treatment for those patients admitted from 1991 to 1998 are shown as summarised by the following tables. (Tables 5.1 to 5.3)

- From 1991 to 1998 the total effective rates and the markedly effective rates, in each year, for the treatment of the primary diseases or syndromes are were shown in Table 5.1.
- In some patients after treatment with CM of their primary diseases the results indicated such treatments were not effective. But the treatment of the secondary diseases obtained was effective. Thus the statistics of the total effective rate and the markedly effective rate of

Table 5.1 The efficacy of treatment of the primary diseases or syndromes in patients admitted to the TCM Klinic, Kotzting, 1991 to 1998

	Total cases	Total effective rate		Markedly effective plus remission rate	
		cases	%	cases	%
1991	580	394	67.93	266	45.86
1992	1043	766	73.44	496	47.56
1993	991	783	79.01	486	49.04
1994	990	808	81.62	477	48.18
1995	986	781	79.21	492	49.90
1996	983	758	77.11	475	48.32
1997	1005	801	79.70	505	50.55
1998	1007	823	81.73	520	51.64
	7585		77.97 (mean)		49.04 (mean)

treating the primary diseases plus the secondary diseases were also calculated., These results are shown in Table 5.2.

- A total of 102 kinds of diseases or syndromes were treated in the hospital. Among them 23 sorts of diseases in which the number of treated patients were over 50 cases. The therapeutic efficacy or otherwise of treating these diseases are shown in Table 5.3.

Table 5.2 Results of total effective rate and markedly effective rate after treatment

	Total cases	Total effective rate		Markedly effective plus remission rate	
		cases	%	cases	%
1991	NS	NS		NS	
1992	1043	871	83.51	560	53.69
1993	991	865	87.29	538	54.29
1994	990	898	90.71	527	53.23
1995	986	889	90.16	557	56.49
1996	983	840	85.45	524	53.31
1997	1005	871	86.67	537	53.43
1998	1007	881	87.49	520	51.49
	7585	6115	87.29 (mean)	3763	53.75 (mean)

Table 5.3 Results of treatment of various types of diseaes in TCM Klinic Kotzting from 1991 to 1998

Diseases	Total cases	Effective cases (%)	Markedly effective cases (%)	Remission cases (%)	Ineffective cases (%)	Aggravation cases (%)
lumbar syndrome	1049	266 (25.36)	535 (51)	35 (3.34)	209 (19.92)	4 (0.38)
migraine	1001	254 (25.38)	563 (56.24)	63 (6.29)	120 (11.99)	1 (0.1)
headache	712	172 (24.16)	326 (45.79)	48 (6.74)	165 (23.17)	1 (0.14)
polyarthralgia	660	246 (37.27)	270 (40.91)	8 (1.21)	136 (20.61)	
cervical syndrome	631	194 (30.75)	333 (52.77)	19 (3.01)	85 (13.47)	
polyneuro-pathy	322	102 (31.68)	114 (35.40)	12 (3.73)	94 (29.19)	
tinnitus	281	76 (23.84)	68 (24.20)	1 (0.36)	145 (51.60)	
asthma	275	77 (28.00)	127 (46.18)	11 (4.00)	60 (21.82)	
trigeminal neuralgia	251	57 (22.71)	117 (46.61)	27 (10.76)	48 (19.12)	2 (0.80)
inflammatory enteritis	236	78 (33.05)	98 (41.53)	9 (3.81)	49 (20.76)	2 (0.85)
postherpetic neuralgia	171	50 (29.24)	69 (40.35)	10 (5.85)	42 (24.56)	
dizziness	165	46 (27.88)	55 (33.33)	19 (11.52)	45 (27.27)	
atypical facial neuralgia	145	47 (32.41)	39 (26.90)	4 (2.76)	55 (37.93)	
chronic bronchitis	132	42 (31.82)	67 (50.76)	8 (6.06)	15 (11.36)	
asthenia syndrome	116	47 (40.52)	47 (40.52)	1 (0.86)	20 (17.24)	1 (0.86)
abdominal pain	114	33 (28.95)	44 (38.60)	10 (8.77)	27 (23.68)	
insomnia	92	40 (43.48)	30 (32.61)	1 (1.09)	21 (22.82)	
chronic stomachache	91	14 (15.39)	51 (56.04)	9 (9.89)	17 (18.68)	

Table 5.3 Results of treatment of various types of diseaes in TCM Klinic Kotzting from 1991 to 1998 (*continued*)

Diseases	Total cases	Effective cases (%)	Markedly effective cases (%)	Remission cases (%)	Ineffective cases (%)	Aggravation cases (%)
chronic sinusitis	82	22 (26.83)	42 (51.22)	5 (6.10)	13 (15.85)	
neurodermatitis	70	17 (24.28)	44 (62.86)	1 (1.43)	7 (10.00)	1 (1.43)
melancholia	69	20 (28.98)	31 (44.93)	3 (4.35)	15 (21.74)	
hemiplegia	64	30 (46.88)	21 (32.81)		13 (20.31)	
abdominal flatulence	62	27 (43.55)	16 (25.81)		19 (30.64)	
cases	6791	1948	3107	304	1420	12
%		28.68	45.75	4.48	20.91	0.18
Markedly effective rate			3411 50.23%			
Total effective rate			5359 78.91%			

Therapeutic Methods Using Chinese Herbal Medicines for some Common Diseases in the Hospital

MIGRAINE

Migraine is a very common complaint in Germany. According to our clinical investigations and the theories of CM, migraine can be classified into two types.

A) *Wind-Cold* type: is caused by the accumulation of the pathogenic *Wind-Cold* in the *Liver*, which attacks the *Stomach* or *Middle-jiao* leading to production of the *Turbid-Yin*. Thus if *Wind-Cold* with *turbid-yin* together up-stir the head, migraine occurs. This headache is also called "*Jue-Yin*-headache".

- Main manifestations: Headache appears on one side of the head which inverses to *Cold* and *Wind*, cold in the limbs, nausea, vomiting or in some cases with diarrhoea, thready or slow pulse, pale and purple tongue with thin whitish coating.
- Principle of treatment: Expelling *Wind*, warming the *Liver* to expel *Cold* and replenishing the *Middle-jiao* to remove *Turbid-Yin*.
- Basic prescription: Modified decoction of *Evodia* and Powder of *Ligustici chuanxiong* mixed with *Camillae sinensis* (Wu zhu yu Tang, Chuan Xiong Cha Tiao San). Details of the herbal ingredients are:

Fructus Evodiae	10 g
Radix Angelicae dahurica	10 g
Rhizoma Ligustici	10 g
Radix Notopterygii	10 g
Herba Asari	3 g
Radix Codonopsis pilosulae	10 g
Rhizoma Ligustici chuanxiong	10 g
Radix Angelicae sinensis	10 g

- Explanation of prescription: *Fr. Evodiae* is pungent in flavor and hot in property. It is used for warming the *Liver* channel to dispel *Cold*, sending down the reversed ascending *Qi* and warming the *Stomach* to stop nausea and vomiting. *R. Angelicae dahuricae* is effective for *Yangming* headache (forehead), *Ligustici chuanxiong* for *Shaoyin* and *Jueyin* headache (bilateral and vertical). *R. Notopterygii* for *Taiyang* headache (occipital), *Ligustici* for vertical headache, *Asari* for expelling *Wind* and *Cold*. *Codonopsis pilosula* is used for replenishing *Middle-Qi* to help the *Liver* to dispel *Wind* and *Cold*, to remove the *Turbid-yin*. *Angelicae sinensis* with *Ligustici chuanxiong* act together for nourishing the *Liver* blood to relieve headache.

● Based on our clinical investigation, it shows that about 75% patients with migraine belong to this type. More than 800 cases of migraine were treated with this prescription and obtained obvious effectiveness. The total effective rate was 88%, markedly effective rate was 62.53%. In the following up of one year, it maintained in 85.4% and 55.6% respectively.

B) *Wind-heat type*: is caused by the hyperactivity of *Liver-Yang* or *Liver-Heat*, which may accompany deficiency of *Liver-Yin* or *Liver-blood*.

● Main manifestations: Migraine with nausea or vomiting, prefers cool, without cold limbs, the tongue is reddened.
● Principle of treatment: Expelling *Wind*, clearing away *Heat* from the *Liver*, nourishing *Yin* or blood and subduing hyperactivity of *Liver-yang*.
● Basic prescription:

Radix Bupleuri	10 g
Radix Scutellariae	10 g
Ram. Uncariae cum Uncis	10 g
Fructus Tribuli	10 g
Radix Angelicae dahuricae	10 g
Rhizoma Ligustici	10 g
Bombyx batryticatus	10 g
Herba Asari	3 g
Rhizoma Ligustici chuanxiong	10 g
Radix Rehmanniae	20 g

Explanation of the prescription: Bupleuri and Scutellariae are used for clearing away heat from the *Liver*, Uncariae cum Uncis and Tribuli are effective for subduing the hyperactivity of *Liver-yang* and expelling *Wind*, Angelicae dahuricae for *Yangming* headache, Ligustici for vertex headache, Bombyx batryticatus and Asari for expelling *Wind* to relieve muscular spasm and headache, Ligustici chuanxiong is an important drug for treatment of headache and acting together with Rehmanniae for nourishing blood of the *liver* to subdue the hyper-activity of *Liver-yang*.

This type is the minority in the patients with migraine.

NEURODERMATITIS

Neurodermatitis is a chronic pruritic, lichenified eczematous eruption that results from constant scratching. It is classified as local and dis-seminated types. For the present presentation, the later type will be described. This disease is called "Neu Pi Xia" in CM

The disease is caused by excessive or persistent stagnation of the *Liver Qi*, which will turn into *Liver fire*. The *Liver fire* produces patho-genic *Wind* and consumes the blood of the *Liver* leading to deficiency of the blood which also gives rise of *Wind*, finally resulting in neuro-dermatitis. The deficiency of the circulating blood produces a thick, dry and rough skin. The *Fire* and *Wind* acting together will cause the pruritic, lichenified eczematous eruption.

Main manifestations: Paroxysmal and severe itching on the affected parts will occur. The affected skin is widespread and can spread over to the whole body, especially on the trunk and limbs. The affected skin is reddish, thick, rough and dry and crowds of papillae appear on it with fine and broken scurf. The conditions may accompany irritability and insomnia. The tongue is reddened, the pulse is thready and rapid.

Principle of treatment: Nourishing the blood and cooling the blood, expelling *Wind* and purging the *Liver Fire*.

Basic prescription: Modified Decoction of Gentianae for purging the *Liver Fire* (Longdan Xieyan Tang)

Herba Gentianae	6 g
Radix Bupleuri	10 g
Radix Scutellariae	10 g
Fructus Gardeniae	10 g
Radix Gentianae macrophyllae	10 g
Radix Ledebouriellae	10 g
Cortex Dictamni radicis	10 g
Radix Sophorae flavescentis	10 g
Radix Angelicae sinensis	10 g
Radix Rehmanniae	20 g
Cortex Moutan radicis	10 g
Radix Glycyrrhizae	10 g

Explanation of the prescription: Gentianae, Scutellariae and Gardeniae have the effect of purging the *Liver Fire*. Bupleuri is used for activating the *Liver* without damaging the *Liver-yin* when it is applied with Glycyrrhizae. Gentianae macrophyllae, Ledebouriellae, Dictamni radicis and Sophorrae flavescentis are used for expelling *Wind* and *Heat* to relieve itching, Angelicae sinensis, Rehmanniae and Moutan are applied for nourishing and cooling the blood to reduce itching and moisten the dryness.

We have treated 70 inpatients suffering from disseminated neuro-dermatitis with this prescription, a good efficacy was obtained; the total effective rate was 88.57%, the markedly effective rate was 64.29%; that was 100% and 71.4% respectively one year after discharge.

BRONCHIAL ASTHMA

The occurrence of brachial asthma is due to congested phlegm and fluid accumulated in the lungs for a long period, that turn into *Heat syndromes*. On the other hand, if the patients contracts external *Cold* or *Heat*, the phlegm and the *Cold or Heat* are locked in the lungs, such conditions will cause the obstruction of the respiratory tract. The flow of *Lung-Qi* is disturbed resulting in the impairment of descending function of *Lung-Qi* leading to adverse rising. Then asthma occurs.

Asthma is mainly classified as the following two-types

A) Asthma of Heat-type: is due to obstruction of Heat-phlegm in the lungs.

Main manifestations: Dyspnea with wheezing, irritable oppressed sensation in the chest, yellowish mucoid sputum or alternating with whitish sputum, reddened tongue with yellow coating, smooth and rapid pulse.

Principle of treatment: Expelling *Heat* and resolving phlegm, sending down abnormally ascending *Qi* and relieving asthma.

Basic prescription: Modified Decoction for Relieving Asthma (Ding Chuan Tang)

Semen Gingko	10 g
Herba Ephedrae	10 g
Fructus Perillae	10 g
Semen Armeniacae amarum	10 g
Fructus Schisandrae	10 g

Herba Asari	3 g
Radix Bupleuri	10 g
Radix. Scutellariae	10 g
Flos. Lonicerae	10 g
Herba Taraxaci	10 g
Radix. Paeoniae alba	10 g
Rhizoma Rehmanniae Preparatae	20 g

Explanation of the prescription: *Ephedrae* and *Asari* can disperse and descend the inhibited and abnormally rising *Lung-Qi* and relieve asthma. *Gingko* serves to eliminate phlegm, stop coughing and act together with *Schisandrae* to astringe *Lung-Qi* for preventing the consumption of *Lung-Qi*, and *Perillae, Armeniacae amarum* lower the abnormally rising *Qi*, eliminate phlegm and enhance the effect of relieving asthma. *Lonicerae* is used for eliminating *Heat* from the lungs, *Bupleuri* can expel *Heat* and regulate the flow of *Liver-Qi* to enhance the effect of descending *Qi* of the other drugs in this prescription, *Scutellaria, Taraxaci* eliminate the *Heat* from the liver to help eliminating the *Lung-heat*. *Paeoniae, Rehmanniae* nourish the blood of the liver to soften the liver. A feature of the prescription is to consider the relationship between the lungs and the liver. Theory of TCM believe that "*Wood fire* impairs *Metal*", therefore in this prescription which regulates the function of the *Liver* to help the *Lungs* to enhance the effect of relieving asthma.

B) Asthma of Cold type: is due to Cold-phlegm obstructed in the lungs.

Main manifestations: A feeling of fullness and distress in the chest, dyspnea with wheezing sound in throat, coughing with thin whitish sputum, without yellowish sputum. A large amount of the thin whitish sputum and preference for warmth are the features of *Cold*-type of asthma. Other symptoms include pale tongue with whitish coating, and smooth pulse.

Principle of treatment: Warming the lungs, eliminating phlegm, descending the abnormally rising *Qi* and relieving Asthma.

Basic prescription: Modified Minor Blue Dragon Decoction with Gypsum Fibrosum (Xiao Qing Long Tang);

The ingredients of the prescription are not shown here as the minority of patients with the asthma treated in the hospital were of the *Cold* type.

A total of 275 inpatients with asthma were treated. The total effect rate was 78.18%, markedly effective rate was 50.18%, one year later after discharge it was 94% and 60.7% respectively.

TRIGEMINAL NEURALGIA

Trigeminal neuralgia is characterized by sudden, lighting-like paroxysms of pain in the distribution of one or more divisions of the trigeminal nerve. It is usually classified as *Wind-cold type* or *Wind-heat type*.

A) *Wind-cold type*: is caused by *Wind-cold* obstructing the channels and resulting in blood stasis. The majority of the patients with trigeminal neuralgia belong to this type.

Main manifestations: The pain is exacerbated by wind and cold, reduced by warm, cold in the limbs, pale tongue with thin whitish coating, thready and/or even pulse.

Principle of treatment: Eliminating wind and warming the channels to expel cold, promoting blood circulation to remove the blood stasis for relieving pain.

Basic prescriptions:

Herba Asari	3 g
Radix Aconiti lateralis prep.	10 g
Radix Angelicae dahuricae	10 g
Rhizoma Ligustici	10 g
Radix Paeoniae rubra	10 g
Rhizoma Ligustici chuanxiong	10 g
Caulis Spatholobi	10 g
Radix Astragali	10 g

Explanation of prescription: Asari and Aconiti lateralis prep. serve as warming the *Channels* to expel *Cold* for relieving pain, Angelicae dahuricae und Ligustici are used for eliminating *Wind* and *Cold* to alleviate pain, Astragali has the action in stabilizing the exterior, it is used in the prescription acting together with other ingredients to enhance the actions of eliminating *Wind* and *Cold* and relieving pain, the other 3 herbs in the prescription used together serve to promote the flow of *Qi* and blood in the *Channels* for alleviating pain.

B) *Wind-heat type*: is caused by wind-heat obstructing the *Channels* leading to blood-stasis. The minority of the patients with trigeminal neuralgia are classified in this type.

Main manifestations: Pain with burning sensation that is exacerbated by warm or heat and reduced by cold; reddened tongue with thin or without coating; smooth and rapid pulse.

Basic prescriptions: In the above mentioned prescription for treatment of *Wind-cold* type R. Aconiti lateralis prep. should be omitted and add R. Bupleuri and R. Scutellariae for expelling heat.

A total of 251 inpatients with trigeminal neuralgia had been treated during this period. The total effective rate was 80.08%, markedly effective rate was 57.37%. One year after discharge the figure was 86.1% and 60.5% respectively.

Results of Following up

In order to further determine the efficacy of CM in patients who were treated in the hospital, a retrospective survey was carried out in 1996. The 2545 patients admitted from 1st February 1994 to 31st July 1996 were followed up after discharge. Follow-up questionnaires were sent out at 2-month, 6-month and 1 year intervals. The results were shown in Table 5.4. The results indicated that the total effective rate immediate after discharge was 88.9%, in which the markedly effective plus remission rate was 50.9%. One year after discharge 84% of cases also remained effective and in some cases the condition of disease was more improved than that of just discharge, the remission rate was increased by 7.3%.

It was interesting to note that before treatment, patients took sick leave averaging at 1.5 month per year (27.1% cases took over 3 months) in the first year of the period studied. After discharge the absence from work was 0.5 month (16.7% cases took over 3 months) in one year after treatment.

Discussion and Conclusion

Orthodox medicine (OM) is an advanced medical science. The practice of OM can treat many diseases with markedly efficacy. But many other diseases after OM treatment without much success. Since 1991 there have been 7585 inpatients receiving treatment with Chinese medicine (CM) in the hospital. Before admission these patients all were treated by OM outside the hospital without getting a good efficacy. During

Table 5.4 Following-up figures for effective rate at discharge and 1 year later for the period 1994 to 1996

(%)	Cases	Effective (%)	Markedly (%)	Remission (%)	Ineffective
headache	214/112	36.0/34.8	38.3/33.0	7.9/10.7	17.8/21.4
migraine	308/178	31.8/29.8	50.3/38.2	11.4/17.4	6.5/14.3
trigeminal neuralgia	84/43	27.4/25.6	50.0/37.2	11.9/23.3	10.7/14.0
polyneuropathy	46/19	43.5/31.6	32.6/26.3	2.2/15.8	21.7/26.3
dizziness	26/15	61.5/33.3	26.9/40.0	3.8/13.3	7.7/13.3
allergic rhinitis	27/10	44.4/30.0	40.7/30.0	7.4/20.0	7.4/10.0
chronic bronchitis	38/15	29.5/33.3	47.4/46.7	5.3/20.0	7.9/0
asthma	101/45	29.7/33.3	51.5/37.8	10.9/22.9	7.9/6.7
Crohn's dis.	24/14	33.3/28.6	41.7/21.4	8.3/28.6	16.7/21.4
ulcerative colitis	53/23	52.8/26.1	37.7/65.2	1.9/4.3	7.5/4.3
neurodermatitis	35/25	42.9/28.6	45.7/35.7	8.6/35.7	2.9/0
cervical syn.	119/52	37.8/23.1	47.1/57.7	11.8/15.4	3.4/3.8
lumbar syn.	268/126	39.9/33.3	43.7/31.0	8.6/18.3	7.8/17.5
other	982/465	39.6/30.1	37.7/36.1	9.1/15.3	13.6/18.5
mean	2325/1131	38./30.6	41.8/37.0	9.1/16.4	11.2/16.0

Total effective rate was 88.9/84.0. *at discharge/ 1 year later.

admission check-up to the hospital many patients say: "The treatment in your hospital is my last hope." The therapeutic results showed that after treatment with CM the average total effective rate was 87.29% and markedly effective rate was 53.75%. After discharge for one year the follow-up study indicated the rates were 84.0% and 53.4% respectively. These figures indicate that the therapeutic efficacy of CM is not temporary and can be maintained for a longer period. The diseases with the markedly effective rate over 50% can be summarised as follows: neurodermatitis (62.53%), migraine (62.53%), trigeminal neuralgia (57.37%), chronic sinusitis (57.32%), chronic stomach (56.93%), chronic bronchitis (56.82%), cervical syndrome (55.78%), lumbar syndrome (54.34%), tension headache (52.53%), asthma (50.18%).

Chinese medicine can be considered as a summation of the experience of China's population in combating illness through centuries. It has played an important role in the prosperity of the Chinese nations, and is still of incalculable value. Our results also show that CM exerts profound effects on the medical service for the patients in the developed countries with all the advantages of orthodox medical technology and treatment. One advantage of CM is that the medical cost is much lower than that of orthodox medicine. CM is warmly welcomed by German patients. Since 1991 the German media often report the news and the knowledge of CM in the magazines, radios, newspapers and TV etc.

The integration of CM with OM for treatment of diseases may reach a higher degree of success. In the hospital we have treated patients with acupuncture, Tuina-massage and Chinese herbal medicine, we can only use decoction of herbal medicine. Other prepared or ready-made Chinese medicine such as pills, tablets etc. are not approved for use by the German government in the hospital. In order to enhance the efficacy by considering the principle of forming the composite prescriptions (Fu Fang) and choice the CM herbs, we often apply the idea of the integration of CM with OM. As a result the treatment effective rate was increased.

For example, the composite prescription for the treatment of asthma, first of all, is derived according to the principles of CM. The expelling of *Heat* and resolving *Phlegm*, and sending down abnormally ascending *Qi*, are achieved by using Gingko, Ephedrae, Perillae, Armeniacae amarum and Asari according to these principles. Meanwhile, we also choose the herbs with consideration of the pathogenesis of orthodox medicine of asthma. It is well known that during immune-reactions within the body some inflammatory cytokines as IL-3, IL-4, IL-5, IL-8, etc. play an important role in the pathogenesis of asthma. We use *Bupleuri, Schisandrae, Lonicerae, Taraxaci, Paeoniae* and *Rehmanniae* to regulate the immune-reactions and inflammation involved in the process of asthmatic attack. The results showed that the effect was better than that of forming prescription only according to the theories of CM.

It must be emphasised that the therapeutic experiences described in this chapter are incomplete and require further exploration and exploitation by using appropriate scientific methods.

We believe that the school of CM set up in the hospital has exerted an active action for providing the knowledge and practical experience of CM in Germany in a rational and professional manner. In the 21st century some orthodox medical doctors who have been trained in CM will become the experts of the integration of CM with OM. They will obtain excellent results in the integrated field. We also believe and welcome the idea that studies of CM will be carried out in some university hospitals in Germany and other European countries.

It is worth mentioning that the study of migraine quoted in this Chapter is a successful example for research into assessing the efficacy of treatment with CM using random, controlled methods with placebo. The study of the assessment of quality assurance of crude Chinese herbs has also produced great results.

One can conclude that the experience of working in the Koetzting TCM Klinic since 1991 has brought "A beautiful spring of Chinese Medicine" to Germany and other advance developed countries.

6 THE PRACTICE OF CHINESE MEDICINE IN THE NATIONAL HEALTH SERVICE ENVIRONMENT IN THE UNITED KINGDOM

John Tindall

General Introduction

Similar to the development of complementary medicine in other developed countries in Europe, the introduction of Chinese medicine into the public health service in the United Kingdom has not been easy. Such development requires professionals with strong self-interest and determination to face the challenge and obstacles along the orthodox medical path. The acceptance of Chinese medicine (CM) as a discipline within a National Health Service (NHS) setting contributing to patient care has taken the author, a Physiotherapist and a Practitioner in CM, a great deal of effort since 1985. The following is a personal account describing how he overcame the difficulties he encountered and succeeded to demonstrate how valuable the Gateway Clinic he has set up since 1990 to the service in the South Western Hospital. He also gives a very positive view on how CM, in particular acupuncture, can be developed to help alleviate medical burdens in areas such as HIV/AIDS, Hepatitis C infection, and drug abuse apart from the more common applications in dermatology, gynaecology, rheumatology etc.

THE EARLY DEVELOPMENT FROM 1983

The author, John Tindall, has been qualified as a Physiotherapist since 1983 at West Middlesex Hospital. His work for the Lambeth Health Care Trust began at Tooting Bec Hospital in 1985 working with Mental Health unit and Drug Dependency programmes. John initiated the use of natural health care in the form of Shiatsu, Reflexology, applied kinesiology, autogenic, Silva mind control, Bach flower remedies, *Qi Gong*, essential oils and creative visualisations. Within two years, it was clear that clients benefited from these treatments. Through practice and observation of outcomes it became apparent to John that he could not treat all the clients himself and that it could possibly be more efficient and effective to use Chinese medicine and its related treatments such as acupuncture and *Qi Gong* as well as herbs. This would demand less help from other disciplines he described. The hospital doctors were not in favour of this and John was expected to come up with some concrete evidence before he could start his new plan.

He discovered the work of Dr. Mike Smith at the Lincoln clinic in the South Bronx in New York utilising ear acupuncture and Chinese medicine in substance abuse and HIV/AIDS treatment. John was given a bursary for three months to visit the Lincoln clinic to study the programme there.

John worked under the direct supervision of Dr. Mike Smith and his colleagues and traveled through the USA, establishing the National Acupuncture Detoxification Association (NADA) treatment programme including such diverse locations as Oglala Sioux Reservation, Pine Ridge, South Dakota. John returned to the U.K. and his Unit General Manager Mr. Ray Rowden was interested in the idea of integrating Chinese medicine and Natural Health care into the Mental Health Unit, drug services and HVI/AIDS treatment. Mr. Rowden gave John his "blessing" to pioneer this work. Unfortunately this did not rest well with other health care professionals and he was not awarded a budget.

John established a daily service with his own finances of ear acupuncture and body acupuncture and *Qi Gong* using the Physiotherapy Department for in-patients' service at the Tooting Bec Hospital. These patients were drug and alcohol dependents and mental health clients. He visited the outpatient drug dependency unit at St. Thomas Hospital and the Stockwell Project Street Agency twice weekly to provide acupuncture. Within one year, he had also established acupuncture at the Landmark (HIV/AIDS Community Centre) and the Phoenix House Rehabilitation Centre and conducted workshops in Sweden and Trinidad outside his NHS work.

On a daily basis he was treating up to 90 clients a day with the assistance of two volunteer colleagues, Andrew Mathews and Phil Sims, whom he had trained.

PROGRESS IN THE 1990s LEADING TO THE FORMATION OF GATEWAY CLINIC

In 1990 John, Andrew, and Phil moved to South Western Hospital and they were assigned an empty Nightingale ward, which they converted into a clinic. This was eventually closed for demolition and they moved to the Porters Security Lodge which was in a bad state of disrepair; but now the service was financed by the Hospital for the areas of Lewisham, Southwark, and Lambeth.

In 1991, the Porters Lodge was revamped to make a modern walk in clinic for clients with drug abuse problems, HIV/AIDS, psychological disorders and general health clients referred by a general practitioner (GP). The programme finally was started off.

In the later part of 1991 John was introduced to Professor WU Bo Ping who subsequently came to stay with John for three months. During this period Professor Wu gave him close personal tuition in Chinese medicine. Since that time Professor WU and John have had continuous exchange and many extended periods of intensive work together. Professor WU has been accepted as one of the patrons of the clinic as is Royston Low, Giovanni Maciocia, Michael McIntyre and Dr. Ke.

Many organisations nationally and internationally recognise the work of the Gateway Clinic and take guidance and consultation from the Clinic practitioners. There are now over 60 drug units and 80 prisons in the UK utilising the National Acupuncture Detoxification Association (NADA) practices for drug abuse. There are now over 6000 NADA practitioners throughout Europe and the Eastern Block.

THE OBJECTIVES AND PHILOSOPHY OF THE GATEWAY CLINIC

John's original aim was to provide TCM on the NHS to those clients that could not afford such care privately and to prove to the medical profession that this approach is effective, efficient and affordable.

The Clinic is modeled after the "open plan Chinese Medicine Clinic", which is practised in China. Meetings are held in a large community space where people are all treated as equals together. It would seem too many that there is no privacy and that case histories are taken and discussed in earshot of everyone. This does not fit in well with the orthodox correctness and thus attracts a lot of criticism from health care professionals and managers. However, healing starts from a position of sincerity in facing the truth. The emphasis of creating the community spirit is essential to this process. The biggest block to mankind's *Qi* flowing smoothly is the ego and all the old internal messages that stop the mind, body and spirit from receiving fresh new messages and functioning properly. These principles are the root to the balance of *Yin* and *Yang* and the manifestation of harmony between the macrocosm (universe) and the microcosm (man). Consequently, clients feel free to be natural and enjoy discovering their natural healing ability.

Physically the Clinic consists of two large rooms where clients receive treatment. In one, thirty to forty people can be seated at any one time. In the other there are ten treatment couches for use at any one time. There is no separate room for private consultation and there are no separate rooms for male and female patients. Screens are available for those who need to remove their clothing. Nevertheless, most of the clients perceive the clinic as a community setting and, although there is no privacy, there are great benefits gained from such environment. If people are listening they only do so passively and actively not listening.

In this open public forum the Chinese medicine is seen for what it is and the results, or failures, or reactions, are in full view. People have to remove the necessary "clothing" and disclose their personal problems, which expose them, such that they have to recognise their conditions. From that point they can then face the goal of raising their ability and reaping the rewards of good health at all levels. A happy, enjoyable and sincere spirit is maintained by the clinicians, no matter how serious or life threatening the health problems may be or how much pressure they may be under.

This arrangement has bought about the desirable results. It has led the clinicians at the Gateway to realise the significance of the "*Qi field*" in organising the healing process of the community. Many people, who have visited the Gateway Clinic, reported a calm "homecoming" experience, which is encouraging to both patients and care providers.

Obviously over the years there have been orthodox medical practitioners, nursing professionals, and physiotherapists and administrators, who maintain strong opinions and refuse to recognise the evidence of the work of nature being done. As time passes on the political climate has had to find new innovations and methods of working, as the allopathic model is too costly and hazardous, incomplete and unpopular.

There is the need for a Gateway Clinic in every hospital in the UK. and it will probably happen in the near future. The general public has welcomed the friendly and sincere attitude and the natural flow of Chinese Medicine, particularly when the results proven to be good. All clients have benefited on some level or another and many have resolved their health issues completely and they went on to learn the

Chinese systems of Longitivity such as Qi Gong, Tai Chi, meditation and food therapy etc.

THE NEED FOR FINANCIAL SUPPORT FROM THE NHS

The Gateway Clinic has always been working on a "shoe string budget". It has had to rely on volunteer practitioners to assist with the immense workload. The practitioners have had to modify what they originally learnt in college to serve the need of the clients according to the conditions they present with. Practically this is most clearly seen in the needle techniques applied and the herbs and medical substances used.

The clinicians are expected to treat acute and chronic health problems and handle all stressful situations smoothly and calmly. This requires that they themselves practise what they preach, consequently all are involved in using *Qi Gong*, herbs, acupuncture for themselves which in itself gives a greater understanding of the truth nature of TCM,

The Gateway staffs are invited to give lectures and see clients nationally and internationally. The innovations made in the field of drug abuse, HIV/AIDS, hepatitis C and cancer have brought considerable interest from the media, medical consultants, pharmacists from many countries particularly from those with minimal financial resources.

John Tindall has been instrumental in establishing a lot of this work and at present is engaged in developing Chinese Herbal Products for Hepatitis C and for dealing with the side effects of interferon and ribovirin. He is continuing to train health care professionals in the drug addiction field in statuary and non-statutory organisations and prisons under the YUAN Traditional Medicine College & Ear Acupuncture Register.

The Hospital now acknowledges the achievements and is at present developing strategies to utilize these skills to obtain more financial resources to extend the service.

This year the Gateway service is absorbed into the main stream HIV Budget and so its future is more secured than before. Previously one had to bid for survival on an annual basis.

It is the consequence of the extremely high work capacity and consistency of the Gateway Team and the emphasis simplicity and proven effectiveness of Chinese medicine that the clinic is now able to look forward to further expansions.

Just from looking at our time table and knowing that we treated 60 clients per day and had a total load of 1000 clients and providing 17,000 treatments last year for a total running cost of £100,000, clearly pointing out that the setting up of a Gateway style Clinic in every hospital in the United Kingdom is justified.

The Present State of Chinese Medicine in the UK Relating to the Development of the Gateway Clinic

Exponential growth for Chinese medicine is possibly the most accurate appraisal at present.

There is the register of Traditional Chinese Medicine for all qualified herbalists and the British Council of Acupuncture for all qualified acupuncturists. These professional bodies represent the profession publicly and to the government. There are isolated independent organisations, which prevent unified view and voice to the government being presented that hold the development process back to some degree. Consistent efforts are being made by those involved to get TCM recognized and accredited.

To this end all of the various Chinese medicine and acupuncture colleges are going through an accreditation process which has succeeded in that several courses have gained university status such as those courses in Chinese medicine offered by Middlesex University and Westminster University in London.

The level of postgraduate education is also gradually rising but there is no continuing education system suggested yet.

There is a huge growth of the use of CM products by the public and there are new private centers opening all the time. The press and medical coverage is mixed. Some set out to ridicule and ruin CM's reputation and other are positive and informative.

More statutory and non statutory organisations are using Chinese medicine particular in the field of HIV/AIDS, hepatitis C and drug abuse. The use of acupuncture in the substance abuse field has had the fastest growth mostly due to the earnest work of The National Acupuncture Detoxification Association (NADA) and many prisons throughout the UK are using this protocol with their inmates.

The number of OM practitioners, nurses, and physiotherapists who utilizes Chinese medicine is growing and many OM GP practices have brought in the services of qualified CM practitioners for such conditions as dermatology, gynaecology and rheumatology, etc.

Unfortunately there are no recognised pay scales for CM practitioners and no professional bodies ready yet to negotiate on such issues with the health authorities. So given the present financial crisis in the NHS those practitioners who have managed to start in hospitals or health clinincs are grossly under paid. This may deter others from promoting existing facilities or introducing Chinese medicine into the NHS.

Acknowledgments

In writing this article I feel the need to acknowledge those teachers from whom I share their wisdom, experience, and practice of Chinese medicine, as their enthusiasm has inspired me in my work. I also acknowledge all those clients who have received treatment under my care for their patience and diligence they have shown in their healthcare.

Ryston Low, The British College of Acupuncture, London; Dr. Michael Smith, Lincoln Clinic, South Bronx, New York; Giovanni Maciocia, London School of Chinese Herbal Medicine; Michael McIntyre, London School of Chinese Herbal Medicine; Dr. Ke, London School of Chinese Herbal Medicine; Professor Wu Bo Ying, Beijing Academy of Traditional Chinese Herbal Medicine and Zhi Xing Wang, Qi Gong Master.

I left the N.H.S in November 1999 to form the Yuan Traditional Medicine College, Yuan Products & Yuan Clinic. I see 30 clients a day, I am actively involved in developing treatment programmes for Hep C, HIV/AIDS and Cancer. I manage the ear acupuncture register to help all drugs workers became fully able and qualified to use ear accupuncture for all aspects related to substance abuse.

I no longer am involed with NADA as our new college and register has gone far beyond the NADA protocol. Myself and my colleagues are actively teaching and treating clients in over 10 countries each year.

Reference

Tindall, J. (1994), The Gateway Clinic Experience: The treatment of HIV and AIDS using traditional Chinese Medicine. *European Journal of Oriental Medicine 1(3), 6–11.*

7 TREATMENT OF IRRITABLE BOWEL SYNDROME USING CHINESE MEDICINE

Lily Cheung

Diagnosis and Treatment of IBS According to Orthodox Medicine

Clinical features: The irritable bowel syndrome (IBS) is the term often used for all other types of functional bowel disease than specifically diagnosed ones. It is a functional disorder of the small and large ntestine. This disorder is characterised by hyperirritability and altered motility and secretion of the gastrointestinal tract, but there is no structural pathology and no specific diagnostic test for the syndrome. The symptoms may be associated with menstruation and the menopause, mental and physical fatigue may be factors influencing the symptoms, and both sexes are affected, more in females than male.

The pain when it occurs is situated in the left iliac fossa and is usually relieved by bowel motion (i.e. defaecation or the passage of wind). The patient may complain of constipation, or diarrhoea with the passage of frequent small volumes of stools, often characterised with mucous, and a feeling of incomplete emptying of the rectum. Palpable tender sigmoid colon may be detected. The length of history of the complaint is usually long, with recurrent episodes and long symptom-free intervals. The patient may have a history of abdominal pain since childhood. Mild episodes of pain occur frequently in the normal population and often go undetected and undiagnosed. The patient with IBS looks well despite frequent episodes of pain.

Aetiology: The exact cause of IBS is not known. As part of the digestive process the intestines move food by the wavelike contraction of peristalsis. IBS occurs when the normal peristalsis becomes irregular and uncoordinatedly disrupting of the normal digestive process. Many authorities consider IBS as a stress-induced illness while others opinion veers towards towards food sensitivities, in particular in the aged. Overeating is known to aggravate IBS. Lactose intolerance, irregular eating habit, smoking may contribute to the worsening of IBS. Other drug-induced aggravations are: antibiotics and sugar substitutes (sorbitol) which induce diarrhoea, antacids, morphine-like drugs, tricyclic antidepressants cause constipation. Psychological factors are important and IBS can be exacerbated by stress.

Examination and diagnosis No specific diagnosis for IBS, but sending stool samples for laboratory test rules out serious diseases. Personal history taking and psychological tests rule out emotional and stress problems. Endoscopy of the rectum and colon will eliminate serious problems.

Treatment   IBS is mainly treated by relieving the symptoms.

Management
- Explain the symptoms and their mechanism to the patients,
- Ressure the patients the benign nature of the conditions and dispel cancer phobia that the patient may have.
- Suggest high bran diet that may help.
- Prescribe mild antispasmodics such as mebeverine.
- Treat underlying stress and depression.

IBS is recognised as a multi-system disorder affecting more than the gastrointestinal tract though the cause of IBS is not known. In a recent Forum held to discuss the role of diet in the management of IBS dietary fibre was considered helpful and that the use of prebiotics and probiotics in the modification of gut flora affecting the micro environment to reduce the production of colonic hydrogen. (Forum, 2000).

Diagnosis and Treatment of IBS According to Chinese Medicine

In Chinese medicine, a holistic approach for diagnosis and treatment of the disease will be followed. The diagnosis of an individual's disease depends on the environmental influence, mental status apart from the organic causes of ill health. It is the imbalance of these that leads to the appearance of signs and symptoms of diseases. Readers may refer to Chapter 2 for philosophical aspects of the concepts. Thus in dealing with IBS the following are considered: emotional factors, uncontrolled eating habits and the six exogenous factors may be involved with IBS. (Zhou and Jin, 1997; Zhu, 1989).

- *Anger and/or depression* can impair the *Liver* causing *Qi* stagnation of *Liver*, which in turn causes constipation and abdominal pain.
- *The uncontrolled eating habits (or improper diet)* lead to deficiency of *Spleen Qi* that impairs the functions of *Spleen* in transportation and transformation. This results in loose stools and diarrhoea.
- *The Exogenous Factors* involved in producing IBS symptoms are: *Wind Cold, Summer Heat* and *Dampness* which impair *Stomach and Spleen Qi*, or the *Spleen* stagnancy resulting from the *Dampness*; can cause lose stools and diarrhoea.

CLASSIFICATION OF IBS ACCORDING TO CHINESE MEDICINE CONCEPTS

Chronic IBS or related diarrhoea often presents with deficiency syndromes as follows:

- Weakness of *Spleen* and *Stomach*: symptoms of intermittent diarrhoea appear possibly with mucous, indigestion, poor appetite; exacerbated by raw food or fatty and spicy food, feeling of tiredness; the tongue appears pale with white coat; pulse is thread and weak
- Disharmony of *Liver and Spleen*: patient usually complains of abdominal pain, which is relieved by bowel motion, stomach distention probable caused by gas; symptoms are usually linked to anxiety, depression and anger; tongue appears pale red with thin white coat; pulse is taut.
- Deficiency of *Yang* of the *Spleen and Kidney*: watery stools with undigested food present, abdominal pain and gaseous distention relieved by bowel motion, the four limbs usually feel cold, presence of low back pain, tongue-pale with white coat, pulse-deep and thread.
- Retention of *Damp* and *Heat*: intermittent abdominal pain with distension, loose bowels with burning bowel motion, usually presence of mucous and slight bleeding; tongue, red with yellow greasy coat; pulse, taut and slippery.

Principles of treatment with chinese medicine approaches

In general treatment involves the administration of acupuncture or the use of decoctions of Fu-Fang (composite formulae containing mixtures of CM herbs) in order to achieve the followings:

- Invigorate and strengthen the *Spleen* and regulate the *Stomach*
- Soothe the *Liver* and regulate the *Spleen*
- Reinforce the *Spleen* and the *Kidney*
- Clear *Heat* and remove *Dampness*.

Case History

Four case histories for the treatment of IBS are described in the following text for discussion.

CASE HISTORY ONE: FEMALE, AGE 30 YEARS

Complaint: Diarrhoea with bleeding

History: Periodical abdominal pain for the past 5 years, leading to diarrhoea and bleeding. Symptoms were worse before periods. Pain was relieved by bowel movements. Pain occurred 2 to 3 times daily. The condition is made worse also by eating bread. Other symptoms included feeling tired; poor appetite; heavy periods and frequent absence from work. Sigmoidscopy; abdominal scan; gastroscopy; stool examination and barium meal were carried out at the hospital. Blood tests showed slight anaemia. Had been on a prescription of fybrogel and colprenrin without any effect.

On Examination Complexion was pale and dull. On the left side of the lower abdomen, a lump was felt which was 3 inches long and tender on palpation. Tongue colour—pale with white coat. Pulse—small and slightly deep.

Diagnosis: Weakness of spleen and stomach.

Treatment: Electro-acupuncture and moxibustion were used to help strengthen spleen and regulate stomach. Table 7.1a summarises the acupuncture points used with.

Electro-acupuncture and moxibustion were supplied. Corresponding Hua-tuo points can be used instead of points on the UB channel. Two treatments were given per week for the next four weeks after which all symptoms were generally reduced. Weekly treatments were given for the next 3 months. At the end of that period, all symptoms have disappeared and no more treatments wer required. Table 7.1b summarises the points used.

Comments: Needling at point Zusanli, balances peristalsis via vagal nerve activity through the anterior fibialis. Some research also shows that this point can strengthen the immune system, reduce mucous

Table 7.1a Electro-acupuncture points used and moxibustion for treating IBS of a 30-year old female patient during the first period

Points Used	Nerves stimulated	TCM explanations
Ab Shih points (pain sensitive points)		
Tianshu (St25)	T7-T12	Front Mu point of the large intestine; regulate Qi flow to strengthen function of spleen and large intestine; specific point for stopping diarrhoea.
Zusanli (St36)	L4-SI	Lower He-sea point of the stomach channel; regulates digestive system.
Shangjux-Xu (St37)	L4-SI	Lower He-sea point of the large intestine channel; regulate Qi flow and functions of stomach and spleen; specific for stopping diarrhoea.
Pishu (UB20)	T11-T12	Back Shu point of the Spleen; regulate and strengthen function of spleen; specific for stopping diarrhoea.
Wcishu (UB21)	T12-L1	Back Shu point of the stomach; nourish digestive system; improve stomach yin; specific for relieving abdominal pain.

Table 7.1a Electro-acupuncture points used and moxibustion for treating IBS of A 30-Yr old female patient during the first period (*Continued*)

Points Used	Nerves stimulated	TCM explanations
Dachangshu (UB25)	L4	Back Shu point of the Large Intestine; regulates Qi flow; specific for reducing diarrhoea, abdominal pain and distension.
Ciliao (UB32)	S2	Clears lower jiao damp heat; improve large intestine function specific for treating abdominal pain and constipation.

The combination of points Dachangshu and Zusanli is effective in regulating the digestive system, relief abdominal spasm and pain. After 5 treatments, the diarrhoea and bleeding and the size of the lump were reduced and bleeding during the last period was less heavy. At end of the fifth treatment car studs were left in on the Stomach and Large Intestine points. The condition remained stable for the next 6 weeks without treatment. Two more treatments were given after the 6-week break, after which her bowel motions returned to normal; bleeding stopped and the lump had disappeared. After an interval of 9 weeks, there was still no abdominal pain, bowel motions remained normal but there was some bleeding and the lump had started to make an appearance. Her period was due in a few days time. At this stage, the TCM diagnosis was changed to Spleen & Kidney Yang Xu.

Electro-acupuncture and moxibustion were applied. Corresponding Hau-tuo points can be used instead of points on the UB channel. Two treatments were given per week for the next four weeks after which all symptoms were generally reduced. Weekly treatments were given for the next 3 months. At the end of that period, all symptoms have disappeared and no more treatments were required. Table 7.1b summarises the points used.

Table 7.1b Electro-acupuncture points used and moxibustion for treating IBS of a 30 year old female patient during the second period

Points used	Nerves stimulated	TCM explanations
Sanyingjiao (Sp6)	L4-SI	Spleen, Liver & Kidney crossing point; strengthens spleen and kidney functions; reinforce yin Qi.
Daheng (Spl5)	8th-12th inter-Costal nerve	Front Mu point; warms middle jiao to improve digestive function.
Taichong (Liv3)	L4-S2	Shu-stream and Yuan-source point and Gate point; soothes liver; regulate Qi and activates blood.
Shenshu (UB23)	L1-L3	Back Shu point of the Kidney; trengthens kidney Qi.
Ciliao (UB32)	S2	Strengthens kidney Qi.

discharge and inflammation. Stimulating Tianshu and Zusanli together has a better effect of regulating digestive function and reducing pain and spasm of the abdomen. Tianshu and Shangjuxu in combination promotes phagocytosis, at the same time increasing serum globulin which in turn has a positive effect on the immune system. Dachangshu and Tianshu seems to together regulate the large intestine function more effectively.

CASE HISTORY TWO: FEMALE, AGE, 34 YEARS OLD

Complaint: Daily diarrhoea for the past 3 years

History: Had been suffering with watery diarrhoea two to three times a day, preceded by abdominal pain and gaseous distension. Felt more comfortable after bowel motions. Had been diagnosed as IBS. Was on a course of steroids with no improvement. Was recently given mesalazine and had been watching her diet carefully. So far there had been no improvement in the symptoms.

On Examination: There was pressure pain on the lower abdomen on the right side. An area of hardening like a sausage can be felt over this area. Her complexion was pale and she looked weary. Tongue—pale with deep teeth marks and a thin white coat. Pulse—fast.

TCM Diagnosis: Spleen and Kidney Yang Xu

Treatment: Acupuncture and moxibustion was given to rein-force spleen and kidney according to the following points used (Table 7.2):

Comments: After the first session, the patient had 4 days of normal bowel motion, twice daily. On the fifth day, bowel motion was loose again twice a day. At the second session the hard area and the area of pain in the abdomen reduced. No change in the tongue. Pulse—slower than before. The same points were used. On the third session, the tongue had less teeth marks. Pulse—small and slow. The same prescription was used and the following herbs were given.

Table 7.2 Electro-acupuncture points used and moxibustion for treating IBS of a 34 year old female patient

Points used	Nerves stimulated	TCM explanations
Daheng (Spl5)	T8-T12	Front Mu point; warms middle jiao to improve digestive glands function
Shangjuxu (St37)	L4-SI	Lower He-sea point of the L1 channel; regulate Qi flow + function of spleen + stomach; specific point for diarrhoea
Zusanli (St36)	L4-SI	Lower He-sea point of the St channel; regulate the digestive system
Pishu (UB20)	T11-T12	Back shu point of the spleen; regulate + strengthens the function of the spleen; specific point for diarrhoea
Weishu (UB21)	T12-L1	Back shu point of the stomach; moisturise the digestive system; improve the stomach yin; specific point for abdominal pain
Shenshu (UB23)	L1-L3	Back shu point of the kidney; strengthens kidney Qi
Ciliao (UB32) Ah Shih point	S2 on right lower abdomen	Strengthens kidney Qi The use of painful points is part of the basic principles of treatment

The patient is also advised to abstain from cold food and food with a very high fibre content.

Bai Shao	(*Radix Paeoniae Alba*)
Bai Zhu	(*Rhizoma Atractylodis Macrocephalae*)
Fang Feng	(*Radix Ledebouriellae*)
Fu Ling	(*Poria*)
Gancao	(*Radix Glycyrrhizae*)
Dang Shen	(*Radix Codonopsis Pilosucae*)

The above prescription was taken daily for 10 weeks with weekly treatment of acupuncture. The patient recovered completely.

CASE HISTORY THREE: FEMALE, AGE 33 YEARS OLD

Complaint: The past 2 weeks. the patient had been suffering with diarrhoea accompanied by some bleeding and mucous.

History: 8 years previous, the patient started having abdominal pain with diarrhoea mucous and breeding. After each bowel motion, she experienced a burning sensation. There was the occasional bout of constipation. Drugs prescribed had no effect. 3 years ago, she tried acupuncture with success. Symptoms started to appear again 2 weeks ago, the diarrhoea gradually increasing in severity for 4 days followed by constipation for the next 3 days then diarrhoea again alternating with constipation. Each bowel motion was accompanied by blood and mucous and a burning sensation at the end There was also a constant feeling of wanting to have a bowel motion.

On Examination: There was pressure pain on the distended abdomen. Tongue—slight red with a yellow coat. Pulse—wiry.

TCM Diagnosis: Retention of damp heat.

Treatment: Clear heat and disperse damp with acupuncture and moxibustion as indicated in Table 6.3.

Comments: A total of 6 weekly treatments were given. The patient recovered fully.

CASE HISTORY FOUR: MALE, AGE 31 YEARS OLD

Complaint: Suffers with alternating diarrhoea and constipation.

History: Had been suffering with the above symptoms for the past 9 years. There was more diarrhoea than constipation. During bouts of diarrhoea, the patient would have at least 3 bowel motions a day. There was no mucous discharge or bleeding. Abdominal pain was present on the right side. The pain is reduced after each bowel motion although the abdomen always felt distended and gassy. These episodes were influenced

Table 7.3 Electro-acupuncture points used and moxibustion for treating IBS of a 33 year old female patient

Points used	Nerves Sstimulated	TCM explanations
Tianshu (St25)	T7-T12	Front Mu point of LI; regulate Qi flow to strengthen the spleen and LI; specific point for diarrhoea
Zusanli (St36)	L4-SI	Lower He-sea point of the St channel; regulate the digestive system
Shangjuxu (St37)	L4-SI	Lower He-sea point of the L1 channel; regulate Qi flow of the stomach and spleen; specific point for diarrhoea
Pishu (UB20)	T11-T12	Back shu point of the spleen; regulate function of spleen; specific point for diarrhoea
Dachangshu (UB25)	L4	Back shu point of LI; regulate Qi flow; specific pint for diarrhoea, (UB25) abdominal pain and distension
Yinlingquan (Sp9)	L3-S2	Reduce heat; remove damp; regulate function of SJ channel

by his emotions of anger and depression. Was diagnosed as IBS. Medication prescribed had not made any difference.

On Examination: Appeared nervous and anxious. Presence of pressure pain on the right side of the abdomen. Tongue—pale red with a thin white coat. Pulse—wiry.

TCM Diagnosis: Disharmony of liver and spleen

Treatment: Acupuncture and moxibustion was prescribed to smooth liver function and regulate spleen according to the points indicated in Table 7.4.

Comments: A total of 10 weekly treatments were given and the patient's bowel motions were more regular and better controlled.

Conclusion

All patients who sought treatment from the Clinic experienced unsuccessful treatment with orthodox medicine. With the exception of the first case of the four cases described all were treated with

Table 7.4 Electro-acupuncture points used and moxibustion for treating IBS of a 31year old male patient

Points used	Nerves stimulated	TCM explanations
Tianshu (St25)	T7-T12	Front Mu point of L1; regulate Qi flow to strengthen spleen and large intestine; specific point for diarrhoea
Zusanli (St36)	L4-SI	Lower He-sea point of the St channel; regulate the digestive system
Pishu (UB20)	T11-T12	Back shu point of the spleen; regulate the function of the spleen; specific point for diarrhoea
Ganshu (UB18)	T9-T10; CrN XI	Regulate function of liver Qi; reduce mental depression; regulate blood circulation
Taichong (Liv3)	L4-SI	Shu-stream and Yuan-source point and Gate point; soothes liver; regulate Qi and activate blood
Fengchi (GB20)	CrN X	Regulate liver Qi to disperse stagnation; refresh the mind

Ear points were needled at Shenmen and Dachang.

acupuncture and CM medicine (mainly as mixtures of several herbs. Depending on the severity of the cases, treatment after 6 to 10 weeks gave improvement.

References

Forum (2000). Irritable bowel syndrome and diet—exploring the controversies. *Pharmaceutical Journal*, **264**, 736.

Zhou, Z.-Y. & Jin, H.-D. (1997) Gastrointestinal Diseases. In: Clinical Manual of Chinese Herbal Medicine & Acupuncture. Churchill Livingstone, P90–101.

Zhu, C.-H. (1989). Clinical Handbook of Chinese Prepared Medicine. Paradigm Publication.

8 THE PROGRESS OF USING CHINESE HERBAL MEDICINES IN CANCER RESEARCH

Jennifer Man-Fan Wan

Introduction

Cancer is currently the second leading cause of death for many developed communities such as those in the United States and Hong Kong and is projected to be the number one cause of early death in the next century, in part because as people live longer the risk of developing cancer increases. There are no successful universal treatments at present. Medical treatments for cancer entail physiologic stress. Results include toxic tissue effects, often damage to cell DNA structure and changes in normal body function. Both the immune system and gastrointestinal tract are often victimized. Anemia and infections associated with bone marrow effects, nausea, vomiting, anorexia, stomatitis, ulcers and diarrhea with gut failure along with hair loss are common symptoms of chemo- and radiotherapy toxicity.

Chinese herbal medicines have been used as remedies for cancer treatment for several thousands of years. However, in many cases there is no consistent opinion or definite conclusion on their curative effects as yet, this because the use of Chinese herbs or folk medicines is the result of a long-term accumulation of clinical experiences rather than scientific merits. After the birth of New China, research in Chinese medicine has made tremendous progress with new experience in preventing and treating of cancers. Several photochemicals with anti-tumor promoting potential have so far been reported. Many experimental studies both *in vivo* and *in vitro* have provided evidence for the possible protective mechanisms underlying the value of antioxidants, immuno-modulatory, enzymes inhibition and cell cycle arrest and the induction of apoptosis. This chapter contains the Western and Eastern physician's concept of tumors and their treatments, and presents latest scientific research evidence on the anticancer mechanisms of Chinese herbal medicine.

Western Concept of Tumors and Their Treatments

Cancers are populations of cells in the body that have acquired the ability to multiply and spread without the normal restraints. Most cancers take the form of tumors, although not all tumors are cancers. A tumor is simply spontaneous new tissue form that serves no physiological purpose. It can be benign like a wart, or malignant, like most lung cancers. Cancer cells can also spread (in a process called metastasis), to distant sites via the blood and lymphatic circulation, thereby producing invasive tumors in almost any part of the body. Malignant tumors affect host functions by compression, invasion, and destruction of normal tissues and also by the elaboration of substances that circulate in the blood stream. The effects of a growing tumor in a patient may include fever, anorexia (loss of appetite), weight loss and cachexia (body weight), infection, anemia, and various hormonal and neurological symptoms. Both genetics and lifestyle are potent forces that influence the risk for development cancer or carcinogenesis.

Current Western dilemmas for physicians managing patients with cancer include surgery, chemotherapy, radiotherapy, and hormone replacement and hormone antagonists. Research in progression includes vitamins and their synthetic analogues, immunotherapy as the use of gamma-interferon and interleukin-2, growth factors as interleukin 3/ganulocyte-stimulating factor, and gene therapy. Many anti-cancer drugs, radiation, hormones, cytokines, transferred gene (gene therapy) exert their cytotoxic effects by inhibiting or disturbing the progression of cells through the cell cycle (Darzynkiewicz et al. 1995, Gorczyca et al. 1993). The cell cycle involves the division of a single eukaryotic cell into two daughter cells via four biologically defended phases namely first gap (G1), DNA synthesis (S), second gap (G2) and mitosis (M). The cells may exist in a quiescent, non-proliferating state at Go phase (Reddy 1994). The two main cell cycle effects of anti-cancer agents are: (i) exert a lethal or apoptoic effect which is maximal in a certain phase or phases of the cycle, (ii) affect the progression of cells through the cycle, by arresting cells at particular point in the cycle. The former increases cell death and the latter results in a slower proliferation of the tumor cells. Chemotherapeutic agents are effective because they disrupt the normal processes in the cell responsible for cell growth and reproduction through the cell cycle. Some agents interfere with DNA synthesis (S-phase), disrupt DNA structure and RNA replication, others prevent cell division by mitosis (G2/M), or cause hormonal imbalances, or make unavailable the specific amino acids necessary for protein synthesis (Go/G1)(Gorczyca *et al.* 1993, Liu *et al.* 1997, Darzynkiewicz *et al.* 1995, Reedy 1994, Traganos *et al.* 1996). This diversity in mode of action provides a basis for grouping drugs into six classes of chemotherapeutic agents: anti-metabolites, alkaloids, alkylating agents, antibiotics, enzymes and hormones. These agents are often used in conjunction with surgery or radiation.

Scientists presently believe that gene therapy is a promising field in oncology. It is believed that chemosensitivity of the cancer cells can be enhanced through genes transfer using the recombinant retroviruses to deliver the specific genes (Rainov *et al.* 1998, Tong *et al.* 1998). Efficient introduction of biologically active genes by intratumoral injection of a replication-defective adenoviral expression vector into tumor cells would greatly facilitate cancer therapy (Zwacka *et al.* 1998). The gene therapy approaches being employed at present fall into three major categories: (1) enzyme/pro-drug systems, (2) tumor suppressor gene replacement therapy; and (3) immune-gene therapy which is based on cytokine or tumor antigen expression to induce tumor immunity (Rainov *et al.* 1998). Although promising, much effort will be required to realize the potential for clinical application of adenovirus-based cancer gene therapy.

Traditional Chinese Physician's Concept of Tumours

In the medical history of China, tumours and cancers are not recent phenomena but quite ancient ones and are mentioned in many of China's oldest medical books. The "tumour" has been recorded as early as 2,000 years ago in the *Canon of Medicine* (Fu, 1985). The book listed tumours of different areas of the body such as tendon tumor, intestinal tumour, breast and lips tumours, and so on. Benign and malignant tumors have been mentioned in many medical books but often by different names. Commonly, a malignant tumor in Chinese Medicine is called "ai"—literally, "rock" since cancer is hard and fixed, and with an uneven surface. Cancer is sometimes called "lost-of-lustre" in Chinese Medicine because at the final stage of the disease the patient often loses all his lustre just like a withering tree with its bark and branches all dried up (Gao Binngjun in the *Comprehension of Ulcers* (Fu, 1985).

Many of the ancient medical books such as *Renzhai Guide to Diagnosis and Prescriptions* of 1264, *Orthodox Manual of Surgery of Chen Shigong* of 1617, *General Records of Effective Cures*, published around 1111–1117, *and Comprehension of Ulcers* published in 1805, discussed the pathology of tumor (Fu, 1985). Many descriptions of the signs, characteristics and symptoms of cancer are also described in the Chinese medical literature through generations. Although some of the discussions offer only conjectures, there are many reasonable explanations. For instance, a specific description of lip cancer can be found *in Orthodox Manual Surgery of Chen Shigong published in 1617*. Lip cancer, as described by the book, may be due to general factors of deep sorrow, or irascibility, or to local factors like irritating the lip by taking fried, crispy or roasted food (Fu, 1985).

According to Traditional Chinese Medicine (TCM), the causes of tumours include excessive tension, external disease factors, senility, or the changing of food and habits, which lead to "Qi" stagnation and blood stasis. In addition, abnormal material obstruction produced in the body, or dysfunction or derangement of the viscera and so on would cause tumours. In the "Inner Canon of Medicine" (*Huang Di Nei Jing*), the obstruction of the esophagus is described to be due to over-anxiety. That is to say, emotion is one of the inducing factors (Fu, 1985). The Chinese believed that the incidence of all the common cancers in humans are determined by various potentially controllable external factors such as their habits, diet, exercise, smoking, and customs rather than by their ethnic origins. In this regard, the TCM theory is very much similar to that of Western medicine.

Although doctors of Chinese Medicine in the past recognized that some of the tumors were incurable, they had no fear of their fierceness. The Chinese physicians believed in treating the human body as a "whole" so as to reinforce the general health, then administrate medicine direct to the tumour and operate it if necessary. The earliest recorded surgical removal of a tumour was as early as the 3rd century. The *Elementary Medicine*, published by *Li Yan* in 1575, mentioned that a very sharp knife was used to remove an adipose tumour. Surgery for cancer treatment described in *Records of Emperor Jing Di* in the History of the Jin Dynasty as "*at first, the emperor got a tumour in his eye and then commanded an operation to be performed*" (Fu, 1985).

The philosophy, thus treatment of diseases, of Chinese Medicine is very different from that of the West. Chinese doctors adopt the principle of differentiating a syndrome according to the individual condition. Chinese Medicine is prescribed to the cancer patients based on not the disease entity but the overall symptoms, signs and health condition. The treatment objectives are to strengthen the host's defense on one hand, and to "weaken" the tumour on the other and to remove the tumours with surgery and radiation if necessary. Today in China, the physicians managing patients with cancer fall into three categories: (1) conventional therapy, (2) Chinese Medicine, and (3) integration of Chinese Medicine and conventional therapy. Chinese techniques of external therapy include acupuncture; acupressure, message, moxibustion, and internal therapy with a wide range of medicines consisting of herbal, animal and mineral products (Cheng 1990, Chi *et al.* 1995, Liu 1990, Li *et al.* 1994a, Wang *et al.* 1994, Zhu 1994, Zhang 1992, Zheng *et al.* 1997). Acupuncture involves the insertion of very thin steel needles into vital-energy points along the meridians. Over 800 such points have been identified (Cheng 1990). Acupressure utilizes the same principles and points as acupuncture, but sharp finger pressure rather than needles is used to effect stimulation, both usually combined in therapy, help to improve the cancer patient blood circulation, immune function and pain reduction (Yang *et al.* 1995, Agliett *et al.* 1990). Chinese herbal medicine is often used in conjunction with chemotherapy and radiotherapy and/or surgery (Cha *et al.* 1994, Chu 1988, Yang *et al.* 1995, Zhu *et al.* 1994, and Zhang 1992).

Recent Evidence on Chinese Herbal Medicine in Cancer Research

Present cancer treatments and development in the West face numerous limitations. The principal aim of cancer chemotherapy is to kill tumor cells selectively without harming normal cells, but this is rarely achieved. A major problem is the limitation of anti-neoplastic drugs resulting from lack of sensitivity of the tumor and from toxicity to normal tissues. Many anti-neoplastic drugs such as the anti-metabolites 5-fluorouracil, methotrexate, the alkylating agents mitomycin C and cisplatin, and the anti-oestrogenic drug tamoxifen, have all been proven to possess certain degrees of toxicity to normal tissues. (Viale *et al.* 1998, Bajetta *et al.* 1998, Ribas *et al.* 1998, Recchia *et al.* 1998, Hansen *et al.* 1996). Clinical side effects include gastrointestinal toxicity, leukopenia, hand-foot syndrome and nutropeni. A number of alkylating agents and/or topoisomerase II inhibitors can also promote the incidence of treatment-related leukemia (Diamandidou *et al.* 1996).

Oral mucositis is a common, dose limiting and potentially serious complication of chemotherapy and radiation (Rumana *et al.* 1998). Head and neck radiation affect the oral mucosa and salivary secretions, as well as the esophagus, influence the taste sensations and sensitivity to food temperature and texture and may induce neurologic symptoms

(Muracciole *et al.* 1998). Abdomen radiation may produce denuded bowel muscosa, loss of villi and absorbing surface area, vascular changes form intimal thickening, and ulcer formation. Various intestinal resections of tumor excisions may cause steatorrhea due to general mal-absorption, fistulas, or stenosis.

Retroviral-mediated gene-labeling protocols have been approved for clinical studies that are designed to gain a better understanding of cancer disease progression and response to therapy. The field is at a very early stage in its evolution, and one concern is that the considerable hurdles that must be overcome are seen as examples of the failure of cancer gene therapy. Some concerns on toxicity related to the use of adenovirus, risks and side effects from transgenes, lack of tumor-specificity of transgene expression, and potential problems with efficient gene delivery to solid tumors (Tong *et al.* 1998, Van Gool *et al.* 1998).

At present, there is an increasing interest in Chinese traditional systems of medicines from non-western societies. The expectation is that at least some of the medicinal products will be efficacious, and hope of that traditional use will be based on products with low toxicity. With the development of sciences and technology in modern times, people are able to extract the effective ingredients of Chinese Medicines and to study their anticancer mechanisms. Guided by the experience of TCM, many naturally occurring products from vegetables, herbs, fungi, animals, and minerals have been considered to exert certain chemo-preventive and treatment properties against carcinogenesis based on scientific research by scientists (Han 1994a, Han 1994b, Rui 1997, Xu 1991, Zheng *et al.* 1997, Zhang *et al.* 1994, Yu *et al.* 1992). Among the plant kingdom, the active ingredients are extracts from leaves as well as seeds, roots and fungus (see Photos). With advanced technologies such as high-performance liquid—chromatography (HPLC), nuclear magnetic resonance, mass spectrophotmetry for isolation, separation and purification; gel electrophoresis, and DNA fingerprinting for species identification, a number of active components of Chinese herbal medicine origin such as indirubin, lycobetaine, hydroxycaptothecin, beta-elemene, irisquinone, oridonine, norcantharidin have been isolated from the parent materials (Xu 1991, Han 1994a, Han 1994b).

Many are now known by their immuno-modulatory, anti-oxidative, enzymatic inhibitory and cell-cycle cytotoxic specific properties (see references on Table 8.1). Han (1994) has also provided a relatively recent report on the current study of anticancer drugs originating from plants and traditional medicines in China, with particular emphasis on camptothecin, tanshinone, taxol, daiden, acetyl boswellic acid, curcumin and ginsenosides. Some of these newly developed drugs such as camptothecin from *Camptotheca accuminata* (Traganos *et al.* 1996, Eder *et al.* 1996, Siter *et al.* 1997) and taxol from *Taxuss chinensis* (Goldhirsch *et al.* 1998, Lee *et al.* 1998, Lilenbaum *et al.* 1995) have been cited in Western scientific literature as chemopreventive and chemotherapeutic agents. They are presently undergoing clinical trials.

It is now known that one of the major applications of Chinese herbal medicine is to promote immune functions. *Coriolus versicolor* (Yun Zhi) (Liu *et al.* 1993, Tsuru *et al.* 1984, Yang 1993a), *Panax ginseng* (Ginseng) (Xiaoguang *et al.* 1998, Rui 1997), *Curcuma longa Linn* (Curcumin) (Anto *et al.* 1996, Hanif *et al.* 1997) have been termed by the Chinese and Japanese as biological modifiers owing to their ability to boost up the host's immunity. "Yun Zhi" of the *Coriolus versicolor spp.* (Figure 8.1) has been known in China as food and medicine for thousands of years (Compendium of Materia Medica by Li Shi Zhen of the Ming Dynasty) and is by far the most extensively researched and best explored in terms of its medical value, in particular, in the treatment of cancer. In 1987, Professor Yang and his co-workers isolated the active ingredient of Yun Zhi from the deep layer cultivated mycelia of *Coriolus versicolor spp.* The active component is a protein bound polysaccharide (PSP) which consists of 6 kinds of monosaccharides: glucose, mannose, galactose, xylose, arabinsoe and rhamnose and they are connected with a small molecular protein-polypeptide (Yang *et al.* 1987, Yang 1993b, and Yang *et al.* 1993a). Several *in vitro* and *in vivo* studies have shown that PSP has a definite anti-tumors function (Dong *et al.* 1996, Wan *et al.* 1998, Sugimachi *et al.* 1995, Liu *et al.* 1993, Yang 1993b, Yang *et al.* 1993a). The anticancer properties of Yun Zhi PSP are said to be attributed to its immuno-modulatory actions such as to promote T-lymphocytes proliferation, interleukin-2, gamma-interferon production (Liu *et al.* 1993, Li *et al.* 1990, Shiu *et al.* 1992, Yang *et al.* 1993, Yang *et al.* 1992b). Yun Zhi PSP used in Asia today is produced by modern biotechnology. It is being sold as over-counter supplement for cancer treatment.

Similar to many anticancer agents, active compounds of Chinese Medicines are now known by their cell cycle specific effects. They can directly affect the cancer cells by either (i) slowing down their proliferation or (ii) increasing death by apoptosis (programmed cell death), or both. The former can be achieved by arresting cells in the cell cycle phase such as Go/G1, S and G2/M, delaying cellular DNA synthesis, inhibiting the mitotic process, or interfering with the expression of cell

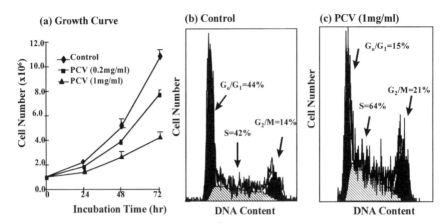

Figure 8.1 The effect of Yun Zhi PCV on the growth and cell cycle distribution of human leukemic HL-60 cells

PCV (purified *Coriolus versiocolor*) inhibited the growth of the HL-60 cells in a dose-dependent manner, after 48 hours ($p < 0.01$) and 72 hours ($p < 0.001$) of treatment (Figure 8.1a). DNA histograms analyzed by flow cytometry showing 72-hours PCV treatment (Figure 8.1b) significantly ($p < 0.001$) reduced cells in G0/G1 phase and arrested cells in S and G2/M phase when compared to Control (Figure 8.1c). Results are expressed as Mean ± SEM, n = 8.

cycle regulatory genes, oncogenes, or apopotic genes. The latter can be achieved by direct induction of DNA strands break, interference of the metabolic process, and suppression of the anti-apopotic genes (see Table 8.1 for references). We have recently discovered that Yun Zhi PSP of *Coriolus versicolor* exhibits S-phase cell cycle arrest specific activity in addition to its immuno-modulatory properties. The PSP used in our experiment has been further purified by HPLC and termed purified *Coriolus versioclor* (PCV). Figure 8.1a shows the growth curve and DNA histograms (Figures 8.1b and 8.1c) of the human promy-oleukemic cells (HL-60) cells without (Control) and with (PCV) 0.2 mg/ml and 1 mg/ml PCV 72-hours culture. DNA flow cytometry revealed that reduction in HL-60 cell growth by PCV was likely to be attributed to the blockage on G1/S or G2/M and/or both checkpoints in the cell cycle. Together with the immunological data, our data provides scientific evidence to support the anticancer properties of Chinese herbal Medicines.

Many Chinese medicine active compounds also known to cause cell death in cancer cells by the induction of apopotsis (i.e. through free

Table 8.1 Current evidence for potential anticancer drugs of Chinese herbal medicine origin

Herbal species and their active components	Anticancer mechanistic actions	References
Camptotheca accuminata (Camptothecin; Topotecan and 9-amino-20(S)-camptothecin (9-AC) are analogs of camptothecin).	Prototypical DNA topoisomerase I interactive agent. Induces S-phase cell cycle arrest, DNA damage and apoptosis; In clinical Phase I & II trails for testing	Traganos *et al.*, 1996; Palissot *et al.*, 1996; Siter *et al.*, 1997; Eder *et al.*, 1996.
Cephalotxus bainanensis (Harringtonine, Homoharringtonine)	Induce apoptosis. Exhibit high chemotherapeutic efficacy on human acute granulocytic leukemia and acute myelocytic leukemia in clinics. Diminish metastasis	Li *et al.*, 1994; Xu *et al.*, 1991.
Curcuma longa Linn (Curcumin, Curcuminoids)	Inhibit both initiation and promotion of cancers in animal models. Act as antioxidant, strong inhibitor of cyclooxygenase and lipooxygenase, induce G2/M cells arrest, induce cell death through Bcl-2, p53, cyclin B expression, inhibit DNA synthesis.	Anto *et al.*, 1996; Hanif *et al.*, 1997; Mehta *et al.*, 1997.
Coriolus versicolor (Polysaccharide Peptide)	Raises human T-helper cells, interleukins (IL-1, IL-2), natural killer cells and interferons. Induces cell cycle arrest, extends DNA synthesis time of HL-60 cells. Reduces toxicity of radiotherapy and chemotherapy.	Liu *et al.*, 1993; Tsuru *et al.*, 1984; Li 1990; Yang 1992a; Yang *et al.*, 1993; Shiu *et al.*, 1992; Yano *et al.*, 1994; Wan *et al.*, 1998.

Table 8.1 Current evidence for potential anticancer drugs of Chinese herbal medicine origin (*continued*)

Herbal species and their active components	Anticancer mechanistic actions	References
Indigofera tinctoria (Indirubin)	Down-regulation of c-myc gene. Induces leukemic cell differentiation. Applied in chronic myelocytic leukemia treatment.	Liu *et al.*, 1996; Han 1994.
Panax ginseng (Ginsenosides)	As antioxidants, enhanced immune function, nitric oxide synthesis. Inhibit DMBA-induced skin papilloma.	Rui 1997; Xiaoguang *et al.*, 1998
Taxuss chinensis (Taxol, Paclitaxel)	Induces apoptosis, down regulates bcl-xL protein, induce interleukin-8 production, activate c-Jun NH2-terminal kinase, induces cell cycle arrest. In Phase I clinical trail (USA).	Goldirsch *et al.*, 1998; Lee *et al.*, 1998.
Radix Salviae Miltiorrhizae (Tanshinone)	Inhibits DNA synthesis, PCNA expression and activity of DNA polymerase delta of leukemic cell line (HL-60). Induces differentiation of human cervical carcinoma cell line ME180. Induces DNA damage by production of reactive free radicals	Wang *et al.*, 1996, Kasimu *et al.*, 1998, Wu *et al.*, 1991.

radicals formation, down-regulating the apopotic genes, affect hormones and ions transport, or cause DNA strands break (Table 8.1). Apoptosis or "programmed cell death" represents a mode of cell death during which the cell activity participates in self-destruction (see review Arends *et al.* 1990, Gorczyca *et al.* 1993). It has been identified by the internucleosomal DNA cleavage, which appears to be associated with endonuclease activation. Camptothecin from *Camptotheca accuminata* is a prototypical DNA topoisomerase I interactive agent which kills cancer cells by breaking the DNA strands leading to cell death by apoptosis (Traganos *et al.* 1996, Palissot *et al.* 1996). Topotecan and 9-Amino-20 (S)-camptothecin (9-AC), the analogs of camptothecin, are now being tested in Phase I clinical trail for leukemia and in Phase II trail for the metastatic breast cancer in the US (Eder *et al.* 1996). Paclitaxel, an analog of taxol from the *Taxuss chinensisspp* (Goldirsch *et al.* 1998, Lee *et al.* 1998), is also being currently tested in clinical trial as an apoptotic drug. Pharmacological studies demonstrated that curcumin is an antimutagen as well as an antipromoter for cancer (Hanif *et al.* 1997, Anto *et al.* 1996). The anticancer effect of curcumin is related to its ability to accumulate cells in the G2/M phase, inhibition on prostaglandin synthesis, as well as antioxidant property (Hanif *et al.* 1997). Cucumin also induces cell death through suppression of the cell death genes such as Bcl-2 and p53 (Mehta *et al.* 1997). Bufalin, an active principal of Chinese medicine Chan-su has been shown to induce cell death of human leukemia U937 by apoptosis (Watabe *et al.* 1997). All fifteen tanshinone analogues isolated from the chloroform extract of Danshen roots (*Salviae Miltiorrhizae Radix*) have showed certain degrees of cytotoxicity to the KB, Hela, Colo-205 and Hep-2 carcinoma cell lines (Wang *et al.* 1996).

It is suggested that the planar phenanthrene ring of the tanshinones may be essential for interaction with DNA molecules whereas the furano-o-quinone moiety could be responsible for the production of reactive free radicals in the close vicinity of the bases to cause DNA damage (Kasimu *et al.* 1998, Wu *et al.* 1991). The antiproliferative effect of tanshinone has also been associated with its ability to inhibiting DNA synthesis, proliferative nuclear antigen (PCNA) expression and activity of DNA polymerase delta (Wang *et al.* 1996, Wu *et al.* 1991).

While it is important for drugs and treatments to be analyzed in modern terms to confirm their therapeutic claims and avoid confusions, one must remember that most highly purified compounds when used alone according to the Western approach will not only be unable to tackle all the heterogeneous cancer cells at once, but often exert side effects which further damage the host's immunity and other vital organs because of their DNA-specificity. Others will gain no further creditability owing to their weak cytotoxicity and non-specificity when used in isolation.

The Integration of Chinese Medicine with Modern Science

Internationally, there is an increasing focus on the protective effects of Chinese medicine on the toxic side effects of anti-neoplastic drugs (Ebisuno *et al.* 1989, Sakagami *et al.* 1991, Tsuru *et al.* 1991, Agliett *et al.* 1990, Siter *et al.*, 1997, Traganos *et al.* 1996). However, the greatest difficulty for the Western physicians to understand Chinese Medicine lies in the tremendous differences between Western and Chinese theory of the human body and disease formation. For instance, Western medicine views the human body in terms of structure and organs, from morphology and anatomy down through histology to molecular biochemistry. Function is seen in terms of structure, as in pathology, and disease tends to refer to structure. In the contrary, Chinese medicine tends to emphasize function rather structure, especially internal structure. The ancient Chinese ideograph for spleen, for instance, does not mean spleen in the modern sense; instead it refers to the entire gastrointestinal system. Likewise, problems with the kidney refer to symptoms arising from the entire endocrine system in the modern sense. In Chinese medicine, the term "tumor" in folk medicine is applied to every wide range of patho-logical manifestation, which sometimes have no relation to the various forms of neoplasia. On the whole, Chinese Physicians perceive a pattern of disharmony in the cancer patient and prescribe Chinese Medicines in such a way as to help the body itself to restore its harmony or "Yin-Yang" balance.

The Theory Of Yin-Yang permeates all aspects of the theoretical system of Chinese medicine. Briefly speaking, yin and yang are a philosophical conceptualization, a means to generalize two opposite principles, which may be observed in all related phenomena within the natural world. The early theory of yin-yang was formed in the Yin and Zhou dynasties (sixteenth century-221 B.C). Chinese view all matters as inter-communicating and inter-dependent. In fact the yin-yang concept applies to modern science. For instance, sense and antisense in molecular biology, helper/inducer cells and suppressor/cytotoxic cells in the immune system, enzymes and anti-enzymes such as trypsin and anti-trypsin, antagonists and agonists, coagulants and anticoagulants in the biological builds, and the sympathetic and parasympathetic nervous systems. Hypothetically, in the yin-yang concept, Chinese does not view the term "balance" with a planar dimension in which two fixed static structures in equilibrium act from opposite ends (Figure 8.3a), but reflecting all forms, elements and characteristics equalizing and proportioning themselves in a circular motion (Figure 8.3b). Cancers or disease occurs when balance, or the relative stability of equilibrium between the interdependent elements being set off by internal and external factors (Figure 8.3c) (i.e. too much heat or cold, dryness or dampness, or sweet and sour, too much joy or sadness). Practitioners of Chinese medicine will not simply isolate a disease agent or a variable and to treat it with aggressive and combative approach like that in the west (Figure 8.3a) but to perceive a pattern of disharmony in the integrated whole (Figure 8.3b). Thus, treatments with Chinese Herbal Medicine is given in formulation or "Fu-Fang", which is tailored to the individual's overall symptoms, signs and health status. Hypothetically, Chinese Medicine is applied to all variables so as to re-adjust their "radius" back to fit the circle or network (Figure 8.3 c).

The prescription or Fu-Fang (composite formulae) contains multiple active constituents given in different dosages and in various combinations. Table 8.2 presents the classical doctor-prescriptions; showing *Radix salviae miltiorrhizae* and *Radix Astrgali* are given in different dosages and combinations for different cancers. Fu-Fang is often used in combination with chemotherapy and radiotherapy. It is unique in a sense since orchestration of the many different biological activities i.e. immunological, pharmacological, haemological, metabolic, or specific cellular and genetic actions offered by each individual active components and their interactions should be able to return the patient back to homeostasis or to yin and yang balance.

In this regard, Yun Zhi PCV helps to give a good scientific illustration to the mechanistic actions of Fu-Fong based on its cell cycle specificity. PCV is not commonly used alone but given in formulations and in conjunction with chemotherapy and radiotherapy to patients in China. Our previous flow data (Figure 8.1c) indicates that PCV is a weak chemotherapeutic agent if used in isolation since it induces no cytotoxicity. We have further tested our hypothesis that by arresting cells in the S-phase, PCV should be able to promote the cell killing

Table 8.2 Classical formulations of Chinese medicine for cancer treatment

Anticancer Herbs	Other herbal components	Dosage (g)
Radix Astragali		
a. For Lung Cancer Treatment	*Radix Astragali* (Milkvetch Root)	12
	Radix Codonopsis (Tangshen)	12
	Nidus Vaspae (Polistes Mandarius Saussure's)	12
	Poria (Indian Bread)	15
	Polyporus (Agaric, Umbellate Pore Fungus)	15
	Semen Coicis (Coix Seed)	15
	Radix Codonopsis Lanceolatae (Lance Asiabell Root)	30
	Herba Hedyotis Diffusae (Spreading Hedyotis Herb)	30
	Herba Houttuyniae (Heartleaf Houttuynia Herb)	30
	Rhizoma Pinelliae (Pinellia Tuber)	30
	Rhizoma Atractylodis Macrocephalae (Langehead Atractylodes Rhizome)	9 9
b. For Liver Cancer Treatment	*Radix Astragali* (Milkvetch Root)	21
	Radix Rehmanniae (Rehmannia Root)	12
	Rhizoma Atractylodis Macrocephalae (Largehead Atractylodes Rhizome)	9
	Radix Ophiopogonis (Dwanf Lilyturf Tuber)	15
	Radix Stephaniae Cephananthae (Oriental Stephania Root)	15
	Fructus Lycii (Barbary Wolfberry Fruit)	3
	Cortex Cinnamomi (Cassia Bark)	6
	Fructus Schisandrae (Orange Magnoliavine Fruit)	6
	Radix Codonopsis (Tanshen)	4.5
	Cornn Cervi Pantotrichum (Hairy Deer Horn, Pilose Antler)	4.5
Radix Salviae miltiorrhizae		
(a) For Liver cancer Treatment	*Radix Salviae Miltiorrhizae* (Danshen Root)	30
	Herba Salviae Chinensis (Chinese Sage Herb)	30
	Spica Pruaellae (Common Selfheal Fruit-spike)	30
	Rhizoma Cyperi (Nutgrass Galingale Rhizome)	15
	Radix Codonopsis (Tangshen)	15
	Herba Verbenae (European Verbena Herb)	15

Table 8.2 Classical formulations of chinese medicine for cancer treatment (*continued*)

Anticancer Herbs	Other herbal components	Dosage (g)
	Rhizoma Panidis (Panis Rhizome)	15
	Herba Glechomae Hederaceae (Ground Ivy Herb)	15
	Herba Centipedae (Centipeda Minima)	9
	Gekko Swinhenis (House Lizard)	9
(b) To Reduce Side Effect of Chemotherapy	*Radix Salviae Miltiorrhizae* (Danshen Root) and its bark	10
	Radix Glehniae (Coasital Glehnia Root)	10
	Ponia (Indian Bread), Radix Ophiopogonis (Dwarf Lilyturf Tuben)	12
	Fructus Lycii (Barbary Wolfberry Fruit)	12
	Rhizoma Polygonati (Polygonatwn Sibinicum)	12
	Radix Astragali (Milkvetch Root)	12
	Radix Codonopsis (Tangshen)	30
	Fructus Ligustni Lucidi (Glossy Privet Fruit)	15
	Radix Glycyrrhizae (Liquorice Root)	15
		3

effect of other cytotoxic S-phase inhibitors among the mixed herbs. Tested by flow cytometry technology, we have shown that PCV pretreatment enhanced the apopotic effect of the S-phase inhibitor, camptothecin (Figure 8.2a-c). The PCV-pretreated HL-60 cells underwent more apoptosis (71.9%) when challenged by the S-phase DNA topoisomerase I interactive agent, chemptothecin, than those without PCV incubation (56.4%). These data not only provide the scientific basis for the clinical observation of tumor regression, but also confirm the unique opportunities of Yun Zhi PCV to be used as a cell-cycle-targeting agent in chemotherapy and radiotherapy.

Current research concentrates on successful outcomes with Chinese herbal medicine for cancer treatment when integrated with other forms of therapies such as chemotherapy, radiotherapy, acupressure and acupuncture (Zhang 1994, Zhang 1992, Zhu 1994, and Yang *et al.* 1995). *Astragalus membranaceus* and *Ligustrum lucidum*, for instance, have been considered as an adjunct in cancer therapy for treatment of liver, lung and rectal cancers (Wong *et al.* 1992). Other Chinese herbal formulations currently gained confidence in anticancer and anti-metas-

tasis include Juzen-taiho-to, a Kampo (Chinese herbal) medicine
(Ohnishi *et al.* 1996), Shikaron, which is a mixture of 8 Chinese herb
extracts (Kurashige *et al.* 1998), and Keishi-ka-kei-to, a TCM composed of a mixture of crude extracts from five medicinal plants
(Cinnamomi cortex, Paeoniae radix, Zizyphi fructus, Zingiberis
rhizoma and Glycyrrhizae radix) (Suzuki *et al.* 1997). This field is at a
very early stage in its evolution in the West. Some concerns are on standardization since the individualized prescription usually consists of a
mixture of a number of herbs and other natural products which is
often decoded before being taken by the patient. Furthermore, the multiple bioactive constituents in the natural compounds used as Materia
Medica present a particularly difficult problem with quality control,
accountability and safety measures.

Conclusion

The continuous search for new anticancer drugs from plants based on
Chinese medicine is believed to be a fruitful frontier in cancer treat-

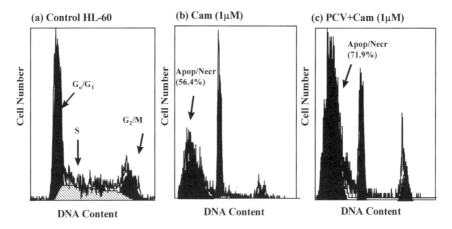

Figure 8.2 PCV potentiates the apopotic effect of camptothecin on the human
leukemic HL-60 cells

DNA histograms of HL-60 cells showing (a) Control with no apoptotic/
necrotic pre-G1 peak, (b) 56.4% apoptotic/necrotic death after 5 hours of
Cam treatment, and (c) 71.9% apoptotic/necrotic death after 5 hours Cam
incubation and 72 hours PCV pre-treatment (p < 0.001 vs. Cam). Results are
expressed as Mean ± SEM, n = 8.

(a) Planer Balance   (b) Circular Balance (Yin[g] and Yang Balance)

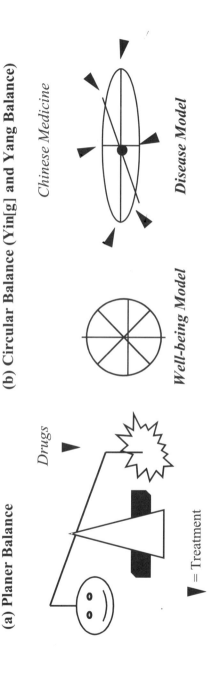

Chinese Medicine

Drugs

Well-being Model   *Disease Model*

▶ = Treatment

Figure 8.3 Hypothetical models for well-being and disease with treatments according to western and Chinese concepts

The West tends to view things in a discrete manner or planar manner and treatment with drugs is specifically targeted at the cancer cells (a). According to the Yin-Yang theory, Chinese view all things as inter-communicating and inter-dependent. All elements are co-existing, equalizing and proportion themselves in a circular manner. Disease occurs when one or more variables are off-balanced (c); treatment of Chinese medicine will be applied to deal with not only on the distorted variable, but also to the other variables so as to re-adjust the individual's entire radius until the balance is regained (b).

ment and chemoprevention. However, one must appreciates the experience of Chinese medicine is essential for researchers to enter into the appropriate direction in the search for the new anti-cancer drugs. The application of chemotaxonomic principles to relate species of those plants used in folk medicine has provided an approach, which can be successfully applied, for the development of new anti-neoplastic agents. Only in such a way can the experience of Chinese medicine be integrated into modern medicine and make its contribution in the advancement of cancer treatment in the world.

References

Agliett, L., Roila, F., Tonato, M., Basurto, C., Bracarda, S., Picciafuoco, M., Ballatori, E., and Del Favero, A. (1990) A pilot study of metoclopramide, dexamethasone, diphenhydramine and acupuncture in women treated with cisplatin. *Cancer Chemotherapy Pharmacology*, 26(3), 239–40.

Anto, R.J., George, J., Babu, K.V., Rajasekharan, K.N., and Kuttan, R. (1996) Antimutagenic and anticarcinogenic activity of natural and synthetic curcuminoids. *Mutation Research*, 370, 127–31.

Arends, M.J., Morris, R.G., and Wyllie, A.H. (1990) Apoptosis: The role of the endonuclease. *The American Journal of Pathology*, 136, 593–608.

Bajetta, E., Biganzoli, L., Carnaghi, C., Bartolomo, M., Spagnoli, I., Cassata, A., Galante, E., Mariani, L., Stampino, C.G., and Buzzoni, R. (1998) Oral doxifluridine plus levoleucovorin in elderly patients with advanced breast cancer. *Cancer*, 83, 1136–41.

Cha, R.J., Zeng, D.W., and Chang, Q.S. (1994) Non-surgical treatment of small cell lung cancer with chemo-radio-immunotherapy and traditional Chinese medicine. *Chung Hua Nei Ko Tsa Chih*, 33(7), 462–6.

Cheng, X. (1990) *Chinese Acupuncture and Moxibustion*. Foreign Languages Press, Beijing 100044, China.

Chi, H., and Li, P. (1995) Therapeutic effects of the combined Chinese and Western medicine on metastatic carcinoma in the supraclavicular lymph nodes-an analysis of 285 cases. *Journal of Traditional Chinese Medicine*, 15, 87–89.

Chu, D.T., Wong, W.L., and Mavlight, G.M. (1988) Immune restoration of local xenogeneic graft-versus-host reaction in cancer patients by fractionated Astragalus membranaceus in vitro. *Journal of Clinical and Laboratory Immunology*, 25, 119–123.

Darzynkiewicz, Z. (1995) Apoptosis in anti-tumor strategies: Modulation of cell cycle or differentiation. *Journal of Cellular Biochemistry*, 58, 151–159.

Diamandidou, E., Buzdar, A.U., Smith, T.L., and Hortobagyi, G.N. (1996) Treatment-related leukemia in breast cancer patients treated with fluorouracil-oxorubicin-cyclophosphamide combination adjuvant chemotherapy: the University of Texas M.D. Anderson Cancer Center experience. *Journal of Clinical Oncology*, **14**, 2722–30.

Dong, Y., Kwan, C.Y., Chen, Z.N., and Yang, M.M.P. (1996) Anti-tumor effects of a refined polysaccharide peptide fraction isolated from *coriolus versicolor: in vitro* and *in vivo* studies. *Research Communications in Molecular Pathology and Pharmacology*, **92**, 140–148.

Ebisuno, S., Hirano, A., Kyoku, I., Ohkawa, T., Lijima, O., Fujii, Y., and Hosoya, E. (1989) Studies on combination of Chinese medicine in cancer chemotherapy: protective effects on the toxic side effects of CDDP and anti-tumor effects with CDDP on murine bladder tumor (MBT-2). *Nippon Gan Chiryo Gakkai Shi*, **24**, 1305–12.

Eder, J.P., Rubin, E., Stone, R., Kufe, D.W. (1996) Trials of 9-amino-20 (S)-camptothecin in Boston. *Annals of the New York Academy of Sciences*, **13**, 247–55.

Fu, W.K. (1985) *Traditional Chinese Medicine and Pharmacology*. Foreign Languages Press, Beijing, China.

Goldhirsch, A., Coates, A.S., Castiglione-Gertsch, M., and Gelber, R.D. (1998) New treatments for breast cancer: breakthroughs for patient care or just steps in the right direction? *Annual Oncology*, **9**(9), 973–6.

Gorczyca, W., Gong, J., Ardelt, B., Traganos, F., and Darzynkiewicz, Z. (1993) The cell cycle related differences in susceptibility of HL-60 cells to apoptosis induced by various anti-tumor agents. *Cancer Research*, **53**, 3180–3192.

Han, R. (1994a) Highlight on the studies of anticancer drugs derived from plants in China. *Stem Cells*, **12**, 53–63.

Han, R. (1994b) Recent progress in the study of anticancer drugs originating from plants and traditional medicines in China. *Chinese Medical Journal (English)*, **10**, 61–9.

Hanif, R., Qiao, L., Shiff, S.J., and Rigas, B. (1997) Curcumin, a natural plant phenolic food additive, inhibits cell proliferation and induces cell cycle changes in colon adneocarcinoma cell lines by a prostaglandin-independent pathway. *Journal of Laboratory and Clinical Medicine*, **130**, 576–84.

Hansen, R.M., Ryan, L., and Anderson, T. (1996) Phase III study of bolus verus infusion fluorouracil with or without ciplatin in advanced colorectal cancer. *National Cancer Institute*, **88**, 668–74.

Jing, Y., Watabe, M., Hashimoto, S., and Nakajo, K. (1994) Cell cycle arrest and protein kinase modulating effect of bufalin on human leukemia ML 1 cells. *Anticancer Research*, **14**, 1193–8.

Kasimu, R., Tanaka, K., Tezuka, Y., Ging, Z., Li, J.X., Basnet, P., Namba, T., and Kadota, S. (1998) Comparative study of seventeen Salvia plants: aldose reductase inhibitory activity of water and MeOH extracts and liquid chromatography-mass spectrometry (LC-MS) analysis of water extracts. *Chemical and Pharmaceutical Bulletin*, 46, 500–504.

Kurashige, S., Jin, R., Akuzawa, Y., and Endo, F. (1998) Anticarcinogenic effects of shikaron, a preparation of eight Chinese herbs in mice treated with a carcinogen, N-butyl-N'-butanolnitrosoamine. *Cancer Investigation*, 16, 166–9.

Lee, L.F., Li, G., Templeton, D.J., and Ting, J.P.Y. (1998) Paclitaxel (Taxol)-induced gene expression and cell death are both medicated by the activation of c-Jun NH2-terminal kinase, *Journal of Biological Chemistry*, 273, 28253–60.

Li, L., Xia, L.J., Jiang, C., and Han, R. (1994) Induction of apoptosis by harringtonic and homoharringtonine in HL-60 cells. *Yao Hsueh Hsueh Pao*, 29(9), 667–72.

Li, Q.S., Cao, S.H., Xie, G.M., Gan, Y.H., Ma, H.J., Lu, J.Z., and Zhang, Z.H. (1994) Combined traditional Chinese Medicine and Western medicine. Relieving effects of Chinese herbs, ear-acupuncture and epidural morphine on postoperative pain in liver cancer. *Chinese Medicine Journal*, 107, 289–294.

Li, X.Y., Wang, J.F., Zhu, P.P., Yang, S.X., Liu, L., and Ge, J.B. (1990) Immuno-modulating actions of PSP. *European Journal of Pharmacology*, 183, 904–908.

Lilenbaum, R.C., Ratain, M.J., Miller, A.A., Hargis, J.B., Hollis, D.R., and Schilsky, R.L. (1995) Phase I study of paclitaxel and topotecan in patients with advanced tumors: a cancer and leukemia group B study. *Journal of Clinical Oncology*, 13(9), 2230–7.

Liu, F. (1990) Application of traditional Chinese drugs in comprehensive treatment of primary liver cancer. *Journal of Traditional Chinese Medicine*, 10, 54–60.

Liu, Q.Y., and Stein, C.A. (1997) Taxol and estramustine-induced modulation of human prostate cancer cell apoptosis via alteration in bcl-xL and bak expression. *Clinical Cancer Research*, 3(11), 2039–2046.

Liu, W.K., Ng, T.B., Sze, S.F., and Tsui, K.W. (1993) Activation of peritoneal macrophages by polysaccaropeptide from the mushroom, *Coriolus versicolor. Immuno-pharmacology*, 26, 139–146.

Mehta, K., Pantazis, P., McQueen, T, and Aggarwal, B.B. (1997) Antiproliferative effect of curcumin (Diferuloylmethane) against human breast tumor cell lines. *Anticancer Drugs*, 8, 470–81.

Muracciole, X., and Regis, J. (1998) Peritoneal metastasis of intracranial glioblastoma via a ventriculoperitoneal shunt preventing organ retrieval: case report and review of the literature. *Clinical Transplantation*, 12, 348–50.

Ohnishi, Y., Fujii, H., Kimura, F., Mishima, T., Murata, J., Tazawa, K., Fujimaki, M., Okada, F., Hosokawa, M., and Saiki, I. (1996) Inhibitory effect of a traditional Chinese medicine, Juzen-taiho-to, on progressive growth of weakly malignant clone cells derived from murine fibrosarcoma. *Japanese Journal of Cancer Research*, **10**, 2039–44.

Palissot, V., Liautaud-Roger, F., Carpentier, Y., and Dufer, J. (1996) Image cytometry of early nuclear events during apoptosis induced by camptothecin in HL-60 leukemic cells. *Cytometry*, **1; 25**(4), 341–8.

Rainov, N.G., Dobberstein, K.U., Sena-Esteves, M., Herrlinger, U., Kramm, C.M., Philpot, R.M., Hilton, J., and Chiocca, E.A. (1998) New pro-drug activation gene therapy for cancer using cytochrome P450 4BI and 2-aminoanthracene/4-ipomeanol. *Human Gene Therapy*, **9**, 1261–1273.

Recchia, F., Frati, L., and Rea, S. (1998) Minimal residual disease in metastatic breast cancer: treatment with IFN-beta, retinoids and tamoxifen. *Journal of Interferon Cytokine Research*, **18**, 41–7.

Reddy, G.P.V. (1994) Cell cycle: regulatory events in G1 to S transition of mammalian cells. *Journal of Cellular Biochemistry*, **54**, 379–386, 1994.

Ribas, A., and Albanell, J. (1998) Cyclophosphadmide, methotrexate, and chronic oral tegafur modulated by flinic acid in the treatment of patients with advanced breast carcinoma. *Cancer*, **82**, 878–85.

Rui, H. (1997) Research and development of cancer chemo-preventive agents in China. *Journal of Cellular Biochemistry (Supplement)*, **27**, 7–11.

Rumana, C.S., and Valadka, A.B. (1998) Radiation therapy and malignant degeneration of begin supratentorial ganglioliomas. *Neurosurgery*, **42**, 1038–43.

Sakagami, H., Aoki, T., Simpson, A., and Tanuma, S.I. (1991) Induction of immunopotentiation activity by a protein-bound polysaccharide, PSK (Review). *Anticancer Research*, **11**, 993–1000.

Shiu, W.C.T., Leung, T.W.T., and Tao, M. (1992) A clinical study of PSP on peripheral blood counts during chemotherapy. *Phytotherapy Research*, **6**, 217–221.

Siter, K., Feldman, E.J., Halicka, H.D., Traganos, F., Darzynkiewicz, Z., Lake, D., and Ahmed, T. (1997) Phase I Clinical and laboratory evaluation of topotecan and cytarabine in patients with acute leukemia. *Journal of Clinical Oncology*, **15**(1), 44–51.

Suzuki, F., Kobayashi, M., Komatsu, Y., Kato, A., and Pollard, R.B. (1997) A traditional Chinese herbal medicine, inhibits pulmonary metastasis of B16 melanoma. *Anticancer Research*, **17**(2A), 873–8.

Tong, X.W., Engehausen, D.G., Kaufman, R.H., Agoulnik, I., Contant, C., Freund, C.T., Oehler, M.K., Kim, T.E., Hasenburg, A., Woo, S.L., and Kieback, D.G. (1998) Improvement of gene therapy for ovarian cancer by using acyclovir instead of ganciclovir in adenovirus medicated thymidine kinase gene therapy. *Anticancer Research*, **18**, 713–718.

Tsuru, S., Nomoto, K., Taniguchi, M., Kitani, H., and Watanabe, M. (1984) Depression of macrophage functions and T-cell-mediated immunity to

Listera infection in tumor-bearing mice and its prevention of PSK. *Cancer Immunology and Immunotherapy*, **18**, 160–163.

Tsuru, S., Shinomiya, Katsura, Y., Gotoh, M., Noritake, M., and Nomoto, K. (1991) Effects of combined therapies with protein-bound polysaccharide (PSK, krestin) and fluorinated pyrimidine derivatives on experimental liver metastases and on the immunologic capacities of the hosts. *Oncology* (Basel), **48**, 498–504.

Traganos, F., Seiter, K., Feldman, E., Halicka, H.D., Darzynkiewicz, Z. (1996). Induction of apoptosis by camptothecin and topotecan. *Annals of the New York Academy Sciences*, **13**, 101–10.

Van Gool, S.W., van den Oord, J., Uyttebroeck, A., and Brock, P. (1998) Cutaneous toxicity following administration of actinomycin. *Medical and Pediatric Oncology*, **31**, 128–132.

Viale, M., Pastrone, I., Pellecchi, C., Vannozzi, M.O., and Szposito, M. (1998) Combination of ciplatin-procaine complex DPR with anticancer drugs increases cytotoxicity against ovarian cancer cell lines. *Anticancer Drugs*, **1**, 457–63.

Vokes, E.E., Drinkard, L.C., Hoffman, P.C., Ferguson, M.F., and Golomb, H.M. (1994) A Phase II study of cisplatin, 5-fluorouracil, and leucovorin augmented by vinorelbine (Naveline) for advanced non-small cell lung cancer: rational and study design. *Seminars in Oncology*, **21**(5) suppl (10) 79:89.

Wan, J.M.F., and Sit, W.H. (1998) "Yun Zhi" extract inhibits human promyelocytic leukemic cancer cells growth by delaying cells transit through the cell cycle. *Asia Pacific Biotech News*, **2**, 30–33.

Wang, G., Sun, G., Tang, W., and Pan, X. (1994) The application of traditional Chinese Medicine to the management of hepatic cancerous pain. *Journal of Traditional Chinese Medicine*, **14**, 132–138.

Watabe, M., Kawazoe, N., Masuda, Y., Nakajo, S., and Nakaya, K. (1997) Bcl-2 protein inhibits bufalin-induced apoptosis through inhibition of mitogen-activated protein kinase activation in human leukemia U937 cells. *Cancer Research*, **57**, 3097–100.

Wong, B.Y., Lau, B.H., Tadi, P.P., and Teel, R.W. (1992) Chinese medicinal herbs modulate mutagenesis, DNA binding and metabolism of aflatoxin B1. *Mutation Research*, **279**, 209–16.

Wu, W.L., Chang, W.L., and Chen, C.F. (1991) Cytotoxic activities of tanshinones against human carcinoma cell lines. *American Journal of Chinese Medicine*, **XIX**, 207–216.

Wang, X., Yuan, S., Huang, R., and Song, Y. (1996) An observation of the effect of tanshinone on cancer cell proliferation by BrdUrd and PCNA labeling. *Hua His Ko Ta Hsueh Hsueh Pao* 27(4), 388–91.

Xiaoguang, C., Hongyan, L., Xiaohong, L., Zhaodi, F., and Rui, H. (1998) Cancer chemopreventive and therapeutic activities of red ginseng. *Journal of Ethnopharmacology*, **60**, 71–8.

Xu, B. (1991) Recent advances in pharmacologic study of natural anticancer agents in China. *Memorias doInstitute Oswaldo Cruz*, **86**, (*suppl*), **2**, and 51–5.

Yang, J., Yu, M., Zhao, R., Chen, G., and Lu, W. (1995) Influence of radio-therapy and chemotherapy on the function of malignant tumor patients and regulation function of acupuncture. *Chen Tzu Yen Chiu*, **20**, 1–4.

Yang, M.M.P., Chen, Z., and Kwok, J.S.L. (1993a) The antitumor effect of a small polypeptide from Coriolus versicolor. *American Journal of Chinese Medicine*, **20**, 221–226.

Yang, Q.Y. (1993) *In Proceedings of International Symposium on PSP*. Q.Y. Yang and C.Y. Kwok (eds). Fudan University Press, Shanghai.

Yang, Q.Y., Jong, S.C., Li, X.Y., Zhou, J.X., Chen, R.T., and Xu, L.Z. (1993b) Anti-tumor and immuno-modulating activities of the polysaccharide-peptide (PSP) of *Coriolus versicolor*. *Ecos. Riv. Immunol. Immunofarm*, **12**, 29–33.

Yang, Q.Y., Yong, S.C., and Yang, X.T. (1987) The physio-chemical characteristics of the polysaccharide-peptide (PSP) of Coriolus vericolor (Yun Zhi). *In Report on the Polysaccharide-peptide (PSP) of Coriolous versicolor*, Landford, China, pp. 1–6.

Yano, H., and Miroguchi, A. (1994) The herbal medicine sho-saiko-to inhibited proliferation of cancer cell lines by inducing apoptosis and arrest at the G0/G1 phase. *Cancer Research*, **54**, 448–452.

Yu, L.J., Ma, R.D., Wang, Y.Q., Nishino, H., Takayasu, J., He, W.Z., Chang, M., Zhen, J., Liu, W.S., and Fan, S.X. (1992) Potent anti-tumorgenic effect of tubeimoside I isolated from the bulb of Bolbostemma paniculatum (Maxim) Franquet. *International Journal of Cancer*, **50**, 635–638.

Zhang. J., Wang, G., Li, H., Zhung, C, Mizuno, T., Mayuzumi, H., Okamoto, H., and Li, J. (1994) Anti-tumor active protein-containing glycans from the Chinese mushroom Songshan lingzhi, *Ganoderma tsugae* mycelium. *Bioscience Biotechnology and Biochemistry*, **58**, 1202–1205.

Zhang, D.Z. (1992) Effects of traditional Chinese medicine and pharmacology on increasing sensitivity and reducing toxicity in tumor patients undergoing radio-chemical therapy. *Chung Kuo Chung His Chieh Ho Tsa Chih*, **12**(3), 135–8.

Zheng, S., Yang, H., Zhang, S., Wang, X., Yu, L., Lu, J., and Li, J. (1997). Initial study on naturally occurring products from traditional Chinese herbs and vegetables for chemo-prevention. *Journal of Cellular Biochemistry (Suppl.)*, **27**, 106–12.

Zhu, B.F. (1994). Observation on 17 patients of radio-ulcer with combined traditional Chinese medicine and Western medicine therapy. *Chung Kuo Chung His I Chieh Ho Tsa Chih*, **14**, 89–91.

9 DNA TECHNIQUES FOR THE AUTHENTICATION OF CHINESE MEDICINAL MATERIALS

Pang-Chui Shaw
Fai-Ngor Ngan
Paul Pui-Hay But
Jun Wang

Introduction

The World Health Organization estimates that 80% of the world's population uses traditional medicine in their primary healthcare. In China and neighboring countries, Chinese medicine (CM) provides a low cost and "natural" approach to health care. Over 1000 species of plants, animals and minerals are used in CM. Substitutes and adulterants are often found introduced intentionally or accidentally to the market and thus seriously interfere with the therapeutic effects of CM, and sometimes even lead to poisoning. Therefore, an efficient identification program to survey traditional Chinese medicinal materials is essential.

Cases of poisoning due to the misuse of Chinese medicinal materials have frequently surfaced in Asia and Europe. In 1989, two persons in Hong Kong suffered serious neuropathy and encephalopathy after consuming the roots of *Podophyllum hexandrum*; a toxic herb commonly called Guijiu. This herb was distinguished as *Gentiana rigescens* (Longdancao) (Ng *et al.* 1991) by a supplier in China. The same herb was also found as a substitute in the samples of *Clematis* species (Weilingxian) leading to 14 cases of neuropathy in Asian countries in 1995–96 (But *et al.* 1996). Four cases of drowsiness were attributed to erroneous dispensing of the anticholinergic Yangjihua (flower of *Datura metel*) as Lingxiaohua (flower of *Campsis grandiflora*) (But 1994). Adulteration was responsible for an epidemic of severe kidney damage (de Smet 1992) in Belgium where the herb *Stephania tetrandra* (Hanfangji) was substituted by the nephrotoxic *Aristolochia fangchi* (Guangfangji).

Traditional Methods of Authentication

The absence of an objective and accurate inspection system is frequently one of the major reasons for herbal poisoning. Classical means of authentication refer to organoleptic characteristics such as texture or the odor of the herb. Its reliability depends heavily on examiners' judgment, which is subjective and error-prone.

Microscopic examination is frequently used to reveal the characteristic cell components or tissues of a medicinal material or its manufactured product. Nevertheless, different medicinal materials, in particular for those related species, may have similar characteristics. Therefore, this approach may not be sufficient to provide an unequivocal means of authentication.

The detection of chemical constituents is a common identification tool as well. Thin layer chromatography (TLC) and high-pressure liquid chromatography (HPLC) provide a more precise means of detection and have become routine procedures in the identification of herbal materials. TLC profiles of several herbs are specified in the Chinese Pharmacopoeia published in 1995. Recently, capillary electrophoresis has been used to infer the botanical sources and to assess the quality of Ephedrae Herba (Liu *et al.* 1993), Coptidis Rhizoma (Liu *et al.* 1994), Ginseng Radix (Chuang *et al.* 1995) and Paeoniae Radix (Chuang *et al.* 1996). Increased sensitivity has been achieved by coupling HPLC or gas chromatography with other analytical systems. For instance, the combination of liquid chromatography and tandem mass spectrometry was efficient to detect co-eluting, closely related substances (Covey *et al.* 1986) and to quantify active components from traditional Chinese medicine over a concentration range of 1 ng/ml to 10 μg/ml (Wang *et al.* 1997).

One of the intrinsic problems in the chemical analysis is that the level of the active components may be affected by physiological conditions, harvesting period and storage conditions. Moreover, closely related species may contain similar chemical components. In addition, the chemical method usually requires a relatively large amount of samples for a proper analysis and some of the instruments such as HPLC; capillary electrophoresis and mass spectrometry are expensive and may not be available in many analytical laboratories.

Classical cytogenetic methods including chromosome counting and karyotyping may also be used to differentiate medicinal materials (Honda *et al.* 1994) and also play a role in assessing hybridity of plants (Magdalita *et al.* 1997). Nevertheless, it is not useful in differentiation of closely related species. Proteins are exploited as identification markers in

Epimedium species (Koga *et al.* 1991), and to differentiate inter- and intra-species of *Panax* (Koren & Zhuravlev 1998; Sun *et al.* 1993). One of the drawbacks of such markers is that the protein patterns vary in different tissues, developmental stages and environment as a consequence of temporal and spatial gene expression. Distinguishable markers may also not be easily detected in closely related species and protein is prone to degradation after prolonged storage of the herbs.

DNA Markers

DNA molecules are reliable markers for informative polymorphisms as the genetic composition is unique for each individual and is less affected by age, physiological conditions as well as environmental factors. Additional advantages of DNA markers include: (1) small amount of sample is sufficient for the analysis, which is particularly relevant for Chinese medicinal materials that are expensive or in limited supply, and (2) detection is not restricted by the physical form of the sample.

POLYMERASE CHAIN REACTION (PCR)

PCR enzymatically multiplies a defined region of the template DNA. The specific multiplication is attributed to the presence of primers, which are single-stranded polynucleotides that recognise and bind to the complementary DNA sequence on template DNA. The amplification process starts with denaturation of the double-stranded template DNA to single-stranded DNA under high temperature, usually between 90°C to 95°C, followed by specific annealing of the primer(s) to the single-stranded template DNA. The annealing condition depends on the length and the GC content of the primers. The annealed primers are then extended by a thermostable polymerase. Repeating the denaturation-annealing-extension step leads to an exponential accumulation of the DNA fragment of defined sequence. Owing to its sensitivity and ability to amplify DNA from a small amount of materials *in vitro*, a variety of PCR-derived methods have been established for detecting polymorphism.

Random-primed PCR
In 1990, two similar approaches, Random Amplified Polymorphic DNA (RAPD) and Arbitrarily-primed PCR (AP-PCR) were invented

(Williams *et al.* 1990; Welsh and McClelland 1990). RAPD uses a single primer of 10 nucleotides and AP-PCR uses approximately 20 nucleotides to amplify the template DNA (Figure 9.1). Another similar approach using 5–8 nucleotides in primer length was attempted by Caetano-Anolles (1991a, b), and is called DNA Amplified Fragments

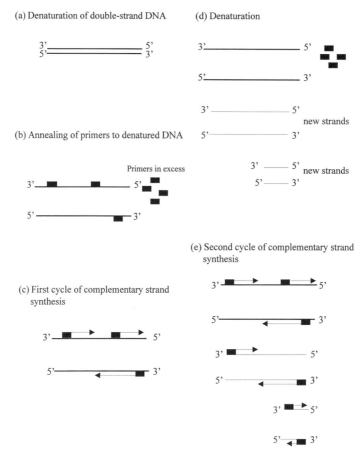

Figure 9.1 Schematic representation of random-primed polymerase chain reaction. (a) A double-stranded DNA molecule is denatured under high temperature (e.g. 94°C) to single-stranded DNA. (b) Arbitrarily chosen oligodeoxyribonucleotide primers (short black boxes) are added to bind to the complementary sites on the template at a lower temperature. More than one complementary sites may exist on the template DNA. (c) The primers are extended by (dashed arrows) thermal stable DNA polymerase to longer DNA molecules. (d) and (e): the steps (a) to (c) are repeated for 30–45 cycles resulting in a pool of different-sized fragments.

(DAF). Amplified DNA fragments are generated if they contain sequences at least partially complementary to the 3″ end of the primer. DNA profiles are variable for different biological samples depending upon the presence or absence and the different locations of annealing sites. Several companies have now marketed RAPD kits, making it a popular fingerprinting method.

Over the years, random-primed PCR has been extensively applied to study genetic similarity in such materials as *Glycyrrhiza*, (Yamazaki *et al.* 1994), *Cannabis* (Gillan *et al.* 1995; Jagadish *et al.* 1996; Shirota *et al.* 1998), *Clematis* (Zhang *et al.* 1996), *Coptis* (Cheng *et al.* 1997), *Indigofera* (Zhang *et al.* 1997), *Liriope* (Wu *et al.* 1998), *Anoectochilus* (Cheng *et al.* 1998), *Perilla* (Ito *et al.* 1998) and snakes (Wang and Zhou 1996; 1997; Wang *et al.* 1996). Random-primed PCR has also been employed to differentiate between cultivated and wild garlic cultivars (Al-Zahim *et al.* 1997). We are one of the first groups in the world to apply RAPD and AP-PCR to authenticate dried Chinese medicinal materials and have successfully distinguished herb samples derived from *Panax* (Figure 9.2), *Taraxacum, Elephantopus, Acorus, Cremastra, Dysosma, Epimedium* and commercial ginseng products (Cheung *et al.* 1994; Shaw and But 1995; Cao *et al.* 1996a, b; Ngan *et al.* 1997). Recently, we have extended the technique to identify *Codonopsis pilosula* from different localities (Zhang *et al.* 1999).

Attention has been drawn to the reproducibility of the random-primed PCR since low temperature is used to anneal a short primer to its target site, in which process perfect match between primers and template does not always occur. Therefore the fingerprints between laboratories and even between different experiments may not always be consistent. Moreover, random-primed PCR can be affected by different PCR machines, different brands of T*aq* polymerase and variation of salt concentration. Careful control of DNA quality and amplification conditions are necessary to obtain consistent banding patterns. Modifications have been made to increase reproducibility and to exploit additional polymorphic markers. For examples, using primers with tRNA gene motifs (McClelland *et al.* 1992), or with a hairpin at the 5″ end (Caetano-Anolles and Gresshoff 1994) and pairwise combination of primers (Welsh and McClelland 1991; Micheli *et al.* 1993; Hu *et al.* 1995). Also, using long primer pairs (LP-PCR) of 18 to 24 nucleotides may facilitate the detection of intra-specific and inter-specific genetic variation and generate more reproducible fingerprints (Gillings and Holley 1997). To avoid the interference of artifactual DNA band, it is prudent to carry out PCR using at least

M 1 2 3 4 5 6 7 M 8 9 10 M

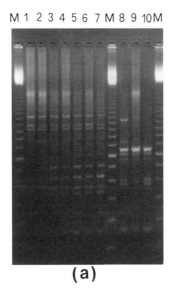

(a)

M 1 2 3 4 5 6 7 M

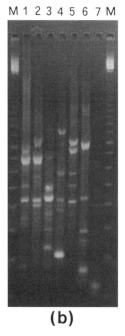

(b)

Figure 9.2 (a) DNA fingerprints of *Panax quinquefolius and P. ginseng* generated by OPC-05: 5″ GAT GAC CGC C 3″. Reaction was performed in 25 μl containing 25 ng plant DNA, 0.1 mM dNTPs, 0.2 μM primer, 1X T*aq* buffer (10 mM Tris-HCl, pH 8.3; 50 mM KCl; 0.001% gelatin), and 0.5 units T*aq* polymerase in a Thermolyne® thermocycler through 45 cycles of 94°C, 1 min; 36°C, 1 min; 72°C, 2 min. The products were resolved onto a 2.5% TBE agarose gel and photographed by polaroid 665 film. Lane 1: *P. quinquefolius*, three-year-old from Canada. 2: *P. quinquefolius*, four-year-old from Canada. 3: *P. quinquefolius* from USA. 4: *P. quinquefolius* from USA. 5: *P. quinquefolius*, four-year-old from China. 6: *P. quinquefolius*, four-year-old from China. 7: *P. quinquefolius*, four-year-old from China. 8: *P. ginseng* root without epidermis from China. 9: *P. ginseng* fresh root from China. 10: *P. ginseng* from China. M: 100 bp ladder marker (b) DNA fingerprints of *P. quinquefolius*, *P. ginseng* and their adulterants by AP-PCR using TCS backward primer: 5″ GGT GGA TCC CTA AGC ATC AAC AAT GGT 3″. Reaction was performed in 50 μl containing 100 ng plant DNA, 0.2 mM dNTPs, 2 μM primer, 1X T*aq* buffer (10 mM Tris-HCl, pH 8.3; 50 mM KCl; 0.001% gelatin), and 2.5 units T*aq* polymerase in a Thermolyne® thermocycler through the following cycles: Cycles 1 and 2: 94°C, 5 min; 40°C, 5 min; 72°C, 5 min. Cycles 3 to 42: 94°C, 1 min; 60°C, 1 min; 72°C, 2 min. Cycle 43: 94°C, 0.5 min; 60°C, 0.5 min, 72°C, 10 min. Lane 1: *P. quinquefolius*. 2: *P. ginseng*. 3: *Platycodon grandiflorum*. 4: *Mirabilis jalapa*. 5: *Talinum paniculatum*. 6: *Phytolacca acinosa*. 7: control without DNA template. M: 100 bp ladder marker. DNA fingerprints specific to the two ginseng species and different from the adulterants are generated.

two concentrations of DNA template; bands that do not reproduce at both concentrations should not be included in data analysis (McClelland and Welsh 1994).

A more specific detection method called Sequence Characterized Amplified Regions (SCARS) is derived by Paran and Michelmore (1993) to overcome some of the drawbacks of RAPD. It is implemented by sequencing the unique bands generated in RAPD. Primers of 24-bp oligonucleotides complementary to the fragment were further made to amplify the sequenced loci. Since longer and specific primers are used, high stringent PCR conditions can be applied to achieve a specific annealing between the primer and the template, leading to more reproducible results.

Microsatellites

Microsatellites or simple sequence repeats (SSRs) such as (AC)n, (TCT)n, (TCTG)n are tandem repeats of less than six base pairs and are ubiquitous in plants (Saghai-Maroof *et al.* 1994; Röder *et al.* 1995) and mammals (Vergnaud 1989). Sequence information can be searched from DNA databases or by screening genomic libraries with oligodeoxyribonucleotides (Cornell *et al.* 1991). They can also be obtained by screening a genomic library enriched with repetitive sequences. The regions flanking the microsatellite loci can be amplified by PCR, thus providing co-dominant sequence-tagged sites (STS) or repetitive sequence to act as a probe to generate DNA fingerprints such as for the differentiation between *Panax ginseng* and *P. quinquefolius* (Leung and Ho 1998). However, the development of such markers may be laborious and expensive as it involves library construction, screening and sequencing of clones.

Modifications have been made to simplify the methods of detection (Heath *et al.* 1993) and isolation of the flanking sequences (Thomas and Scott 1993; Rowe *et al.* 1994; Refseth *et al.* 1997). Recently, a new system named Random Amplified Hybridization Microsatellites (RAHM) (Cifarelli *et al.* 1995), Random-amplified Microsatellites Polymorphisms (RAMPO) (Richardson *et al.* 1995), or Random-amplified Microsatellites (RAMS) (Ender *et al.* 1996) that combines microsatellite DNA detection and RAPD amplification has been developed. This method detects second-level amplification products that are useful as molecular markers. RAPD or PCR using microsatellite primers is performed and the products are resolved on an agarose gel. A microsatellite-complementary oligonucleotide is used as a probe to hybridize the gel. Fragments with microsatellite loci will give a signal that may differentiate different species. More informative molecular markers are exploited to discriminate between intra- and inter-specific *Dioscorea* species by using mono-, tri- and tetra-nucleotides repeat probe (Ramser *et al.* 1997). The results are highly reproducible as the minor RAPD bands could also be detected by the method. RAMPO seems more reliable than RAPD in the studies of genetic relatedness as the size and intensity of two bands have to be identical for co-migration to be detectable. It reduces the risk of misinterpretation of co-migrating bands as homologs (Rieseberg 1996). Additional information can be obtained by reprobing the blot with more than five different probes without obvious loss in pattern quality (Ramser *et al.* 1997). This demonstrates the robustness of the method.

Amplified fragment length polymorphism (AFLP)

AFLP is a newly emerged DNA marker technology based on the selective amplification of restriction fragments (Vos *et al.* 1995). Total genomic DNA is digested with appropriate restriction enzymes, ligated to synthetic adaptors and amplified using primers complementary to selective sequence on the adaptor. The complexity of the AFLP profiles is dictated by the primers chosen and the composition of the genomic DNA. Results are reproducible as specific primers and high stringent amplification conditions are used. This technique has been widely employed in the analysis of genetic diversity in bacteria (Lin and Kuo 1996; Janssen *et al.* 1997), fungi (Muller *et al.* 1996; Leissner *et al.* 1997), plants (Lu *et al.* 1996; He and Prakash 1997), insects (Reineke *et al.* 1998) and human (Latorra and Schanfield 1996), as well as in the studies of genetic relatedness (Travis *et al.* 1996; Ellis *et al.* 1997) and gene mapping (Otsen *et al.* 1996).

The power of AFLP in the analysis of genetic diversity is highly appreciated. It has been found that the number of polymorphic loci per assay in soybean varieties detected by AFLP is 12 times higher than that with RAPD (Vogel *et al.* 1994). Moreover, the time needed for data generation is only a fraction of that required in RFLP. Meanwhile, the speed of analysis can be increased further by automated scoring of AFLP loci. Apart from its high efficiency, reliability is another virtue of the technique. The most critical step in AFLP is the complete digestion of genomic DNA; however, partial digestion products are obvious, and can be readily excluded in the detection. Moreover, artifactual polymorphisms resulted from primer mismatch or differential primer sites competition (Lamboy 1994) would be greatly reduced as the results of the increased gel resolution and using fully complementary primers except at the few 3″ end bases. Better separation of fragments on a polyacrylamide gel will reduce miscoring of fragments with similar sizes. Longer primer length in AFLP, usually 19 bases, and matching at 5″ end of primers reduces the occurrence of band competition and "false" polymorphisms (Lamboy 1994; Rieseberg 1996).

Our laboratory has adopted this method in the studies of the Chinese herbal materials. We have successfully discriminated between *Panax quinquefolius* and *P. ginseng* as well as between various cultivars of *P. quinquefolius* from different farms. We note that intact DNA is prerequisite for generating useful AFLP profiles. It is sometimes difficult for Chinese medicinal materials as some of them are processed or stored for a long time leading to DNA degradation.

Direct amplification of length polymorphisms (DALP)

This method resembles random-primed fingerprinting and can detect a larger number of polymorphic loci in one step (Desmarais *et al.* 1998). Multi-loci DNA fingerprint is produced using a pair of universal M13 forward and reverse sequencing primers, with additional bases at the 3″ end of the forward primer. Bands of interest can be isolated from polyacrylamide gel and directly sequenced with the universal primers. No prior knowledge of the flanking region of the loci is required. The method is effective in producing polymorphic markers in vertebrates, invertebrates and viruses. It is also useful for defining sequence tagged sites. The value of this technology for medicinal materials is under evaluation in our laboratory.

RESTRICTION FRAGMENT LENGTH POLYMORPHISM (RFLP)

Traditional RFLP analysis is not suitable for Chinese medicinal materials as it demands large amount of intact DNA. Therefore, PCR-RFLP, a method requiring small amount of DNA for analysis is used. In this method, a defined DNA fragment is first amplified by PCR and then digested with a restriction endonuclease to generate restriction polymorphic profiles unique to the concerned species. It is desirable that the region for PCR-RFLP analysis is flanked by sequence conserved across species so that it can be readily amplified by using "universal" primers. Two of the suitable candidates for such regions are ribosomal DNA (rDNA) and large subunit of ribulose-1,5-bisphosphate carboxylase L (rbcL) gene. The PCR-RFLP of rDNA has been carried out on *Glehnia* and *Atractylodes* (Mizukami *et al.* 1993; 1996; Cheng *et al.* 1997) and we have also successfully used this approach to discriminate *Panax* species from their adulterants (Figure 9.3) (Ngan *et al.* 1998) and

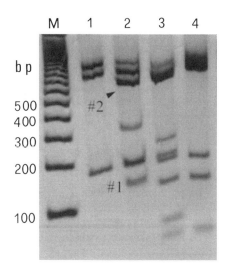

Figure 9.3 The PCR-RFLP pattern of the rDNA for *P. quinquefolius*, *P. ginseng* and their adulterants generating by digestion with *Sau*3A1. A 900-bp fragment containing 18S-ITS1-5.8S-ITS2-26S rDNA was generated by PCR amplification of the template DNA using primers 18d: 5″ CAC ACC GCC CGT CGC TCC TAC CGA 3″ and 28cc: 5′ ACT CGC CGT TAC TAG GGG AA 3″. The PCR products were digested by *Sau*3A1, resolved on a 5% polyacrylamide gel and stained with silver reagent. Lane 1: *P. quinquefolius*. 2: *P. ginseng*. 3: *M. jalapa*. 4: *Ph. acinosa*. M: 100 bp ladder marker. Fragments #1 and #2 are the polymorphic bands of *P. ginseng*. The band of about 320 bp in lane 2 is the product of incomplete digestion of fragments #1 and #2.

obtained a patent for this technology (Wang *et al.* 1999). Various *Epimedium* species have also been differentiated by the PCR-RFLP of the rbcL region (Nakai *et al.*1996).

PCR-RFLP is a precise authentication tool, which circumvents the problem of the reproducibility in random-primed PCRs. The number of bands and patterns are definite and unique to each taxon. It can also be used to detect polymorphism between different individuals of the same species. This approach is therefore convenient and accurate for the authentication of medicinal materials.

DNA SEQUENCING

By selecting an appropriate region for sequencing, different levels of sample discrimination can be achieved. An ideal target locus contains a variable region and two conserved regions where primers can flank to the variable region. For example, intron is a good candidate for such analysis, as it is normally more variable than coding exon. Two species may share a conserved region for a given gene, which allows the primer annealing, but differs significantly in the sequences of its intron, which permits differentiation. ITS regions of the rDNA, rbcL, tRNA gene and cytochrome b meet the above criteria.

The above sequences have been used for authentication purpose. The spacer region of 5S rDNA is sequenced to confirm the crude drug "Angelica root" was derived from *Angelica autiloba* but not *Bupleurm falcatum* or *Glehnia littoralis* (Mizukami 1995). Several ginseng drugs are identified by sequencing the 18S rDNA (Fushimi *et al.* 1996). Our laboratory has sequenced the rDNA for six *Panax* species and two adulterants, *Mirabilis jalapa* and *Phytolacca acinosa* (Ngan *et al.* 1998; Wang *et al.* 1999). High sequence identity exits among the *Panax* species, ranging from 91–99.6%, but lower sequence identity of about 55–63% in the two adulterants have been found. rbcL has also been employed to discriminate "Banxia" and "Tiannanxing" as well as "Banxia" related natural medicines (Kondo *et al.* 1998). The 12S ribosomal RNA and cytochrome b genes have been used to identify two species of *Hippocampus* (Wu *et al.* 1998b), 21 species of turtles shells (Wu *et al.* 1998a) and to authenticate crude drugs of snakes (Wang and Zhou 1996, 1997). Nowadays, an average laboratory can easily generate more than a few thousand base pairs of DNA per day on an automatic DNA sequencer. In couple to further decline in the price of the consumable materials and equipment used in sequencing, we expect that DNA sequencing will become a more common means for the authentication of Chinese medicinal materials.

Comments

As described above, the DNA authentication techniques for the authentication of Chinese medicinal materials can be approximately divided into two types: random-primed PCR based and DNA sequencing. The first type including AP-PCR, RAPD, AFLP, DALP and RAMPO examines multiple markers on the whole genome and may differentiate closely related species or even different individuals. Its power of detection can be further improved by using polyacryalmide gel and radioisotope. The second type of techniques for authentication is to focus on certain well-defined regions such as ITS or cytochrome b by

PCR-RFLP and DNA sequencing. DNA sequences of these regions have been determined for many species, and can be used as guidance to design suitable primers for PCR amplification of relevant DNA fragments in the species to be examined.

We found that sometimes contaminant fungal DNA is preferentially amplified in dried plant samples presumably because the primers used share high degree of homology with fungal species. Therefore, care must be taken when handling herbal samples. Surface sterilization is necessary to reduce fungal or bacterial contamination. For plants, removal of outer epidermis can reduce the risk of DNA contamination of other species. For animals, organs like intestines or stomach must be avoided or removed, and tissues used for DNA extraction must be disinfected thoroughly. With the proper management and appropriate approach, DNA technique is no doubt one of the most sensitive and definitive tools for the authentication of Chinese medicinal medicines.

Acknowledgements

Thanks are due to collaborators at various institutions in China for medicinal samples. Work in our laboratory has been supported by grants from the Research Grants Council (CUHK 19/93M), the Chinese University of Hong Kong, the Environment and Conservation Fund of Hong Kong and the National Research Institute of Chinese Medicine, Taiwan.

References

Al-Zahim, M., Newbury, H.J. and Ford-Lloyd, B.V. (1997) Classification of genetic variation in garlic (*Allium sativum* L.) revealed by RAPD. *Hortsci.*, **32**, 1102–1104.

But, P.P.H. (1994) Herbal poisoning caused by adulterants or erroneous substitutes. *J. Trop. Med. Hyg.*, **97**, 371–374.

But, P.P.H, Tomlinson, B., Cheung, K.O., Yong, S.P., Szeto, M.L., Lee, C.K. (1996) Adulterants of herbal products can cause poisoning. *Brit. Med. J.* **313**, 117.

Caetano-Anolles, G., Bassam, B.J. and Gresshoff, P.M. (1991a) DNA amplification fingerprinting using very short arbitrary oligonucleotide primers. *Bio/technology*, **9**, 553–557.

Caetano-Anolles, G., Bassam, B.J. and Gresshoff, P.M. (1991b) DNA amplification fingerprinting: a strategy for genome analysis. *Plant Mol. Biol. Rep.*, **9**, 292–305.

Caetano-Anolles, G. and Gresshoff, P.M. (1994) DNA amplification fingerprinting using arbitrary mini-hairpin oligonucleotide primers. *Biotechnology*, **12**, 619–623.

Cao, H., But, P.P.H. and Shaw, P.C. (1996a) Authentication of the Chinese drug "Ku-Di-Dan" (Herba Elephantopi) and its substituents using random-primed polymerase chain reaction. *Acta Pharm. Sinica*, **31**, 543–553.

Cao, H., But, P.P.H., and Shaw, P.C. (1996b) A molecular approach to identification of the Chinese Drug "Pu Gong Ying" (Herba Taraxaci) and six adulterants by DNA fingerprinting using random primed polymerase chain reaction (PCR). *J. Chin. Pharma. Sci.*, **5**, 186–194.

Cheng, H.F., Lai, B., Chan, S.C., Chou, C.P., Yang, T.H., Huang, W.H., Liao, C. H. and Lin, C.P. (1997) Molecular differentiation of *Atractylodes* drugs by PCR-restriction fragment length polymorphism and PCR-selective restriction analysis on the 18S-5.8S rDNA intratranscribed spacer 1 gene. *J. Food Drug Anal.*, **5**, 319–328.

Cheng, K.T., Chang, H.C., Su, C.H. and Hsu, F.L. (1997) Identification of dried rhizomes of *Coptis* species using random amplified polymorphic DNA. *Bot. Bull. Acad. Sinica* (Taipei), **38**, 241–244.

Cheng, K.T., Fu, L.C., Wang, C.S., Hsu, F.L. and Tsay, H.S. (1998) Identification of *Anoectochilus formosanus* and *Anoectochilus koshunensis* species with RAPD markers. *Planta Med.*, **64**, 46–49.

Cheung, K.S., Kwan, H.S., But, P.P.H. and Shaw, P.C. (1994) Pharmacognostical identification of American and Oriental ginseng roots by genomic fingerprinting using arbitrarily-primed polymerase chain reaction. *J. Ethnopharmacol.*, **42**, 67–69.

Chuang, W.C., Wu, S.K., Sheu, S.J., Chiou, S.H., Chang, H.C. and Chen, Y.P. (1995) A comparative study on commercial samples of Ginseng Radix. *Planta Med.*, **61**, 459–465.

Chuang, W.C., Wu, S.K., Sheu, S.J., Chiou, S.H., Chang, H.C. and Chen, Y.P. (1996) A comparative study on commercial samples of the roots of *Paeonia vitchii* and *P. lactiflora. Planta Med.*, **61**, 459–465.

Cifarelli, R.A., Gallitelli, M. and Cellini, F. (1995) Random amplified hybridization microsatellites (RAHM): isolation of a new class of microsatellite-containing DNA clones. *Nucl. Acid. Res.*, **23**, 3802–3803.

Cornell, R.J., Atiman, T.J., Hearne, C.M. and Todal, J.A. (1991) The generation of a library of PCR-analyzed microsatellite variants for genetic mapping of the mouse genome. *Genome*, **10**, 874–881.

Covey, T.R., Lee, E.D. and Henion, J.D. (1986) High-speed liquid chromatography/ tandem mass spectrometry for the determination of drugs in biological samples. *Anal. Chem.*, **58**, 2453–2460.

De Smet, P.A.G. (1992) *Aristolochia* species. In P.A.G. De Smet, K. Keller, R. Hansel, and R.F. Chandler, (eds.), *Adverse Effects of Herbal Drugs.* Volume 1, Springer-Verlag, Berlin, pp. 79.

Desmarais, E., Lannelue, I. and Lagnel, J. (1998) Direct amplification of length polymorphisms (DALP) or how to get and characterize new genetic markers in many species. *Nucl. Acid. Res.*, **26**, 1458–1465.

Ellis, R.P., McNicol, J.W., Baird, E., Booth, A., Lawrence, P., Thomas, B. and Powell, W. (1997) The use of AFLPs to examine genetic relatedness in barley. *Mol. Breed.*, **3**, 359–369.

Ender, A., Schwenk, K., Stadler, T., Streit, B., and Schierwater, B. (1996) RAPD identification of microsatellites in Daphnia. *Mol. Ecol.*, **5**, 437–441.

Fushimi, H., Komatsu, K., Isobe, M. and Namba, T. (1996) 18S ribosomal RNA gene sequences of three *Panax* species and the corresponding ginseng drugs. *Biol. Pharm. Bull.*, **19**, 1503–1532.

Gillan, R., Cole, M.D., Linacre, A., Thorpe, J.W., Watson, N.D. (1995) Comparison of *Cannabis sativa* by random amplification of polymorphic DNA (RAPD) and HPLC of cannabinoids: a preliminary study. *Sci. Justice*, **35**, 169–77.

Gillings, M. and Holley, M. (1997) Amplification of anonymous DNA fragments using pairs of long primers generates reproducible DNA fingerprints that are sensitive to genetic variation. *Electrophoresis*, **18**, 1512–1518.

He, G. and Prakash, C.S. (1997) Identification of polymorphic DNA markers in cultivated peanut (*Arachis hypogaea* L.). *Euphytica*, **9**, 143–149.

Heath, D.D., Iwama, G.K., Devlin, R.H. (1993) PCR primed with VNTR core sequences yields species specific patterns and hypervariable probes. *Nucl. Acid. Res.*, **21**, 5782–5785.

Honda, G., Yuba, A., Kojima, T. and Tabata, M. (1994) Chemotaxonomic and cytogenetic studies on *Perilla frutescens* var. *citriodora* ("Lemon Egoma"). *Nat. Med.*, **48**, 185–190.

Hu, J., van Eysden, J. and Quiros, C.F. (1995) Generation of DNA-based markers in specific genome regions by two-primer RAPD reactions. *PCR Meth. Appl.*, **4**, 346–351.

Ito, M., Kato, H., Oka, Y. and Honda, G. (1998) Phylogenetic analysis of Japanese *Perilla* species by using DNA polymorphisms. *Nat. Med.*, **52**, 248–252.

Jagadish, V., Robertson, J. and Gibbs, A. (1996) RAPD analysis distinguishes *Cannabis sativa* samples from different sources. *Foren. Sci. Intl.*, **79**, 113–121.

Janssen, P., Maquelin, K., Coopman, R., Tjernberg, I., Bouvet, P., Kersters, K. and Dijkshoorn, L. (1997) Discrimination of *Acinetobacter* genomic species by AFLP fingerprinting. *Intl. J. Syst. Bacteriol.*, **47**, 1179–1187.

Koga, S., Shoyama, Y. and Nishioka, I. (1991) Studies on *Epimedium* spp.: Flavonol glycosides and isozymes. *Biochem. Syst. Ecol.*, **19**, 315–318.

Kondo, K., Terabayashi, S., Higuchi, M., Komatsu, Y. and Okada, M. (1998) Discrimination between "Banxia" and "Tiannanxing" based on rbcL sequences. *Nat. Med.*, **52**, 253–258.

Koren, O.G. and Zhuravlev, Y.N. (1998) Allozyme variations in two ginseng species *Panax ginseng* and *P. quinquefolius*. Advances in Ginseng Research. *Proc. 7th* Intl. Symp. on ginseng, Korea, September, 1998.

Lamboy, W.F. (1994) Computing genetic similarity coefficients from RAPD data: the effects of PCR artifacts. *PCR Meth. Appl.*, **4**, 31–37.

Latorra D., and Schanfield, M.S. (1996) Analysis of human specificity in AFLP systems APOB, PAH, and D1S80. *Foren. Sci. Intl.*, **83**, 15–25.

Leissner, C.E.W., Niessen, M.L. and Vogel, R.F. (1997) Use of AFLP technique for the identification and discrimination of *Fusarium graminearum*. *Cereal Res. Commun.*, **25**, 555–556.

Leung, F.C. and Ho, I.S.H. (1998) Isolation of novel repetitive DNA sequences as DNA fingerprinting probes for *Panax ginseng*. *Proc. 1st* European Ginseng Congress., Marburg, December, 1998.

Lin, J.J. and Kuo, J. (1996) AFLP™: A novel PCR-based assay for plant and bacterial DNA fingerprinting. *Focus*, **17**, 66–70.

Liu, Y.M., Sheu, S.J., Chiou, S.H., Chang, S.H. and Chen, Y.P. (1993) A comparative study on commercial samples of *Ephedrae* Herba. *Planta Med.*, **59**, 376–378.

Liu, Y.M., Sheu, S.J., Chiou, S.H., Chang, S.H. and Chen, Y.P. (1994) Capillary electrophoretic analysis of alkaloids in commercial samples of *Coptidis* Rhizoma. *Phytochem. Anal.*, **5**, 256–260.

Lu, J., Knox, M.R., Ambrose, M.J., Brown, J.K.M. and Ellis, T.H.N. (1996) Comparative analysis of genetic diversity in pea assessed by RFLP and PCR-based methods. *Theor. Appl. Genet.*, **93**, 1103–1111.

Magdalita, P.M., Drew, R.A., Adkins, S.W. and Godwin, I.D. (1997) Morphological, molecular and cytoplasmic analyses of *Carica papaya* x *C. cauliflora* interspecific hybrids. *Theor. Appl. Genet.*, **95**, 224–229.

McClelland, M., Peterson, C. and Welsh, J. (1992) Length polymorphisms in tRNA intergenic spacers detected using the polymerase chain reaction can distinguish streptococcal strains and species. *J. Clin. Microbiol.*, **30**, 1499–1504.

McClelland, M., and Welsh, J. (1994) DNA fingerprinting by arbitrarily primed PCR. *PCR Meth. Appl.*, **4**, S59–65.

Micheli, M.R., Bova, R., Calissano, P. and D'Ambrosio, E. (1993) Randomly amplified polymorphic DNA fingerprinting using combinations of oligonucleotide primers. *Biotechniques*, **15**, 388–390.

Mizukami, H. (1995) Amplification and sequence of a 5S-rRNA gene spacer region from the crude drug "Angelica root". *Biol. Pharm. Bull.*, **18**, 1299–1301.

Mizukami, H., Ohbayashi, K., Umetsu, K., Hiraoka, N. (1993) Restriction fragment length polymorphisms of medicinal plants and crude drugs II.

Analysis of *Glehnia littoralis* of different geographical origin. *Biol. Pharm. Bull.*, **16**, 611–612.

Mizukami, H., Shimizu, R., Kohda, H., Kohjyouma, M., Kawanishi, F. and Hiraoka, N. (1996) Restriction fragment length polymorphisms of rDNA and variation of essential oil composition in *Atractylodes* plants. *Biol. Pharm. Bull.*, **19**, 577–580.

Muller, U.G., Liparis, S.E. and Milgroom, M.G. (1996) Amplified fragment length polymorphism (AFLP) fingerprinting of symbiotic fungi cultured by the fungus growing ant *Cyphomyrmex minutes*. *Mol. Ecol.*, **5**, 119–122.

Nakai, R., Shoyama, Y. and Shiraishi, S. (1996) Genetic characterization of *Epimedium* species using random amplified polymorphic DNA (RAPD) and PCR-restriction fragment length polymorphism (RFLP) diagnosis. *Biol. Pharm. Bull.*, **19**, 67–70.

Ng, T.H, Chan, Y.W, Yu, Y.L, Chang, C.M, Ho, H.C, Leung, S.Y, But, P.P.H. (1991) Encephalopathy and neuropathy following ingestion of a Chinese herbal broth containing podophyllin. *J. Neurol. Sci.*, **101**, 107–13.

Ngan, F.N., Wang, J., But, P.P.H. and Shaw, P.C. (1997) Application of arbitrarily primed polymerase chain reaction (AP-PCR) in commercial ginseng products. *5th* Intl. Congress. Plant Mol. Biol., Singapore, September, 1997.

Ngan, F.N., Shaw, P.C., But, P.P.H. and Wang, J. (1998) Molecular authentication of *Panax* species. *Phytochem.*, **50**, 787–791.

Osten, M., Den-Bieman, M., Kuiper, M.T.R., Pravence, M., Kren, V., Kurtz, T.W., Jacob, H.J., Lankhorst, A. and Van-Zutphen, B.F.M. (1996) Use of AFLP markers for gene mapping and QTL detection in the rat. *Genomics*, **37**, 289–294.

Paran, I. and Michelmore, R.W. (1993) Development of reliable PCR-based markers linked to downy mildew resistance genes in lettuce. *Theor. Appl. Genet.*, **85**, 985–993.

Ramser, J., Weising, K., Chikaleke, V. and Kahl, G. (1997) Increased informativeness of RAPD analysis by detection of microsatellite motifs. *Biotechniques*, **23**, 285–290.

Refseth, U.H., Fangan, B.M. and Jakobsen, K.S. (1997) Hybridization capture of microsatellites directly from genomic DNA. *Electrophoresis*, **18**, 1519–1523.

Reineke, A., Karlovsky, P. and Zebitz, C.P. (1998) Preparation and purification of DNA from insects for AFLP analysis. *Insect Mol. Biol.*, **7**, 95–99.

Richardson, T., Cato, S., Ramser, J. Kahl, G. and Weising, K. (1995) Hybridization of microsatellites to RAPD: a new source of polymorphic markers. *Nucl. Acid. Res.*, **23**, 3798–3799.

Rieseberg, L.H. (1996) Homology among RAPD gragments in interspecific comparisons. *Mol. Ecol.*, **5**, 99–105.

Röder, M.S., Plaschke, J., König, S.U., Börner, A., Sorrells, M.E., Tanksley, S.D. and Ganel, M.W. (1995) Characterization of PCR-amplified microsatellite loci in wheat. *Mol. Gen. Genet.*, **246**, 327–333.

Rowe, P.S., Francis, F., Goulding, J. (1994) Rapid isolation of DNA sequences flanking microsatellite repeats. *Nucl. Acid. Res.*, **22**, 5135–5136.

Saghai-Maroof, M.A., Biyashev, R.M., Yang, G.P., Zhang, Q. and Allard, R.W. (1994) Extraordinarily polymorphic microsatellite DNA in barley: species diversity, chromosomal location and population dynamics. *Proc. Natl. Acad. Sci. USA*, **91**, 5460–5470.

Shaw, P.C. and But, P.P.H. (1995) Authentication of *Panax* species and their adulterants by random-primed polymerase chain reaction. *Planta Med.*, **61**, 393–492.

Shirota, O., Watanabe, A., Yamazaki, M., Saito, K., Shibano, K., Sekita, S. and Satake, M. (1998) Random amplified polymorphic DNA and restriction fragment length polymorphism analyses of *Cannabis sativa*. *Nat. Med.*, **52**, 160–166.

Sun, F., Cao, Y.Q, Liu, L.X. and Xu, S.M. (1993) Isozymatic patterns for Chinese ginseng and American ginseng. *Chin. Trad. Herb. Drugs*, **24**, 148–149.

Thomas, M.R. and Scott, N.S. (1993) Microsatellite repeats in reveal DNA polymorphisms when analysed as sequence-tagged sites (STS). *Theor. Appl. Genet.*, **86**, 985–990.

Travis, S.E., Maschinski, J. and Keim, P. (1996) An analysis of genetic variation *Astragalus cremnophylax* var. cremnophylax, a critically endangered plant, using AFLP markers. *Mol. Ecol.*, **5**, 735–745.

Vergnaud, G. (1989) Polymers of random short oligonucleotides detect polymorphic loci in the human genome. *Nucl. Acid. Res.*, **17**, 7623–7630.

Vogel, J.M., Powell, W., Rafalski, A., Morgante, M., Tudo, J.D., Taramino, G., Biddle, P., Hanafey, M. and Tingley, S.V. (1994) Application of genetic diagnosis to plant genome analysis: comparison of marker systems. *Appl. Biotechnol. Tree Cult.*, **1**, 119–124.

Vos, P., Hogers, R., Bleeker, M., Reijans, M., Lee, T., Hornes, M., Frijters, A., Pot, J.,Peleman, J., Kuiper, M. and Zabeau M. (1995) AFLP: A new technique for DNA fingerprinting. *Nucl. Acid. Res.*, **23**, 4407–4415.

Wang, J., Ngan, F.N., But, P.P.H. and Shaw, P.C. (1999) Polymerase chain reaction-restriction fragment length polymorphism tests for the authentication of herbal Chinese medicines. US Patent 5, 876, 977.

Wang, X.M., Xue, Y., Zhou, T.H. and Sakuma, T. (1997) Characterization of traditional Chinese medicine by liquid chromatography/atmospheric pressure ionization mass spectrometry. *J. Food Drug Anal.*, **5**, 337–346.

Wang, Y.Q. and Zhou, K.Y. (1996) Study on randomly amplified polymorphic DNA of 10 species of snakes in Colubridae. *Chin. J. Appl. Environ. Biol.*, **2**, 273–279.

Wang, Y.Q. and Zhou, K.Y. (1997) A preliminary study on the identification of crude snake drugs by molecular genetic markers. *Acta Pharm. Sinica*, **32**, 384–387.

Wang, Y.Q., Zhou, K.Y. and Qin, S.Z. (1996) Genomic DNA polymorphisms in six species of serpents using randomly amplified polymorphic DNA (RAPD) markers. *Acta Zool. Sinica*, **42**, 172–181.

Welsh, J. and McClelland, M. (1990) Fingerprinting genomes using PCR with arbitrary primers. *Nucl. Acid. Res.*, **18**, 7213–7218.

Welsh, J. and McClelland, M. (1991) Genomic fingerprinting produced by PCR with consensus tRNA gene primers. *Nucl. Acid. Res.*, **19**, 861–866.

Williams, J.G.K., Kubelik, A.R., Livak, K.J., Rafalski, J.A. and Tingey, S.V. (1990) DNA polymorphisms amplified by arbitrary primers are useful as genetic markers. *Nucl. Acid. Res.*, **18**, 6531–6535.

Wu, P., Zhou, K.Y., Xu, L.S. and Teng, J.C. (1998a) Molecular identification of the Chinese drugs turtle shells. *Acta Pharm. Sinica*, **33**, 304–309.

Wu, P., Zhou, K.Y., Zhang, Z.H. and Xu, L.S. (1998b) Molecular identification of Traditional Chinese drug Hippocampus. *Acta Pharm. Sinica*, **33**, 226–233.

Wu, T., Wang, Y.Q., Yu, B.Y., Hu, B.Y. and Zhou, K. (1998) Classification of four species of plant genus *Liriope* (*Liriope* Lour.) using RAPD. *Chin. Trad. Herbal Drugs*, **29**, 37–40.

Yamazaki, M., Sato, A., Shimomura, K., Saito, K. and Murakoshi, I. (1994) genetic relationships among *Glycyrrhiza* plants determined by RAPD and RFLP analyses. *Biol. Pharm. Bull.*, **17**, 1529–1531.

Zhang, R., Shao, J., Tian, X., Yang, J., Zhang, B. and Ye, H. (1996) Identification of seven species of *Clematis* (*Clematis* L.) by RAPD analysis. (in Chinese). *Chin. Med. Mat.*, **27**, 686–687.

Zhang, R., Zhang, B. and Ye, H. (1997) Use of RAPD to authenticate *Indigoferae* plants. (in Chinese) *J. Chin. Med. China*, **22**, 72–73.

Zhang, Y.B., Ngan, F.N., Wang, Z.T., Ng, T.B., But, P.P.H., Shaw, P.C. and Wang, J. (1999) Random primed polymerase chain reaction differentiated *Codonopsis pilaos*ula from different localities. *Planta Med.*, **65**, 157–160.

SECTION THREE
PROGRESS OF CHINESE MEDICINE AND RELATED PRACTISE IN SOME COUNTRIES AND REGIONS

10 THE PROGRESS OF CHINESE MEDICINE IN AUSTRALIA

Qian Li
Colin C. Duke
Basil D. Roufogalis

Introduction

Chinese medicine (CM) is an important component of the herbal and complementary medical profession and industry in Australia. For the first time in a Western country, the Victorian Government recently announced a comprehensive proposal to regulate the CM practice. What is the implication of the new legislation? In this chapter we intend to present the background and current issues of CM in Australia, and make recommendations on issues such as regulation of practice and products, education and research on CM in Australia.

Development of Chinese Medicine in Australia

Chinese Medicine has an established history in Australia and has expanded rapidly in recent years. CM was introduced into Australia at the time of the gold rush period as early as the 1850's. At Ballarat town in Victoria, a tourist spot where the history of gold mining is maintained, the old clinic of Chinese medicines called Bao Kan Tang is one of the major attractions. This reflects the significance of CM in health care in the early history of Australia.

The major development of CM starts around 20 years ago. During the early 1980s immigrations from South East Asia brought experienced CM practitioners into Australia. In late 1980s till early 1990s a large number of graduates of traditional Chinese medicine (TCM) universities from China came to Australia. During the last few years, many new clinics, herbal shops and CM associations were established. The Therapeutic Goods Administration (TGA) in Australia and the State Administration of Traditional Chinese Medicine in China started to exchange ideas in the area of GMP (Good Manufacturing Practice) for herbal manufacturing.

In CM education, the establishment of CM courses at the Royal Melbourne Institute of Technology (RMIT) has attracted significant publicity in the country. The establishment of Herbal Medicines Research and Education Centre (HMREC) at the University of Sydney in 1997 was regarded as an important development of CM in Australia.

A survey in South Australia carried out by Maclennan (1996) has concluded that alternative medicine is a major industry in Australia. There are increased numbers of medical and pharmaceutical professionals interested in the development of traditional medicine. An interview of 43 doctors was carried out in a large hospital in Sydney in 1995, 56% of them believed that there is a place for CM as an adjunct to orthodox therapy (Wiesner 1995). Because more and more herbal products are sold in pharmacies, community pharmacists proposed to include the subject of herbal medicine in the new Four-Year (Bachelor of Pharmacy) Course that commenced in 1997 at the Department of Pharmacy, the University of Sydney.

On the other hand, the adverse effects and adulteration of Chinese medicines are major concerns of the medical professionals (Bury 1987, Bowron et al. 1991, Wiesner 1995). Asthma and anaphylaxis was observed in seven subjects following ingestion of royal jelly (Thien et al. 1996). Women with breast cancer receiving chemotherapy or hormonal therapy frequently experience menopausal symptoms as a consequence. Some of these patients used the Chinese herb, Dang gui (*Angelica sinensis*), as a supplement. It was warned that there is potential for unopposed oestrogenic agents in the herb that may stimulate breast cancer (Boyle 1997). Cases of poisoning and death caused by aconite (Fu Zhi, *Aconitum*) were reported (Bensoussan et al. 1996). In addition, some problems were identified in a survey of Chinese over-the-counter drugs in the Sydney market (Wong 1993).

Although it is getting popular, like other complementary medicine CM is not recognised by the representative body of medical practitioners, the Australian Medical Association. The principles and scientific aspects of Chinese medicine are not understood by the majorities of the medical and pharmacy professionals. CM is not generally covered by the compulsory medical insurance service of government, Medicare. The exceptions are medically trained general medical practitioners performing acupuncture in their clinic. Only some private health funds such as National Mutual Health Insurance cover acupuncture and Chinese herbal medicine.

In August 1995 the Victoria Government took a major step to set up a Review Committee on Chinese Medicine and allocated a research grant for a review of CM which resulted in the publication of the report, *Towards a Safer Choice* in 1996. The report provides the first comprehensive review of the practice of CM in Australia and recommended occupational registration by statute. In August 1998, the Victorian Government announced a registration system and the policy is expected to be adopted by other states of the country (Victorian Ministerial Advisory Committee, 1998). It is expected that the registration Act will be submitted to the Victorian Parliament for approval in 1999. The CM registration is considered as a milestone of CM development in Australia. CM practitioners take it as government recognition of the profession.

The Chinese Medicine Profession and Industry in Australia

THE CHINESE MEDICINE PROFESSIONALS

There are about 4500 CM practitioners in Australia, and 1000 students are expected to enter the work force by year 2000. About 1500 practitioners are non-medical CM practitioners, defined as primary professionals in that they spend the majority of their time in CM practice. The other 3000 practitioners are the non-primary professionals, who are mainly general practitioners, and a small number of physiotherapists, chiropractors, naturopaths and nurses (Bensoussan *et al.* 1996).

The 1996 Report also indicates that there are more medical acupuncturists than Chinese herbal medicine practitioners. It was found that 54% of CM practitioners in Australia use acupuncture only; 3% use herbs only; and 28% use both together. Only 24% of the non-primary practitioners use CM theory, which means most medical acupuncturists do not use CM theory (Bensoussan *et al.* 1996).

There are over 23 TCM associations in Australia, representing different interested groups of practitioners. The larger ones are Australian Acupuncture and Chinese Medicine Association (764 members), Australian Medical Acupuncture Society (653), Australian Natural Therapist Association (551), Australian Traditional Medicine Society (305), Federation of Chinese Medicine and Acupuncture Societies of Australia (300), Australian Traditional Chinese Medicine Association (237) (Bensoussan *et al.* 1996). The last two were formed by Chinese speaking practitioners.

THE CHINESE MEDICINE INDUSTRY

It was estimated that the Australian population spent about A$621 million on freely available alternative medicines, and for alternative therapists about A$309 million in 1993. About 48.5% of the Australian population purchased alternative medicines, 1.8% purchased (about A$23 million) Chinese medicines (Maclennan *et al.* 1996). More recent estimation of the total sales to consumers of herbs in Australia was A$200 million (Daffy 1997).

Annual turnover of CM was estimated to be approximately A$84 million dollars including patient visits (Bensoussan *et al.* 1996). If the total expenses on complementary medicine including vitamins in Australia are 1 billion dollars, A$84 million is around 8% of total turn over of complementary medicine. The popular herbal products manufactured in Australia originating from Chinese herbs are ginseng, ginger, ginkgo, and Dang Gui.

Regulation of Chinese Medicine Practice in Australia

REGULATION OF CHINESE MEDICINE PRACTITIONERS

Currently, like other complementary medicine practice, CM practice is not regulated by government. CM associations are actively seeking government recognition through registration to ensure long term development of the profession. At the same time, governments need to address safety issues in response to a rapid expansion of the practice and demand for CM and concerns expressed by consumers, practitioners and professional groups. The recommendation of CM regulation received broad support. After three years review, a comprehensive proposal was announced by Victoria Department of Human Services in August 1998.

It is proposed that "protection of title" will be sufficient to regulate the profession, which means the use of certain titles is restricted to practitioners who have the accredited qualifications and are registered under the relevant Act. Unqualified practitioners would be able to continue their practice of acupuncture, Chinese herbal medicine, but would not be able to use the titles associated with the profession (Carlton 1998).

It was proposed to restrict the prescribing of identified toxic herbs to practitioners qualified in Chinese herbal medicine. Currently, ephedra (*Ephedra sinica*, Mahuang) and aconite are not accessible by CM practitioners or dispensers as they are scheduled herbs under Australian regulations. Most submissions supported access to scheduled herbs for suitably trained practitioners, but this did not include those trained only in the use of ready-made herbal products and/or acupuncture. It is likely that additional regulatory measures will be required to complement statutory registration for practitioners to prescribe scheduled herbs (Victorian Ministerial Advisory Committee, 1998).

The Herbal Medicines Research & Education Centre (HMREC) suggested that safe use of scheduled herbal products requires specialised training in this area. Registration of practitioners could lead to the introduction by State and Territory governments of appropriate systems to allow practitioners to be properly equipped to prescribe these substances safely. HMREC could assist in providing such education suitable for accreditation. HMREC could also assist in the classification of the various categories of herbs through its involvement with appropriate scheduling committees.

REGULATION OF DISPENSING OF CRUDE HERBS

At present, crude herbs can be dispensed legally over the counter with no requirements related to safety issues and herbs are usually dispensed by the practitioner who prescribes them. It has been proposed that a CM registration Act could include powers for a Board to establish standards for dispensing and ensure that those who dispense scheduled herbs are appropriately trained (Victorian Ministerial Advisory Committee, 1998).

HMREC pointed out that it is not the accepted practice in the Australian context for practitioners to have both prescribing and dispensing functions. It seems reasonable that dispensers should have sufficient training, equivalent to that found in pharmacy in Australia and CM pharmacy in China, in order to dispense herbal products safely and with best practice. This would require training in pharmaceutical aspects of herbal medicines.

Chinese Medicine Education in Australia

CHINESE MEDICINE EDUCATION PROGRAMS

CM education in Australia started from the 1970s. Currently there are some 10 private colleges and three universities offering diploma or bachelor degree programs in CM (Bensoussan *et al.* 1996). University of Western Sydney and University of Sydney are planning to introduce courses in CM and Chinese herbal medicines respectively.

RMIT has offered Master of Applied Science in Clinical Practice (Acupuncture), Bachelor of Applied Science (Human Biology) with a Chinese Medicine Major, and Bachelor of Applied Science (Chinese Medicine) since 1995. The later is a five years program that commenced in 1996, and Nanjing University of Traditional Chinese Medicine in China conducts year 5 of the course.

University of Technology, Sydney has offered four-year courses of Bachelor of Health Sciences in Acupuncture, and Bachelor of Health Sciences in Chinese Herbal Medicine since 1996, and Master of Health Science in Chinese Herbal Medicine since 1997.

The educational background of CM practitioners in Australia is variable. The length of undergraduate or first CM qualification for practitioners ranged from 50 hours to 8 years, with an average for primary CM practitioners of 43.6 months, and for non-primary CM practitioners, 8 months. Eleven percent obtained a primary CM qualification from overseas, which indicates that only small number of practitioners, have a TCM university background from China. The majority of CM practitioners hold an acupuncture rather then Chinese herbal medicine qualification (Bensoussan *et al.* 1996).

Taking the above points into consideration, postgraduate and continuing education programs are needed to provide the practitioners with systematic knowledge in CM and modern science in Australia. It was pointed out that education and research in herbal and complementary medicines are needed by the Alternative Medicines Summit held in Canberra (Department of Health and Family Services 1996), and by the Review of the Therapeutic Goods Administration (KPMG Management Consulting 1997, Department of Health and Family Services 1997).

POSTGRADUATE AND CONTINUING EDUCATION

Postgraduate and continuing education programs are proposed as follows.

CM practitioners

The CM practitioners in a modern society are required to understand basic modern medical knowledge. Postgraduate studies and continued education are effective ways to provide practitioners with up to date knowledge and scientific data on Chinese herbs, in particular pharma-

Table 10.1 Chinese medicine education programs in Australian universities

Institution	Course
Royal Melbourne Institute of Technology	Master of Applied Science in Clinical Practice (Acupuncture) Bachelor of Applied Science (Human Biology) with a Chinese Medicine Major Bachelor of Applied Science in Chinese Medicine
University of Sydney	Master of Herbal Medicines Short Course on Chinese Herbal Medicines (continuing education)
University of Western Sydney	Bachelor in Chinese Medicine
University of Technology, Sydney	Bachelor of Health Sciences in Acupuncture Bachelor of Health Sciences in Chinese Herbal Medicine Bachelor of Health Sciences in Acupuncture Bachelor of Arts in International Studies Graduate Diploma in Clinical Acupuncture Master of Health Science in Chinese Herbal Medicine
Victoria University of Technology	Bachelor of Health Science—Traditional Chinese Medicine (Acupuncture) Bachelor of Health Science—Traditional Chinese Medicine (Herbal Medicine)

cology of Chinese herbal medicines. Pharmacology is not only essential for the study of CM pharmacy, but is also important for CM practitioners as modern medicine technology is integrated into CM practice. Pharmacology is a bridge between CM and modern medicine.

CM pharmacists

CM pharmacists equivalent to pharmacists in Australia and CM pharmacists in China will need to understand not only basic Chinese materia medica, but also the pharmaceutical aspects of herbal medicines, such as pharmacology of Chinese herbs, chemistry of Chinese herbs, identification of herbs, pharmaceutics, pharmacy practice and regulations.

Medical acupuncturists

There is a need for medical acupuncturists to extend their knowledge of CM principles and herbal medicines. Courses to be developed will contain subjects such as Chinese materia medica, and Chinese herbal formulary.

Pharmacists

Pharmacists are increasingly involved in the sale of products and the provision of information on herbal medicines. There is a growing need and demand for basic and continuing education in this area. Recently, the pharmacy profession has brought in overseas experts to run herbal medicines courses for practising pharmacists (Farnsworth *et al.* 1997).

Herbal Medicines Research and Education Centre

HMREC was established at the Department of Pharmacy, the University of Sydney. The Department has a long tradition in teaching aspects of therapeutic natural products and in research on pharmacological active substances from herbal medicines. It has expertise and facilities in pharmaceutical chemistry, complemented by strengths in pharmaceutics and pharmacy practice. HMREC has already established education and research projects in CM. The first education program is the Short Course on Modern Chinese Herbal Medicines with emphasis on pharmacology of Chinese herbs. HMREC plans to offer a Master in Herbal Medicines for CM practitioners, pharmacists and general practitioners.

The Regulation of Chinese Herbal Medicinal Products in Australia

THE THERAPEUTIC GOODS ACT IN AUSTRALIA

There is no general standard laid down for controlling herbal substances in Australia, although the regulation of herbs as medicines means that standards here are much higher than say the USA, where they are sold as dietary supplements.

The Therapeutic Goods Administration (TGA) under the Commonwealth Department of Health is the national therapeutic goods control authority. It enforces the Therapeutic Goods Act 1989 and the Therapeutic Goods Regulations that align with the documents of the Commission of the European Communities. The object of the legislation is to establish and maintain a national system of controls relating to the quality, safety and efficacy of therapeutic goods in Australia. The Act requires that therapeutic goods imported or manufactured for supply in Australia must be included in the Australian Register of Therapeutic Goods (ARTG) as registered goods or listed goods depending on their contents and intended purpose of use.

The Complementary Medicines Evaluation Committee (CMEC) was established in October 1997 by the Federal Government to provide advice to the TGA. CMEC is to make evaluation of complementary medicinal products, which are intended to be included in the Australian Register of Therapeutic Goods. A new schedule (Schedule 14) has been proposed to include therapeutic goods with complementary or traditional use, or have a use associated with the maintenance of health or prevention of disease.

Listed products

Listed drugs undergo evaluation with emphasis mainly on quality and safety. This applies to most herbal medicines used for minor ailments. No therapeutic claims for serious diseases can be made for such drugs. Drugs eligible for listing are vitamin, mineral, and amino acid supplements, herbal preparations, uncompounded BP substances, such as cinnamon powder or oil (Therapeutic Goods Administration, 1995b).

Products whose indications for use are amongst those prohibited by clause 4 of the Therapeutic Goods Advertising Code (TGAC) are not eligible for listing in the ARTG and must be registered.

Products that fall within the Standard for the Uniform Scheduling of Drugs and Poisons (SUSDP) schedule are not eligible for listing in the ARTG. SUSDP is a Commonwealth document that lists all drugs and poisons into 9 schedules; each has different requirements in labeling and retailing. Most pharmaceutical drugs fall within Schedule S2, S3, and S4. S2 and S3 are over the counter drug and available only from pharmacy, S4 is prescription drug (Table 10.2) (Australian Health Ministers' Advisory Council, 1995, Dash 1997).

Registered drugs

Registered drugs undergo intensive evaluation to ensure quality, safety and efficacy. They are divided into two categories for assessment: prescription drugs and non-prescription drugs (over the counter drugs), and the latter includes traditional medicines (Therapeutic Goods Administration 1995a).

Table 10.2 Schedules of drugs and poisons in Australia

Schedule	Description	Example
S1	Dangerous Poisons	No longer exist
S2	Medicinal Poisons, Pharmacy only	Chlopheniramine Paracetamol
S3	Potent Substances, Pharmacy only	Quinine
S4	Restricted Substances, Prescription only	Aminophylline Ephedrine Amoxycillin Adrenocortical hormones
S5	Domestic Poisons	
S6	Industrial and Agricultural Poisons	
S7	Special Poisons	
S8	Drugs of Addiction	Morphine
S9	Drugs of Abuse	Heroin

Requirements applied to all drugs

Manufacturers of all therapeutic goods must have a license and comply with the Australian Codes of Good Manufacturing Practice. Where a product has an overseas manufacturer, sponsors need to obtain prior clearance of that manufacturer from the TGA's GMP Audit and Licensing Section (GMPALS). In countries where the manufacturing standard is less well known, evidence could consist of a plant master file for the manufacturing site followed by a GMP audit of the factory at the sponsor's cost (Therapeutic Goods Administration 1991). GMP is the major step limiting import of Chinese herbal products into Australia.

All goods must have labels in English about the active ingredient, indication, dosage, instruction and other information. It must declare the presence of all therapeutically active ingredients and contain warning or cautionary statements necessary for proper usage of the product.

The legislation contains requirements for published advertisements about therapeutic goods to ensure that therapeutic goods are promoted in a balanced and truthful way, and that people are not encouraged to self-medicate for conditions that need expert advice. Advertisements for products whose indications for use are among AIDS, gastric, peptic or duodenal ulcer, neoplastic diseases are prohibited (National Coordinating Committee on Therapeutic Goods, 1997).

Additional legislation, which may be relevant to importation or supply of drugs, includes: Customs Act 1901, the Quarantine Act (1908), and the Wild Life Protection (Regulation of Imports and Exports) Act 1982 of Australia.

ISSUES OF REGISTRATION OF CHINESE HERBAL MEDICINES

A number of issues have been identified to be associated with Chinese herbal products.

The dried herbs

Products readily packed and sold direct to the public and indirectly, via a practitioner, should be entered on the ARTG. Therapeutic dried herb products are exempt from the need to be on the ARTG if they are supplied to licensed manufacturers as starting materials or to practitioners as raw material for extemporaneous dispensing. Most Chinese dried herbs can be listed on ARTG except those specified by the Regulations or included in the SUSDP such as *Abrus precatorius*, *Aristolochia, Ipomoea, Senecio, Prunus dulcis (P. amygdalus)var. amara, Aconitum, Ephedra.*

Herbal preparations containing pharmaceutical drugs

The registration of Chinese herbal preparations is a major problem. 130 tons of unregistered drugs were seized by Australian Costumes in 1995. Inspectors continue to find unregistered Chinese medicines in Sydney in 1998. One of the problem was that herbal preparations contained synthetic drugs which are non-prescription or even prescription drugs including Aminophylline (S4), Ephedrine (S4), Glibenclamide (S4), Paracetamol (S2), Chlopheniramine (S2, S3), Ferrous sulphate (S2), Quinine hydrochloride (S3). These drugs must be entered into the ARTG as registered drugs (Wong 1993).

Chinese herbal medicines containing heavy metals

Recently, high contents of heavy metals in Chinese herbal medicines were reported in a survey of herbal medicines in New Zealand. It was found that 30% of the herbal products tested were unsafe either with regard to microbiological contamination or with toxic levels of heavy metals. A high degree of manufacturing inconsistency was observed especially for Chinese herbal products (Waring *et al.* 1997).

It was not unexpected that some Chinese herbal products contained much higher concentration of mercury and arsenic. Toxic minerals used in CM include realgar composed of As_2S_2, and cinnabar (*cinnabaris*) composed of HgS. The herbal product Niuhuang Jiedu Pian contains realgar, and Niuhuang Qingxin Wan contains cinnabar (Pharmacopoeia of P R China 1995). These medicines are known to be toxic and should be used with caution. The issues of risk-benefit quality and regulating status are critically important for the safe and effective use of these products.

Research on Chinese Medicine in Australia

Research is another important component for development and modernisation of CM. The significance of scientific research in CM is as follows.

1. It narrows the gap between CM and orthodox or Western medicine.
2. It provides evidence to explain CM principles and scientifically establish efficacy of Chinese herbs. *Ephedra sinica* is a famous example.
3. Import of Chinese herbal products requires assessment of quality, safety and efficacy. Analytical data, pharmacology and clinical trial results are required for registration and marketing of herbal products.

RESEARCH PROJECTS ON CHINESE MEDICINE IN AUSTRALIA

Research projects on CM in Australia have already attracted much interest from the community and professionals. For example, the clinical trial on hepatitis C at John Hunter Hospital attracted much media coverage. HMREC was established to carry out modern scientific research and education in herbal and complementary medicines. Following is a summary of research projects carried out by HMREC and other centres in Australia.

Characterisation and development of herbal medicines in Australia
There is an acknowledged need by industry and government for local cultivation and production of herbal medicines in Australia. There are over 160 herbs used in Chinese medicines growing locally in Sydney. They may be evaluated for local production and export. HMREC has

recently introduced an herb from China for cultivation and product development.

Drug discovery from Chinese herbal medicines

The pharmacology of Chinese herbal medicines is well documented with extensive ethnopharmacological information, which provides an extensive source of information for new drug discovery. During the last ten years, the Department of Pharmacy of the University of Sydney has been working on drug discovery for cardiovascular agents, and anti-cancer agents from Chinese medicinal plants.

Efficacy of Chinese herbal medicines

Chinese medicine is clinically orientated. Herbs are used in response to patient's needs and efficacy is carefully evaluated and explained systematically with CM theory and methodology. However, clinical trials are required to substantiate any medical claims for herbal and therapeutic natural products in Australia. There are a number of clinical trials of herbal medicines carried out in Australia as Ph.D. projects.

A clinical trial for the use of a herbal formula in the management of perennial allergic rhinitis is being carried out at Concord Hospital in 1998. Other Ph.D. projects include: clinical trial on Chinese herbal preparation for hepatitis C by Yi Fang Yang at Newcastle University; study on Chinese medicine for cancer treatment by Henry Liang at RMIT; treatment of irritable bowel syndrome with Chinese medicine by Alan Bensoussan at University of Western Sydney; and the treatment of osteoporosis using Chinese herbal medicines by Ming Xu at University of Western Australia.

Quality and safety of Chinese herbal medicines

In China 28 toxic herbs and minerals are listed as *Controlled Poisonous Chinese Medicines* which are controlled by strict regulations (Table 10.3) (Guo 1992). These medicines need to be strictly regulated in Australia. The availability of these herbs in Australia remains a subject for further investigation.

Quality control of Chinese herbal medicines includes identification of herbal materials with organoleptic, microscopic and chemical methods, and quality testing of herbal products with chemical methods. The laboratories of HMREC are equipped with state-of-the-art analytical instrumentation and are among the best in Australia. HMREC staffs are experienced in chemical analysis of herbal products.

The Centre is building up a reference library, reference herbs and standard compounds for identification and testing of Chinese herbal medicines.

Integration of Chinese Medicine and Orthodox Medicine

There is a debate between primary CM practitioners and medical acupuncturists in Australia. CM practitioners pointed out that it is dangerous to substitute traditional theories and diagnostic principles with the bio-science model of medicine and/or by practising it without reference to a valid underpinning theory where CM is no longer available (Flowers 1998).

Medical acupuncturists emphasised the importance of understanding the medicine system in Australia. Patients should be assessed at the earliest possible stage to recognise severe and potentially life threatening diseases such that timely action may be taken. Additionally many patients who seek treatment from CM practitioners have a serious disease and are on medications which themselves may have serious side effects and which may interact with herbal preparations adversely (Chow 1998).

Table 10.3 Some controlled poisonous Chinese medicines

Botanical name	Chinese pinyin name
Aconitum brachypodum Diels (Raw)	Sheng Xue Shang Yi Zhi Hao
A. carmichaeli Debx. (Raw)	Sheng Chuan Wu
A. kusnezoffii Rehb. (Raw)	Sheng Cao Wu, Bai Fu Zhi, Fu Zhi
Arisaema consanguineum Schott (Raw)	Sheng Nan Xing
Croton tiglium L. (Raw)	Sheng Ba Dou
Datura metel L.	Sheng Yang Jin Hua
Euphorbia kansui Lou (Raw)	Sheng Gan Sui
Euphorbia lathyris L. (Raw)	Sheng Qian Jin Zhi
Garcinia morella Desv. (Raw)	Sheng Teng Huang
Hyoscyamus niger L. (Raw)	Sheng Tian Xian Zhi
Pinellia ternata (Thunb.) Breit. (Raw)	Sheng Ban Xia
Rhododendron molle (Bl.) G. Don (Raw)	Sheng Nao Yang Hua
Stellera chamaejasme L. (Raw)	Sheng Lan Du
Strichnos nux-vomica L. (Raw)	Sheng Ma Qian Zhi

The CM theory is the foundation of safety, quality and efficacy of CM. At the same time, it is a basic requirement for a practitioner to understand modern medicine for the protection of the public. Therefore, it is advantageous for practitioners to learn both CM and Western medicine as in China and Japan. The integration approach will help CM practitioners to raise their education standard and promote the recognition of CM by the mainstream health care professionals.

Conclusion

CM is expanding rapidly in Australia as indicated by the number of CM practitioners, and the establishment of CM courses in universities. However, qualifications of CM practitioners are variable and poisoning from Chinese herbs has occurred. The safe practice of CM is a concern in Australia. On the other hand, the restriction of CM practitioners to access scheduled herbs such as *Ephedra* and *Aconitum* causes difficulty for CM practitioners in Australia.

Regulation of CM practitioners is proposed to protect the public and to enable the practitioners to access toxic and scheduled Chinese herbs. Introduction of the regulation will provide both opportunity and challenge to CM professionals. It is obvious that to raise the qualification standard of CM practitioners, advanced education programs are needed. Postgraduate and continuing education programs will help CM practitioners to upgrade their knowledge and help other health care professionals to learn more about CM. Integration of CM and Western medicine is beneficial to CM development in Australia.

Chinese herbal medicines have been regulated as medicines in Australia. Major issues related to imported Chinese herbal medicines are that they may contain synthetic drugs, scheduled herbs, and heavy metals. In addition, GMP requirement of manufacturers is a barrier for the import of Chinese medicines from China. To raise the quality standard of Chinese herbal medicines, research on safety, quality and efficacy is required. It may be concluded that education and research will play an important role in the progress of CM in Australia.

References

Attorney-General's Department (1995) *Therapeutic Goods Regulations*, Australian Government Publishing Service, Canberra.

Australian Health Ministers' Advisory Council (1995) *The Standard for the Uniform Scheduling of Drugs and Poisons, No. 10*, Australian Government Publishing Service, Canberra.

Bensoussan, A. and Myers, S.P. (1996) *Towards a Safer Choice, the Practice of Traditional Chinese Medicine in Australia*, University of Western Sydney, Macarthur and Southern Cross University, Sydney.

Bowron, P. and Lewis, J.H. (1987) Possible contamination of a herbal product with a prohibited substance. *Medical Journal of Australia*, **146**, 325.

Boyle, F.M. (1997) Adverse interaction of a herbal medicine with breast cancer treatment. *Medical Journal of Australia*, **167**, 286.

Carlton, A.-L. (1998) Victoria review of traditional Chinese medicine. *Chinese Medicine Forum—Modernisation of TCM in Australia*, Sydney, May 1998.

Chow, R. (1998) Is integration of Chinese and Western medicine possible, feasible and necessary? *Chinese Medicine Forum—Modernisation of TCM in Australia*, Sydney, May 1998.

Daffy, P. (1997) Herbal medicines—an industry perspective. *Herbal Medicines, Current Issues and Future Directions*, Sydney, November 1997.

Dash, R. (1997) *Guide to New South Wales Poisons Schedules*, Pharmacy Guild of Australia NSW Branch, Sydney.

Department of Health and Family Services (1996) *Final Report of the Alternative Medicines Summit*, Canberra.

Department of Health and Family Services (1997) *Government Response to Recommendations Arising from the Therapeutic Goods Administration Review*, Canberra.

Farnsworth, N.R. *et al.* (1997) *UIC Herbal Medicine Courses for Pharmacists*, Sydney.

Flowers, J. (1998) A philosophical view of modernisation of TCM in Australia. *Chinese Medicine Forum—Modernisation of TCM in Australia*, Sydney, May 1998.

Guo, X.Z. (1992) *A Dictionary of Poisonous Chinese Herbal Medicines*, Tianjin Science and Technology Translation Publisher, Tianjin.

KPMG Management Consulting (1997) *Review of Therapeutic Goods Administration*, Department of Health and Family Services, Canberra.

Maclennan, A.H., Wilson, D.H. and Taylor, A.W. (1996) Prevalence and cost of alternative medicine in Australia. *The Lancet*, **347**, 569–573.

National Coordinating Committee on Therapeutic Goods Australia (1997) *Permissible and Prohibited Advertising Claims to the Public for Therapeutic Goods*, Therapeutic Goods Administration, Canberra.

Pharmacopoeia Committee, Department of Health, P.R. China (1995) *Pharmacopoeia of P R China* (Vol 1), Guangdong Science and Technology Publisher, Guangzhou.

Therapeutic Goods Administration (1991) *Australian Code of Good Manufacturing Practice for Therapeutic Goods-Medicinal Products*, Commonwealth Department of Health, Housing and Community Services, Canberra.

Therapeutic Goods Administration (1992) *Australian Guidelines for the Registration of Drugs, Vol. 1, Prescription and Other Specific Drug Products*, Commonwealth Department of Health, Housing and Community Services, Canberra.

Therapeutic Goods Administration (1995a) *Australian Guidelines for the Registration of Drugs, Vol. 2, Non-Prescription Drugs Registered via Compliance Branch*, Commonwealth Department of Human Services and Health, Canberra.

Therapeutic Goods Administration (1995b) *Guidelines for Applicants, Listing Drug Products in the Australian Registrar of Therapeutic Goods for Supply in Australia*, Commonwealth Department of Human Services and Health, Canberra.

Thien, F.C., Leung, R., Baldo, B.A., Weiner, J.A., Plomley, R. and Czarny, D. (1996) Asthma and anaphylaxis induced by royal jelly. *Clinical & Experimental Allergy*, **26**, 216–22.

Victorian Ministerial Advisory Committee (1998) *Traditional Chinese Medicine, Report on Options for Regulation of Practitioners*, Victorian Government Department of Human Services.

Waring, J. and Richardson, R. (1997) Herbal medicines in New Zealand, *Australasian Pharmaceutical Science Association 1997 Conference*, Sydney, Nov 1997.

Wiesner, D.M. and Lloyd, P.J. (1995) The history and practice of Chinese herbal medicine in Sydney: a preliminary review. *Australian Pharmacist*, **4**, 19–96.

Wong, S.C.C. (1993) *Evaluation of Chinese Over the Counter Drugs in the Sydney Market*, Graduate Diploma Thesis, The University of Sydney.

11 THE PROGRESS OF CHINESE MEDICINE IN MAINLAND CHINA

Kelvin Chan
Xin-Min Liu
Yong Peng
Pei-Gen Xiao
Wei-Yi Yang

Introduction

The practice of Chinese medicine has a very long history and is closely related to the development of the culture and life-style of the Chinese people (See Chapter 1). It is remarkable that this tradition of medical practice has survived the test of time. The introduction of orthodox medicine to China in the early 1930s when her weakened government was exposed to western influence had nearly removed the practice of traditional Chinese medicine. Its survival since the mid 1950s when the People's Republic was established has something to do with curing diseases in the traditional ways but also a great deal to do with economics, politics, and culture as well as necessity. Chapter 1 has given a concise account of the historical evolution of Chinese medicine from ancient times up to the 1970s. From then onward, modernisation of healthcare was started by rationalising the Regulations and Acts for all uses of medicinal products (both orthodox medications and Chinese medicinal products) and related practices. This chapter deals with the subsequent progress of Chinese medicine in Mainland China up to the present time. The chapter is divided into three separate parts. Part 1 gives a "General Observation of the Progress of Chinese Medicine in Mainland China" since the 1970s, Part 2 concentrates on the "The Progress in the Development of Chinese Materia Medica" and Part 3 describes "Some Aspects of Progress in Acupuncture in Mainland China". Some of the information had been collected when the project on "Critical Assessment of Traditional Chinese Medicine" was carried out in 1995 by one of us (KC) during the Churchill Travelling Fellowship (Chan, 1996) under the sponsorship of the Winston Churchill Memorial Trust.

Part 1 General Observation of the Progress of Chinese Medicine Since the 1970s

Kelvin Chan & Xin-Min Liu

INTEGRATION OF CHINESE MEDICINE AND ORTHODOX MEDICINE

Twenty years after organised-training of doctors, who were qualified with orthodox medicine (OM), to acquire the knowledge of traditional Chinese medicine (CM), the benefit of joint-experience (both CM and OM) in healthcare had been gradually observed. In the experience of product-related treatment of diseases, it is widely recognised in China that some Chinese medicinal materials (CMM) can be even more effective when used in combination with OM drugs and vise versa (Cheung & Chan, 2000). Beneficial effects were also obtained by the combination of acupuncture treatment with CMM products or OM drugs in certain diseases. The principle of integration of OM and CM begun in the 1970's is now being applied in almost all areas of medicine aside from surgery. However management of post-operative pain consequential to surgical operations can also be controlled and relieved by CM practice of acupuncture. It is particularly appropriate with chronic diseases where OM drugs can be used to control the most acute symptoms of diseases and CMM products are used in conjunction, or as a follow-up treatment. The general concept of integrating both medical practices has been that CMM acts to re-establish the body's own ability to fight the disease by strengthening the immune system by the presence of active agents in the CMM and/or the use of acupuncture. CMM can also be used to overcome the side effects of OM drugs, which are used for acute treatment of the disease. For example CMM products have been used in conjunction with anti-cancer drugs for treating some neoplastic diseases. (See Chapter 18 for details). Indeed it is remarkable how these two systems of medicine can work together and enhance the success of each other.

Such integrated practice needs plenty of practitioners who should be qualified with both CM and OM experience and training (see subsequent sections for details). Academicians and professionals in both CM and OM fields have been continuously debating the possibility and effectiveness of such integration over nearly a decade since the mid 1970s after the "Cultural Revolution" that had nearly stopped any progress of medical science. The formation of the *Yan Jiu Hui* (meaning the association for research interests) in 1981 marked the beginning of such follows-up by the practitioners and professionals. This organisation was initially attached to the China Academy of Traditional Chinese Medicine. After the approval of the Ministry of Science & Technology in 1990 the organisation was referred to as the **Xue Hui** (meaning an academically and professionally recognised association with more prestige than Yan Jiu Hui). Same English name, Chinese Association of Integration of Traditional and Western Medicine (CAIM), was used.

The Aim of the CAIM has been to rally numerous professionals of integrated medical science and technology for the promotion and development of integrated medical practice and to promote such activities. CAIM helps to promote, cultivate and raise the level of the quality of personnels involved in the development of integrated medicine and to be involved with the counseling and teaching of the integrated discipline. It also contributes to the betterment of economical construction of the nation by helping the government to carry out various policies as follows:

- To implement policies on medical science & technology, health and hygiene, professional practices of various aspects of traditional Chinese medicine;
- To implement the policy of Chinese Integrated Medicine;
- To carry out academic activities for the key state scientific research and public health tasks of various stages; these include:
  - To raise standards of all aspects of Integrated Medicine
  - To combine the basic theory with health care and preventive medical practice;
  - To insist on democracy in academic activities
  - To establish the devoting, innovating, and co-ordinating spirit for the integrated medical research;
  - To inherit the traditional medical legacy without restriction by its limitation for improvement;
  - To develop the legacy of traditional Chinese medicine scientifically without deviating from the origin;
  - To formulate the characteristic Chinese Integrated Medicine.
  - To foster international and domestic activities of academic exchange

The CAIM also started 33 academic specialised committees throughout China for carrying out the various activities. It sponsors the publication of the Chinese Journal of Integrated Traditional and Western Medicine with Chinese, English, Japanese and Korean editions, Chinese Journal of Integrated Surgery, Integrated Journal of Practical Clinical First Aid, and Chinese Orthopedics & Traumatology. Its academic specialised committee and several provincial organisations co-sponsor other national journals, which publish articles concerning various aspects of integrated medical practice.

In addition to CAIM, there are others such as Chinese Association of TCM, Chinese Association of Doctor of TCM, Chinese Pharmaceutical Association, and their province branches of CM in China. Several key Journals on CM and CMM are published in China per year. These are Chinese Traditional and Herbal Drugs (*Zhong Caoyao*), in Tianjing; its web site is at http://www. Chinainfo.gov.cn/periodical; Chinese Journal of Chinese Materia Medica (*Zhong Guo Zhong Yao Za Zhi*), in Beijing; Journal of Traditional Chinese Medicine (*Zhong Yi Za Zhi*); Journal of Beijing University of Traditional Chinese Medicine) and more than 30 province journals etc.

GOVERNMENT ADMINISTRATIVE STRUCTURE FOR CHINESE MEDICINE IN CHINA

Since the founding of the People's Republic of China, a series of principles and policies, administered by the State Council through the Ministry of Public Health, have been formulated in China to protect the welfare of patients and promote Chinese medicine (CM). The policy of "Developing orthodox medicine and traditional Chinese medicine" was officially written down in the Constitution. CM was officially incorporated in the healthcare system for the nation at the First National Conference of the Peoples Republic in 1950. Thus CM has become an integral part of the healthcare system playing a role at both micro and macro level. From the 1970s to 1990s its role in the healthcare system has been further consolidated. To meet the needs of developing CM, the State Council established the State Administration of Traditional Chinese Medicine (SATCM) in 1987. After adjusting the organizational structure of the State Council in 1998, the Government Administrative Structure of CM in China is as follows:

State Administration of Traditional Chinese Medicine (SATCM, 1987) and Ministry of Health (MOH, 1949):
SATCM is responsible to the State Council through the MOH. The most important functions of SATCM include:

- Developing and implementing government policy for CM research and education;
- Managing CM hospitals; financing projects relating to CM research and education;
- Encouraging international co-operation.

State Drug Administration (SDA, 1997):

SDA reports directly to State Council. Its responsibility includes:

- Examining and approving of Chinese medicinal materials and products (CMM);
- Working out and enforcing regulation of CMM products;
- Supervising quality control of CMM and products.

Ministry of Science and Technology (MST, 1978):

MST reports to the State Council. Its main function in CM includes:

- Drafting and set up of government policy in CM research plans in conjunction with MOH and SATCM;
- Leading to coordinate science and technological research plans on CM with Ministries and Commission of State Council, and other non-governmental organizations.

State Administration for Examination and Quarantine of Import & Export Goods (SAEQIEG, 1997).

SAEQIEG reports directly to the State Council. It is responsible for

- Carrying out health examination and quarantine;
- Verifying, supervising the management when Chinese medicinal materials (CMM) are imported and exported.

LEGISLATION AND REGISTRATION OF CHINESE MEDICINAL MATERIALS (CMM) PRODUCTS

Over the last decades the Chinese government has introduced a comprehensive legislative system controlling the CMM pharmaceutical industries as well as manufacturers for orthodox medicinal (OM) drugs. The aim of this legislation is to increase the level of control on the production and marketing of all medicines in order to bring

CMM products up to international standards and to ensure safety for healthcare.

Central to this legislative system is the "Law of Drug Administration of People's Republic of China" which has been passed since 1985. Updated Laws and Regulations about CMM have been introduced in China since then. Special attention was formulated to introduce the "Plan of Modernization of the Practice and Use of CM" (Gan *et al.* 1998). This was made by 15 ministries and approved by State Council in 1998. The project has been led by the Ministry of Science and Technology, joint with the Ministry of Health, State Administration of TCM, State Administration of Drug, and National Foundation Committee of Nature Science etc.

The main aims, based on inheriting and carrying forward the advantageous and distinguishing features of Chinese medicine (CM), of the plan are to develop and modernise various aspects of the practice and use of CM by:

- Utilizing modern science and methodology measures
- Drawing lessons and experiences from international standards and regulations for registration of products manufactured from natural Materia Medica;
- Developing CMM products that can be admitted to enter international medicinal markets, and
- Increasing the contest of CMM products on the global markets

NEW DRUG CLASSIFICATION OF CMM PRODUCTS

There are five categories of CMM products in the "Law of Drug Administration of People's Republic of China". (Provision 1985, 1992) Each category has different information requirements for the new drug application. These categories are:

Category 1:
- CMM materials which have been synthesised;
- Newly found materials or new parts for medicinal use.

Category 2:
- CMM with new dosage forms affecting the system of delivery;
- Active principles extracted from natural medicinal substances and their preparations.

Category 3:
- New CMM composed according to either ancient prescription, secret prescription, proved prescription or modified traditional prescription

Category 4:
- CMM whose dosage form is changed but not the system of delivery.

Category 5:
- CMM with a new indication

NEW DRUG APPROVAL REQUIREMENTS FOR CMM PRODUCTS

According to the "Law of Drug Administration of People's Republic of China", the production and clinical application of any new drug must be examined and approved by the MOH (SDA takes over this role with start from 1999). This approval procedure is specified in the "Regulations for New Drug Examination and Approval" Guide which covers orthodox drugs, CMM and biological products.

More recently, the "Amendment and Supplement to CMM Products" has been further developed to cover legislation.

The key points in this amendment are:

- That the examination and approval procedures need to be perfected to improve standards of new CMM products;
- That CMM products should be developed according to modern standards so they can meet the needs of the world market;
- That raw materials and the preparations made from them need to be assessed for quality control purposes; and
- That CM theory should be used for guidance.

Summary of Data Needed for New Drug Application of CMM Products: The following headings indicate contents of the data sheet that are required for completion for the application of product licenses.

- Drug name
- Botanical research
- Function, indication, explanation of use, efficacy
- Data on technical procedures
- Clinical pharmacokinetic, pharmacodynamic investigation

- Bioavailability or dissolution tests, dosage advice
- Specification for manufacturing
  - Analytical reports of 3–5 batches
  - Analysis of chemical components
  - Physical and chemical research results
  - QC (Quality Control) criteria
  - Stability data
  - Experimental methods used
  - Conclusions (should include specimens of packing, labeling and pack insert.)

Category 1,2 and 3 medicinal products have to be tested clinically in more than three hospitals and in more than 300 cases in the 2nd and 3rd phase of clinical trials. Control groups are also required. Category 4 and 5 medicinal products should be clinically tested on more than 100 patients.

THE ISSUES OF QUALITY CONTROL (QC) OF CMM PRODUCTS

The Chinese authorities controlling CMM products are well aware of the importance of quality control and anxious to reach international standards. Consequently at stages ranging from processing, production and distribution there are specific QC requirements, which have to be met, and which are checked by QC departments.

To improve standards of QC, China has developed clinical research guiding principles for all medicinal products, both OM drugs and CMM products. China has also set up a comprehensive organisational structure to monitor and guarantee quality control standards. These include 1600 drug administration organisations, 1953 drug examination and inspection institutes and 11200 drug supervisors.

GAP, GLP, GCP AND GMP ISSUES

The Chinese authorities have placed great emphasis on the importance of Good Agricultural Practice (GAP), Good Laboratory Practice (GLP), Good Clinical Practice (GCP) and Good Manufacturing Practice (GMP) in the production of CMM products. It is seen as a means by which China can reach international standards for pharmaceutical production (MST, 1993; MOH, 1988; SDA 1999).

The Ministry of Science & Technology (MST) approved and promulgated "Management Rules of Experimental Animals" in 1988 and "Good Laboratory Practice (GLP) for Non-Clinical Laboratory

Studies" in 1993. The MOH lay down "The implementation of detailed rules and regulations of managing medical experimental animals" in 1988 and promulgated "the Guidelines on Good Manufacturing and Quality Control for Drugs" in 1982. The government is also placing further pressure on CMM manufacturers to achieve GMP standards. To speed up the process, it was declared that, by 30th June 1998, the authorities would not handle any new drug applications from enterprises that have not passed the GMP certification. Meanwhile, the GAP for the cultivation of CMM natural products and "Good Clinical Trial Practice" (GCTP) are being worked out.

BASIC INFORMATION ON THE MEDICAL SYSTEMS IN CHINESE MEDICINE

Medical system in Chinese medicine

Recent statistical data estimated that there were 2,629 specialized traditional Chinese medicine (CM) hospitals including 53 CM-OM integrated hospitals and 129 ethnic-nationality medicine hospitals in 1998. CM hospitals have been established in 75% of the counties across the whole nation. The difficulty of seeking CM treatment in rural areas has been preliminarily solved. Throughout the country, the CM hospitals have 260,386 ward beds and 397,235 CM-doctors; and they have trained a large number of senior CM-OM doctors and ethnic-nationality medicine doctors. The hospitals annually treated 150,000,000 outpatients and 2,870,000 inpatients in 1998. (SATCM, 1999).

Some hospitals and specialists have demonstrated certain great breakthroughs in the treatment of cardio-cerebro vascular diseases, haematopathy, immunologic diseases, cataract, fractures, acute abdomens, calculus of urinary system, tumors, dermatopathy, anorectal diseases, gynaecological diseases and paediatric diseases. The practice of CM has not only applied systematic theory but also therapeutic methods including medical *Qigong* and diet-therapy. It is warmly welcomed by the Chinese people, and has attracted much attention from the people all over the world.

EDUCATIONAL AND RESEARCH SYSTEMS OF CHINESE MEDICINE

Presently there are 29 universities and colleges of traditional Chinese medicine and pharmacology (TCMP) and other ethnic-nationality medicines. There are over 37,000 undergraduate students reading the degree courses for Chinese medicine (5-year) or Pharmacy of Chinese

Materia Medica (4-year). Along with furthering the education development, 14 professional postgraduate courses have been set up. These enable academic departments to offer postgraduate training for doctorate degree and masters degree as well as implementing the seven-year training system. Up to 1998, 150,000 graduates of university or college level and 6000 postgraduates have been sent to medical practices. There are 53 secondary TCMP schools and basic units with an enrollment of 29,0000 students engaged in training medical personnel for countryside and rural regions. In addition, qualified staffs have been cultivated through in-service training, correspondence courses, evening schools, tutorial education, etc. International TCM education has also made great progress. Many Asian, European, American and Oceanic countries/regions and organizations invite TCMP specialists to give lectures abroad. Among all foreign undergraduate students and postgraduate students studying natural science in China, the number of those majoring in TCM is on top of the list. The TCM universities in Beijing, Chengdu, Guangzhou, Nanjing and Shanghai and Tianjing College of TCM have become main bases for training foreign undergraduate students and postgraduate students. The International Examination Center of Acupuncture and Moxibustion has been set up in Beijing by the SATCM, to cope with demand.

There are now 514,380 people engaged in CM, including 350,743 in Chinese medicine and 163,637 in Chinese Materia Medica. There are 77 national research institutes and about 100 new drug development units on CM with about ten thousand specialists and technicians. The government authorities have set up 4 research centers for the development of engineering technology for CMM products. Modern new and high technology such as computer-aided auto-control technology, image analysis and processing technology, and KDD (Knowledge Discovery in Database) is being used in researching CM (Liu, 1997).

ETHNIC NATIONAL MEDICINE

Ethnic-nationality medicine and pharmacology is a part of traditional Chinese medicine. Many Chinese minority ethnic groups have their own medical theories and practices that have made great contribution to the protection of their people's health and the enrichment of traditional Chinese medicine. In order to promote the ethnic-nationality medicine, the Chinese government has set up many therapeutic, educational and scientific research institutions of ethnic- medicine in minority nationality regions of Xizang (Tibet), Qinghai, Neimenggu, Xinjiang, Yunnan, Guangxi and Guizhou provinces.

CMM Industry and Pharmaceutical Production

There are over 600 manufacturing bases and 13 thousand farms specialized in production of Chinese medicinal materials (CMM). Following the development of rural sideline production and diversified economy, the number of households specialized in the production of CMM is over 340,000, with a total planting area of 180,000 mu (mu is the Chinese measurement of areas, 1.1 million acres). The total CMM planting area is over 11,500,000 mu (7.7 million ac). In 1998, there were 1020 CMM industrial enterprises in China. The annual value of output was 33.49 billion Renminbi (3.4 billion US$). About 124 TCM pharmaceutical factories have been recognized as big- or middle-size state enterprises. Some factories and workshops have come up to the GMP standards. Of these manufactured CMM products, 15 medicines won state golden medals, 77 medicines were awarded silver medals and 215 products got ministerial or provincial prizes (YYJM 1999).

INTERNATIONAL EXCHANGE

China has established cooperative relations with about 100 countries and regions in the field of medical treatment, scientific research and academic exchange. Chinese medicines have been exported to 120 countries and regions. In China, 7 collaborating centers for traditional medicine have been set up by the World Health Organisation (WHO). The World Federation of Acupuncture and Moxibustion Societies (WFAS) which has participants from about 100 countries and regions and is composed of about 50,000 members was established in Beijing in 1987. Participants from 29 countries and regions joined the World Medical *Qigong* Society founded in Beijing in 1989. In 1991, delegates from 40 countries and regions attended the International Congress on Traditional Medicine sponsored by China, and jointly drafted the "Beijing Declaration", which gave an impetus to the development of traditional medicines in the world.

Several dozen joint ventures of scientific research centres for CMM have been established at home and abroad with overseas institutes. Economical and technological cooperative relationships in the field of TCM have been set up between China and Japan, the United States, Germany, Britain, Switzerland, Australia, France, Austria, the Netherlands, Spain, Russia and Tanzania.

Part 2 the Progress in the Development of Chinese Materia Medica

Yong Peng, Pei-Gen Xiao, Kelvin Chan & Xin-Min Liu

Introduction

The prescribing and use of Chinese medicinal materials (CMM) plays a very important role in the general health service, and is by no means inferior to prescribing orthodox drugs in medical practice in China. The present CMM products market have reached 4,000 items, CMM crude substances along with their preparations are estimated to account for around 40% of the total medicament consumption in the whole country (Xiao and Peng, 1992). Thus, much attention has been paid recently to the research and development of CMM for both the source materials and manufactured products.

The development of science and technology for research of CMM has progressed rapidly over the past 30 years. The research of Qinghaosu with the consequent discovery of a series of synthetic Artemisinin derivatives has opened up a new road to treat pernicious malaria. The national general survey of resources of natural CMM has provided reliable data on the distribution and reserves of the medicinal herbs and other natural medicinal substances. The researches on the varieties of crude CMM substances have provided scientific proposal for revising the national standards. Encouraging progress has been made in treatment of tumors, cardio-, and cerebro- vascular diseases and hepatitis. By means of modern scientific technology, researchers have also made remarkable progress in the study of the implications and the therapeutic methods to understand the principle of Zheng-syndrome in CMM.

Investigation and Systematisation of the Resources on CMM

Table 11.1 summaries the finding of the latest nation-wide survey on natural substances that are used for medicinal purposes. The survey reveals that 12,694 items of CMM substances including herbs, animals and minerals are being used as ingredients in CMM (CTHM, 1994)

China has a great resource of CMM supply. The total reserve of 320 common medicinal herbs is about 850,000,000 kg. The area of land for providing CMM from plant source is more than 45,000 ac. There are over 600 CMM medicinal plant bases. These figures have been generated from several series of studies in the past. Details of the results can be obtained from the following publications, which were complied mainly in the Chinese language over a period of time.

- "The Chinese Materia Medica": is regarded as a modern version in this field. The revised editions include 6 volumes that were published in 1979, 1982, 1985, 1988, 1994 and 1998 (IMPLAD, 1979–1998).
- "A Pictorial Encyclopaedia of Chinese Medicinal Herbs": was compiled under the chief editorship of Professor XIAO Pei-gen with many other editors. The book contains 6,000 coloured illustrations and concise descriptions of Chinese medicinal herbs in twelve volumes (1988–1997) (Xiao, 1988–1997).
- "The New Compendium of Chinese Herbal Medicine": was published under the editorship of Professors WU Zhen-yi, ZHOU Tai-yan and XIAO Pei-gen as the chief-editors. It contains 7,221 species of Chinese medicinal plants arranged in three volumes (1988–1991).

Table 11.1 A survey on the natural substances used as CMM sources

Type	Item	Percentage
Medicinal herbs	11,020	86.8%
Medicinal animals	1,590	12.5%
Medicinal minerals	84	0.7%
Total	12,694	100%

- "A Compendium of the Resources on Chinese Materia Medica": was published under the chief editorship of the China National Corporation of Traditional & Herbal Medicine (1994) (CTHM, 1994).

In addition, 35,000 items of ethnopharmacological data of Chinese medicinal plants have been collected and subsequently systematized by electronic computer and published in 1986 and 1989 (Xiao, *et al.* 1986, and 1989)

Acclimatization and Cultivation

In order to guarantee the continuous supply of CMM substances, some 100 medicinal plants (See Table 11.2) have been cultivated by means of ethnobiology and modern agronomic technology.

The cultivating area has reached 330,000 hectares, with the yield per annum around 250,000 tons. More than 3,500 species of Chinese herbal medicines have been introduced in ten Chinese major botanical gardens. Among the 389 rare and endangered species listed in the "Chinese Red Data Book, volume 1", there are 77 typical traditional Chinese medicinal herbs, of which more than 50 species have already been introduced and acclimatized. Many important exotic species such as *Panax quinquefolium, Amomum kravanh, Amomum compactum, Syzygium aromaticum, Crocus sativus, Sterculia lychnophera, Cassia acutifolia, Strychnos nux-vomica* and *Rauvolfia vommitoria,* have already reached the farm productive level. At the same time several wild-growing medicinal plants are now being introduced and culti-vated; these included *Glycyrrhiza uralensis, Fritillaria unibracteata, Buplerum chinense, Cistanche deserticola and Schisandra chinensis* etc. Studies on the cultivation of the most important Chinese medicinal plants have also been carried out. For examples, *Panax ginseng, P. notoginseng, Gastrodia elata, Coptis chinensis, Amomum villosum, Dendrobium nobile, Fritillaria thunbergii, Corydalis yanhusuo and Macrocarpium officinalis* etc. have been attempted. The research pro-jects consist of determination of agro-technical parameters, genetic improvement and control of the main mycological and entomological pathogens.

In order to improve the quality of CMM, non-polluted technology has already been developed, *Crataegus pinnatifida var. major* and some

Table 11.2 List of major cultivated medicinal plants in China

Acacia catechu (st), Achyranthes bidentata (rt), Aconitum carmichaeli (rhz), Alpinia oxyphylla (fr), Alisma orientale (rhz), Allium tuberosum (sd), Amomum villosum (fr), Angelica dahurica (rt), A. sinensis (rt). Andrographis paniculata (pl), Areca catechu (sd), Artabotrys hexapelatus (fl), Artemisia argyi (l), Asparagus cochinchinensis (rt), Aster tataricus (rt), Astragalus mongholicus (rt). Atractylodes macrocephala (rhz), Atropa belladonna (l), Aucklandia lappa (rt), Biota orientale (sd), Brassica juncea (sd), Carthamus tinctorius (fl), Cassia acutifolia (l), C. obtusifolia (sd), Celosia cristat (fl), Chaenomeles speciosa (fr). Cinchona ledgeriana (l), C. grandis (exocarp), Citrus aurantium (fr), C. Medica var. sarcodactylis (fr), C. reticulata (exocarp), Codonopsis pilosula (rt), Coix lacryma-jobi var. ma-yuan (sd), Coptis chinensis (rhz), Cornus officinalis (fr), Corydalis yanhuosu (rhz), Crataegus pinnatifida (fr), Crocus sativus (stigma), Curcuma aromatica (rhz). C. domestica (rhz), C. zedoaria (rhz), Cymbopogon citratus (l), Datura metel (fl), D. innoxia (fl), Dendranthema morifolium (fl), Dendrobium morifolium (fl), Dendrobium nobile (pl), Digitalis lanata (l), Dioscorea opposita (rhz), Dolichos lablab (sd), Eriobotrya japonica (l), Eucalyptus globulus (l), Eucommia ulmoides (bk), Euphorbia longan (aril), Eupatorium fortunei (l), Eurya leferox (sd), Evodia rutaecarpa (fr), Foeniculum vulgare (fr). Ganoderma lucidum (fr-bd), Gardenia jasminoides (fr), Fritillaria thunbergu (bulb), Gardenia jasminoides (fr), Gastrodia elata (rhz), Ginkgo biloba (l, sd), Gleditsia sinensis (fr), Glehnia littoralis (rt), Illicium verum (fr). Impatiens balsaminea (sd), Isatis indigotica (l,rt), Jasminum officinale var. grandiflorum (fl), Lilium brownii var. viridulum (bulb), Lonicera japonica (fl, bud), Lycium barbatum (fr). Magnolia officinalis (bk), M. biondii (fl), Melia toosandan (fr, rt-bk), Mentha haplocalyx (pl), Michelia alba (fr), Morinda officinalis (rt), Morus alba (bk,l), Nelumbe nucifera (l), Ophiopogon japonicus (rt), Paeonia lactiflora (rt), P. suffruticosa (rt-bk), Panax ginseng (rt), P. notoginseng (rt), P.quinquefolium (rt), Perilla fructicosa (l,sd), Phellodendron amurensis (bk), Piper nigurm (fr), Pogostemon cablin (l), Polygonatum cyrtonema (rhz), Poria cocos (pl), Prunus armeniaca (sd), P. mume (fr), P. persica (sd), Pseudostellaria heterophylla (rt), Psoralea corydifolia (fr), Pyrethyrum cinerariifolium (fl), Raphanus sativus (sd), Rehmannia glutinosa (rhz), Ricinus communis (sd), Rosa rugosa (fl), Salvia miltiorrhiza (rt), Schizonepeta tenuifolia (pl), Scrophularia ningpoensis (rt), Sesamum indicum (sd), Sinapis alba (sd), Siraitia grosvenorii (fr), Sophora japonica (fl-bud), Stephania tetrandra (rt), Stevia rebandianum (pl), Styrax tonhinensis (resin), Tremella fuciformis (fr-bd), Trigonella foenum-graecum (sd). Tussilago farfara (fl-bud), Vanilla planifolia (fr), Zingiber officinale (rhz), Ziziphus jujuba (fr).

Key: bk = bark, fl = flower, fr = fruit. l = leaf, pl = plant, rt = root, Sd = seed, St = Stem, Rhz = rhizome, fr-bd = fruit-body others have been granted the National Green-food documentation. An additional study of the "Dao-di" (Genuine) Crude Herbs has also been initiated with much attention. More recently, a scientific publication entitled "The Agronomy of Chinese Medicinal Plants" came into being in 1991 (IMPLAD, 1991).

Quality Control

Quality control has been considered nationally as an important measure for the further development of CMM. A national research project has been set up on "Species Systematisation and Quality Evaluation of Commonly Used CMM Products". It consists of the following aspects: herbology study, resource investigation, plant taxonomic identification, morphological and histological identification, physico-chemical analysis, chemical constituents, collection and processing, and pharmacological and toxicological evaluation. More than 100 commonly used CMM have been thoroughly investigated. By means of UV, IR, NMR, MS, GC-MS and computer softwares, CMM substances could be evaluated in a more scientific basis. From these data guidelines on quality control of source materials will be updated and modified as monographic references (Peng and Xiao, 1993; Xiao and Peng, 1994).

Chemical and Pharmacological Studies

About 200 types of CMM have been studied and screened chemically and pharmacologically. They include a series of the most commonly used ones, such as *Radix Ginseng, Radix Sanchi, Radix et Rhizoma Rheii, Radix Glycyrrhizae, Rhizoma Coptis, Rhizoma Atractylodis Macrocephala, Radix Salviae Miltiorrhizae, Rhizoma Cimicifugae, Bulbus Fritilariae, Herba Epimedii, Radix Paeoniae, Radix Ophiopogonis, Radix Codonopsis Pilosulae, Rhizoma Ligustici, Radix Aconiti, Radix Scutellariae, Rhizoma Anemarrhenae, Radix Lithospermi, Radix Saposhnikoviae, Rhizoma Notoperygii, Radix Trichosanthis, Ructus Corni, Fructus Amonmi, Herba Pogostemonis, Cortex Cinnamomi cassiae, Herba Ephedrae, Herba Cistanches, Cortex Magnoliae officinalis, Cortex Acanthopanacis, Moschus* etc. Some 761 pharmacologically active principles have been found (Table 11.3) (Xiao and Peng, 1994; Xiao and Fu, 1987).

Table 11.3 Some pharmacologically active principles isolated from Chinese medicinal plants

Chemical type	Number of compounds isolated
Alkaloids	213
Terpenes	
● Monoterpenes	36
● Sesquiterpenes	39
● Diterpenes	49
● Triterpenes	65
● Cardiac glucosides	25
Phenolic compounds	
● Quinones	34
● Chromones	9
● Flavonoids	49
● Coumarins	34
● Lignans	42
● Phenyl propanoids	25
● Others	75
● Acids, amides and Miscellaneous	66
Total	**761**

The Research on Processing of Crude CMM Substances

The purposes of processing of CMM are to eliminate or reduce the toxicity or side effects, and to increase the therapeutic efficacy of the ingredients....(See Chapter 4 for further details).

The processing technology for over seventy kinds of ingredients has been studied. For instance, the unprepared root of *Aconitum carmichaeli* is extremely poisonous, due to its highly toxic diesterified alkaloids, aconitine, mesaconitine and hypaconitine. After the traditional method of processing, the diesterified alkaloids are degraded to monoesterified ones, benzoylaconine, benzoylmesaconine and benzoyl-hypaconine respectively through partial hydrolysis, and further to amines, alcohols, i.e., aconine, mesaconine and hypaconine by way of complete hydrolysis. The toxicity is reduced dramatically to the degree of the processed aconite root known as a commonly used CMM "Fu-Zi" (*Radix Aconiti lateralis preparata*) and then its cardiovascular property can play its role.

As a result of these studies, several rules for processing CMM have been discovered. For example, those CMM containing alkaloids are often processed with vinegar, where neutralization takes place between the acid and the alkali, forming water-soluble salt to enhance the efficacy of its decoction.

In addition, based on the processing experience of more than 500 kinds of CMM, two collected works entitled the "Compilation of the Processing Experience on Traditional Chinese Drugs" and the "Compendium of Processing Experience on Traditional Chinese Drugs in past Dynasties" have been published (Xiao and Peng, 1994).

Biotechnology Application

The biotechnological methods have attracted much attention in the field of CMM. Since they provide not only new methods for the creation of better plant varieties but also for the improved productions of plant raw materials. The in vitro cultures of some 100 Chinese medicinal herbs have been carried out. Some of these are *Panax ginseng, Panax quinquefolium, Angelica sinensis, Lycium barbarum, Rehmannia glutinosa* and *Momordica grosvenori* etc. By means of callus or suspension cultures for the production of desirable secondary metabolites, *Panax ginseng* and *Lithospermum erythrorrhizon* could be cited here as good examples toward manufacturing scale in China.

With respect to genetic engineering, like the infection of plant material with *Agrobacterium rhizogenes* carrying modified Ri-plasmids, it has been successfully applied in the studies of *Salvia miltiorrhiza, Fagopyrum dibotrys* and *Scopolia tangutica* etc.(Peng and Xiao, 1993)

New Drug Development

Since 1985 the Ministry of Public Health, PRC has set up a Committee for New Drug Evaluation. There have been about 700 items of new CMM drugs registered up to date. Table 11.4 gives some examples from this list (Xiao, 1992; Xiao and Peng, 1994; Xiao and Peng 1998).

In recent years, Chinese government has laid emphasis on systematizing traditional Chinese medicine by means of modern science and technology for the sake of raising it to a higher level. Consequently, attempts of combining medicinal ingredients from traditional Chinese medicine and

Table 11.4 Examples of new drugs or medicinal products developed from CMM sources

New drug	Originated clue	Usage
Biphenyl dimethoxy dicarboxylate (BDD)	*Schisandra chinensis* (fr)	lowering SGPT
Anisodamine and Anisodine	*Scopolia tangutica* (rt)	anticholinergic effects
Artemisinine (Qing-Hao-Su)	*Artemisia annua* (pl)	anti-malaria
Agrimophol	*Agrimonia pilosa* (winter bud)	antitaenia
Huperzine A	*Huperzia serrata* (pl)	improving memory, for myasthesia gravis
Yu-feng-ning xin-pian (total isoflavonoids)	*Pueraria lobata* (rt)	relieving the symptoms caused by hypertensive diseases
Composite Dan-shen Tablet	*Salvia miltiorrhiza* (rt) and *Panax noto-ginseng* (rt)	for cardiovascular illness
Essence-Retarding Decoction	A composite prescription	as anti-senility agent

orthodox medicine have been initiated for the development of new forms of integrated medications. There are 40 kinds of this form of integrated medications containing CMM developed for use. Such an approach is also reflected in the pharmaceutical industry (Fig. 11.1).

In recent years, the Chinese government has put emphasis and major effort on systematizing traditional Chinese medicine by means of modern science and technology for the sake of raising it to a higher level. As a result the mutual infiltration between Chinese medicine and orthodox medicine has developed a medical practice of integration. There are 40 kinds of this form of integrated medications containing CMM developed for use. Such an approach is also reflected in the pharmaceutical industry (Fig. 11.1).

Clinical Studies of CMM and their Prescriptions

Clinical studies are of the utmost importance in demonstrating efficacy and safety of CMM products, many clinical observations have been carried out as illustrated in Table 11.5 (Xiao and Chen, 1987; Liu and Xiao, 1993).

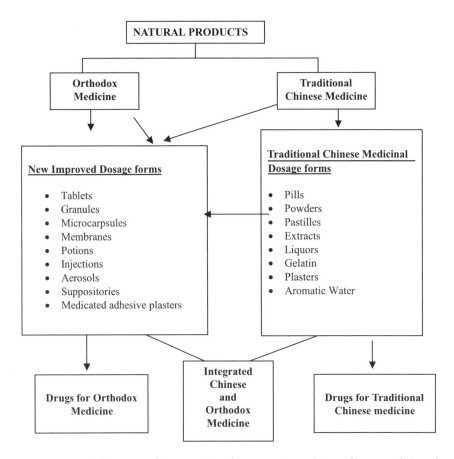

Figure 11.1 The mutual integration between ingredients from traditional Chinese medicine and orthodox medicine in Chinese Pharmaceutical Industry.

Conclusion

The use of CMM products as part of the practice of Chinese medicine has made a great impact to the healthcare of the Chinese people since time immemorial. It has been observed in recent years that the growing use of CMM in other developed countries will demand more CMM products with high quality and guaranteed efficacy and safety. In general the practice of Chinese medicine will continue to make great

Table 11.5 Clinical studies of CMM products and their prescriptions

Disease	CMM products or prescription
Coronary heart disease	Coronary Heart II – Sodium tanshinone IIA sulfonate – *Ligusticuin* (Chuanxiong (rhz) – *Puerarza lobata* (rt) – *Ilex pubescens var. glabra* (l)
Thombotic disease	– *Angelica sinensis* (rt) – *Nao-Xue-Kang* (mainly consists of Hirudo) – Scutellarin
Hyperlipidemia	– *Rheum palmatum* (rt,rhz) – *Polygonum multiflorum* (rt) – *Polygonum cuspidatum* (rhz) – *Typha angustata* (pollen) – *Crataegus pinnatifidus* (fr) – "Jiangzhilin granule"
Hypertension	– *Uncaria rhynchophylla* (st) – *Apocynum venetum* (l) – Baicalin from *Scutellaria baicalensis* (rt)
Cancer	– Indirubin – *Sophora tonkinensis* (rt) – *Hedyotis diffusa* (pl) – Decoctum of *Fructus Ligustri lucidi* and *Radix Astragali*
Nervous system	– Baogonqteng A from *Erycibe obtusifolia* – Huperzine A from *Huperzia serrata* (pl) – *Gastrodia elata* (rhz)
Hepatitis	– *Schisandra chinensis* (kernels) – *Sarmentosin* from *Sedum sarmentosum* – "DahuangZhechong Pill"
Bronchitis	– Vitex Oil and caryophyllene "Wan-Yang-Tablet" – Ginseng-Gecko powder and Ginseng-walnut decoction
Leucopenia	– Berbamine from *Berberis poiretii* (rt) – *Epimedium saggitatum* (pl)
Rheumatoid arthritis	– *Tripterygium wilfordii* (rt)
Indigestion	– "Xiao Jiangzhong decoction" – "Xiangsha Lizhong decoction" – "Huangqi Jianzhong decoction"

contributions to the people's health care within China and other countries. The vast experience as well as the abundant resources of CMM will also be valued for new drug development. The research and development of various aspects of the CMM industry should be continuously reviewed, evaluated and progressed in order to contribute to the healthcare for all mankind.

Part 3 Some Aspects of Progress of Acupuncture in Mainland China

Wei-Yi Yang And Kelvin Chan

Introduction

Acupuncture has been practiced in China for more than 2500 years (See Chapter 1). Because of the wide indication of its therapeutic properties, the simplicity of its application, and its low cost and usually rapid results for treatment of many disorders, it has great value for health care in China, and its use has been spread worldwide in recent years.

MECHANISM OF ACUPUNCTURE

Contemporary acupuncture creates bridges between acupuncture and classical medicine and modern science. Acupuncture acts, from a clinical point of view, particularly through the following forms of action:

a) Regulation of the physiological functions such as relaxing action on striated muscle, anti-inflammatory action and promote immunological effects, and
b) Regulation the mental activities and emotion, producing such actions as antidepressant and anxiolytic effects.

In China, during the recent decades, acupuncture has become very popular in clinical practice, its influence has led the discipline be integrated as part of treatments in different areas of disease. In order to improve its efficiency and expound the mechanism, scientific research has also developed rapidly.

CLINICAL PRACTICE OF ACUPUNCTURE

In recent years, acupuncture has been used to treat a lot of diseases and illnesses, including almost all the areas of clinical practice. The examples are as follows:

Stroke and cerebro-vascular, neurological and psychiatric diseases

The advancement of acupuncture therapy has been demonstrated for effective treatment of stroke and cerebro-vascular, neurological and psychiatric diseases. In reviewing the traditional and contemporary acupuncture prescriptions for "wind-stroke" or cerebro-vascular accident (CVA) and its sequelae, specific emphasis has been given to acupuncture points of the "Central System of Yang Meridians" and the "Eye System of Collaterals", but overlooked the traditional meridian theory. Due to the fact that Chinese medicine (CM) practitioners in the past had not recognized the brain's central functions, the relationship between brain and meridians had never been emphasized. But now, CM doctors accept the value of brain, and these two systems have been integrated for consideration for diagnosis and treatment of CVA diseases. Subsequent volumes in this series will review the Scalp, Ear, Eye (Orbit) and Tongue acupuncture treatments as derivatives of these subsystems. Any recommendations for improved results should be thoroughly explored. Also forthcoming are acupuncture prescriptions for prevention of transient ischemic attack, hypertension, cerebral arteriosclerosis, hyperlipidaema, hyperlipoproteinemia and stress, as well as emergency treatments for coma and shock.

Acupuncture treatment of stroke patients in the sub-acute and rehabilitation stage gave additive therapeutic benefit. The Motor Assessment Scale (MAS) for stroke patients, Sunnaas Index of Activity of Daily Living (ADL) and Nottingham Health Profile (NHP) were used to evaluate the efficiency of acupuncture treatment. The results showed that the acupuncture group improved significantly more than the controls, both during the treatment period of six weeks, and even more during the following year. Although the mechanism of the effects is debatable, there seems to be a positive long-term effect of acupuncture given in the subacute stage post stroke.

Attention on multidisciplinary research in the treatment and rehabilitation of head injuries; developmental disabilities; paralysis; speech perceptual, emotional and other cognitive impairment has focused on and acknowledged the profound technological revolution now underway in the brain sciences. Acupuncture plays an important role in these areas.

Anaethesia and pain management

Acupuncture-drug anaesthesia: In operation with combined acupuncture (body acupuncture & ear acupuncture)-drug anaesthesia in cerebral functional area, satisfactory effects were obtained in all the 80 patients, including 20 cases in language center and 60 in sensory and motor center. The anaesthesia grade 1 rate was 100%. After operation, no aggravations in dysphasia or dysfunction were found. Five cases showed aggravation on myasthenia and dysesthesia, but all recovered within 2–4 weeks. It might result in high tumor resection rate and low incidence of disability, and could be regarded as one of the routine anaesthesia methods (Yan *et al.* 1998).

Continuous electro-acupunture (EA): Acupuncture plays an important role in today's multidisciplinary approach to the treatment of pain. Continuous electro-acupunture (EA) stimulation for several hours leads to a gradual decrease of the analgesic effect, a phenomenon described as "EA tolerance". Attempts were made to change the parameters and mode of stimulation in order to avoid, or at least postpone such development. Such EA tolerance can be avoided by the use of alternating mode (between two legs or hands, for an intermittent duration of ten minutes per limb) rather than simultaneous mode for treating chronic pain patients. The benefit of postponing or avoiding EA tolerance without affecting the potency of the EA-induced analgesia can be achieved.

Acupuncture analgesia for painful diabetic neuropathy: Applying acupuncture analgesia to determine its efficacy and long-term effectiveness could be used to relieve chronic painful peripheral neuropathy in diabetic patients. Some of these patients were already on standard medical treatment for painful neuropathy. Most patients completed the study showing significant improvement in their primary and/or secondary symptoms. These data suggest that acupuncture is a safe and effective therapy for the long-term management of painful diabetic neuropathy, although its mechanism of action remains speculative.

Acupuncture-drug combination for pain relief: Acupuncture analgesia sometimes fails to give sufficient pain relief that may be overcome by appropriate combination of non-narcotic analgesics. The concentration of beta-endorphin (beta-EP) and cortisol in patients (12 cases) after thyroidectomy were measured by RIA technique during acupuncture analgesia. Another 12 thyroidectomised patients who received both acupuncture anesthesia and tetrahydropalmatine were also monitored with the same assay procedure. The results showed that the increase of beta-EP and cortisol in the latter group was less than that of the former, which proved that terahydropalmatine exerted a potentiating effect on acupuncture analgesia. (Zhu *et al.* 1996)

Acupuncture on Myofascial pain dysfunction (MPD): The *He Gu* and *Min Yin* acu-points are sensitive points for the treatment of MPD. After acupuncture, high temperature was detected of the skin in the regions treated, enlarged blood vessels and increased blood flow of the Nail Fold capillary loops in the treatment group were observed, with elimination of pain and increase of mouth opening as compared with the control group. The effective rate of the acupuncture treatment of 477 cases of MPD is 93.1% (Wang, *et al.* 1998).

Acupuncture in Paediatrics: Acupuncture is also an effective treatment of pain in children. Children with migraine headaches and failed in conventional treatment may receive acupuncture. It leads to an increase in activity of the opioidergic system, a significant increase in beta-endorphin levels is observed after acupuncture.

Other acupuncture applications

Acupuncture in Obstetrics and Gynaecology: Prenatal acupuncture treatment significantly reduces the duration of labour and may be a valuable tool in prenatal preparation. Acupuncture reduces the need for other methods of analgesia in childbirth and produces no major side effects. Many women (more than 90%) given acupuncture reported that they would reconsider acupuncture during childbearing period. Of the 122 patients with postpartum breast stasis 50 were treated with acupuncture 72 received ultrasonic irradiation. The results showed a statistically significant difference between the treatment groups with the curative rates after one time therapy in these two groups being 80% and 40.27% respectively. (Xu *et al.* 1996)

Acupuncture treating urinary tract disorders: Acupuncture is a worthwhile alternative in the prevention of recurrent lower urinary tract infection in adult women. It also might be beneficial in the management of neurogenic bladder due to spinal cord injury. It was demonstrated that the earlier the patient received electro-acupuncture therapy, the sooner the bladder would become balanced. On the other hand, acupuncture has no use in the management of neurogenic bladder due to complete spinal cord injury (Cheng *et al.* 1998)

Acupuncture treating some disorders of stomatology: Acupuncture may be indicated for some of these cases. For examples, xerostomia (dry mouth) can be treated successfully with acupuncture. The increase of saliva secretion lasts often for at least one year. Some neuropeptides have been found to influence the secretion of saliva. The sensory stimulation-induced increase in the release of CGRP, NPY and VIP in the saliva could be an indication of their role in the improvement of salivary flow rates in xerostomic patients who had been treated with acupuncture.

Facial acupuncture anaesthesia affecting bile secretion: People become more adventurous to try acupuncture in ways other than following the conventional practice. New treatments are developed continuously and rapidly. For example, the face acupuncture point (Liver point through gallbladder point) has significant effect of promoting bile secretion on the patients of cholecystectomy and choledochotomy and drainage. Special different points stimulation of face acupuncture has a very obvious effect compared with other body acupuncture groups. The result of face acupuncture anesthesia is better than body acupuncture anesthesia during the ligation of oviduct and subtotal gastrectomy. In some instance, trigeminal ganglion may be the main afferent way of stimulation information of face acupuncture (Zhang *et al.* 1996).

He-Ne laser acupuncture in cholelithiasis: The efficacy of He-Ne laser acupuncture, a non-surgical therapy, had been shown effective in the treatment of cholelithiasis in 310 cases. The cure rate was 35.2%, improvement rate 54.5% and invalid rate 10.3%. The stone discharge rate was 60%. The therapeutic effects of laser irradiation group were better than those of control group treated by electric acupuncture in 120 patients (P<0.01). The discharge rate of one piece of stone smaller than 1 cm was higher in the laser acupuncture group than in the electric acupuncture group. In 30 healthy volunteers He-Ne laser acupuncture induced apparent constriction of the gallbladder and dilatation of the common bile duct, observed under ultrasonography examination. It was believed that the therapeutic action of this treatment was mainly achieved by modulating the functions of sympathetic and parasympathetic nervous systems (Bian *et al.* 1998).

Acupuncture in treatment of herpes zoster: Patients with herpes zoster during the first 1–4 days of eruption were treated by drugs combined with (experimental group, 30 cases) or without He-Ne laser irradiation (control group, 30 cases). The sex, age, disease conditions of patients in both groups were comparable and all patients received the same doses of medicaments. The acu-point "Dagukong" at both right and left thumbs was irradiated by He-Ne laser at 25 mW for 5 min per day for not longer than 7 days. T cell sub-populations in the peripheral blood were examined before treatment and at the 15th or the 16th day after eruption. It was found that CD+4 and CD+4/CD+8 were apparently declined (P<0.01) and CD+8 was prominently increased (P<0.01) in both groups before treatment. After treatment the T cell sub-populations in the experimental group recovered with almost complete sub-populations and significantly shorten the abnormal period of T cell sub-populations in patients with herpes zoster (Sun *et al.* 1999).

Acupuncture in treatment of suprapatellar bursitis: To explore a more effective treatment for suprapatellar bursitis, 40 cases of supra-patellar bursitis were treated with ultrashort wave and acupuncture therapy, another 40 cases as a contrast group were only injected with prednisone and procaine in patellar bursae. The effect was compared in two groups after treatment. The near-excellent and cure rate of treat-ment group was higher than that of contrast group. The relapse of the former was also lower than the latter. There was a significant difference (P<0.05) (Wang *et al.* 1998).

Photo-acupuncture in treatment of child obesity: Two hundred and two child-patients of simple obesity were treated with self-produced photo-acupuncture apparatus (101 cases) or ear pressing (101 cases), and the treatment effects were observed and compared. Effects of both methods were satisfactory. The photo-acupuncture showed a better result than that of the ear pressing. After treatment, the obesity indexes were lowered significantly and levels of blood lipids, glucose, cortisol and triiodothyronine were all improved markedly. Therefore, photo-acupuncture is a safe, painless, non-traumatic and effective method for treatment of simple obesity, and it is easy to be accepted by children. (Yu *et al.* 1998).

Research in Acupuncture

Although acupuncture has been widely used for treating disorders, its therapeutic mechanism remains unclear. Following the growing interest in acupuncture, clinical and laboratory research on its effectiveness has been carried out by acupuncturists and other researchers in China. It is also recognised that research activities on acupuncture in other countries where the practice of acupuncture is not based on classical acupuncture would also help to elucidate mechanisms of acupuncture for treatment of diseases.

SOME PROBLEMS ENCOUNTERED IN ACUPUNCTURE RESEARCH

Scientific data on acupuncture have been accumulating over the years, but further adequately designed clinical studies are necessary to provide additional validity for this treatment modality. The problem which acupuncture research has to face is the concept of a control group. If, in control groups, non-acu-point needling is done, some physiological acupuncture effects may be observed or implied. Therefore the effects shown in this group are often close to those shown in the test acupuncture group. In other trials, control groups have received obviously different treatments, such as transcutaneous electrical nervous stimulation (TENS), or TENS-laser treatment; it is not clear if the effects of acupuncture are due only to the local stimulation or psychological effects of the treatment. Someone developed a placebo acupuncture needle, with which it should be possible to simulate an acupuncture procedure without penetrating the skin. In a crossover experiment with volunteers, the placebo needle is sufficiently credible to be used in investigations of the effects of acupuncture.

Other problems which produce difficulties in applying common scientific principles to clinical research on acupuncture have not yet been solved. For example, double-blind trial for acupuncture research in the clinical practice is almost impossible. It may be solved in the future, by using well-designed case studies.

SOME EXAMPLES OF RESEARCH IN ACUPUNCTURE MECHANISMS

General consideration

The techniques of molecular biology and other modern sciences have been applied for research in acupuncture mechanisms relating to its actions on physiological and biochemical systems of the body. These approaches are applied because the mechanisms by which acupuncture works may involve different physiological systems, which are controlled by the actions of endogenous neurotransmitters, hormones and gene expressions, etc. For example, calcitonin gene-related peptide (CGRP) is a very potent vasodilator in the nervous system. Flushing post-menopausal women had higher urinary excretion of CGRP before successful treatment with acupuncture on their flushes. In a rat model, CGRP increased significantly only in the cerebrospinal fluid, after an electro-acupuncture. Manual acupuncture did not change CGRP concentrations in any compartment.

Electro-acupuncture produced an increase in pain threshold that was paralleled by a transient increase in muscle sympathetic nerve activity. During acupuncture, there was a small increase in heart rate and mean arterial pressure, but there was no post-acupuncture hypotension. The placebo control procedure did not change pain threshold or sympathetic nerve traffic. The findings suggest that electro-acupuncture produces moderate hypoalgesia in humans paralleled by a significant increase in muscle sympathetic nerve activity.

Mechanisms of pain relief by acupuncture

Acupuncture plays an important role in today's multidisciplinary approach to the treatment of pain. To date, there are flaws in the conventional, scientific, clinical research methods applied to the evaluation of acupuncture practice for treatment of pain. Some guidelines and suggestions for future clinical trials are presented. Furthermore, in search of more scientific data, a review of several basic and clinical research articles was undertaken to evaluate a possible scientific basis for the mechanism of acupuncture analgesia. For example, several lines of evidence support the endorphin-mediated mechanism of acupuncture analgesia. High or low frequency stimulation induced by electrical acupuncture has been shown to release different types of endorphins. But, problems and limitations of adequately designed clinical trials were also addressed.

With the use of potassium iontophoresis induced tail-flick for measuring the pain threshold, the effects of injecting neurotensin (NT), naloxone (NX), anti-met-enkephalin serum (AMEKS), anti-k-endorphin serum (AEPS) and anti-dynorphin A1–13 serum (ADYNS) into periaqueductal gray (PAG) on electro-acupuncture (EA) analgesia in rats were investigated. NT administration enhanced EA analgesia remarkably. Pre-injection of NX, AMEKS and AEPS into PAG could significantly attenuate the enhancement of EA analgesia induced by NT, but not by administration of ADYNS. The results indicated that NT in PAG is responsible for the enhancement of EA analgesia. The effect of NT may be partly mediated by met-enkephalin and B-endorphin. (Bai, 1999)

Mechanism of regulating rhythm of digestive system by acupuncture

In order to explore the regulating function of acupuncture at the rhythm of digestive system, researchers observed circadian changes of mitotic index of digestive epithelium of the tongue and crypt cells of the jejunum in experimental rats. It was found that both of these cell types had circadian variations. These circadian variations could be changed to inversion of rhythm by the acute phase shift. Needling the Zhusanli (S36) could accelerate the inverse rhythm to recover to the level of the control-animal. This study gave some basis about the affects of acute phase shift on the rhythms of digestive system, and the regulating function of acupuncture on the some abnormal rhythms of digestive system was testified (Zou, 1999).

Mechanisms of acupuncture and moxibustion using cortical infrared thermography (CIT)

To explore the possibility of using cortical infrared thermography (CIT) and temperature variation in studying the principle of acupuncture and moxibustion, the changes of the cerebral cortical temperature during electro-acupuncture (EA) as measured by CIT in twenty cats were observed. By opening the skull before experiments, the cortex of animals was revealed. The distribution of the cortical temperature of the awakened animals was monitored by AGA infrared thermovision, and the thermograms were analysed by computer software package. Results were recorded:

- (1). The thermograms of the profile of the cortex could be displayed clearly, the temperature was higher in the ante and lower post-cortex than that in other regions.
- (2). No tendency of cortical temperature ascending within 30 minutes in cats without EA.
- (3). After EA, the temperature of cortex generally increased by 0.3 to 1.7 degrees centigrade, and 5 min after EA, the increment of temperature was the highest. The normal cortical temperature recovered 10 min after stopping the stimulation.
- (4). The temperature increment was more obvious in the regions of anterior ectosylvian, anterior supra-sylvian and anterior sylvian than that in other regions. The temperatures increased in the cortex were mainly in the somatosensory regions. The extent and position of temperature response of cortex after EA could be displayed with CIT directly by picture. The display of the temperature response could be taken as the indication of the nervous activity.

CIT could be used to conduct the studies of the acupuncture and the brain (Zhang, *et al.* 1998).

Possible physiological mechanism for effects after stimulating the traditional acu-points:

Although acupuncture has traditionally used the acu-points formula to treat diseases, the physiological mechanisms involved and the effectiveness of therapy remain unclear. Taiwan experts investigated the physiological mechanism(s) and response to acupuncture stimulation using the acu-points formula. Scalp-recorded potentials P300 were evoked by auditory stimulation of non-target and target in 13 normal adult volunteers. Latencies and amplitudes were measured. Three assessments were performed in each subject over a period of at least one-week. Each assessment was divided into a control period with no acupuncture stimulation, followed by an acupuncture period and then a post-acupuncture period. Acupuncture needles were inserted into the body as follows:

1) Non-acu-point: Needles were inserted 2 cm lateral to both Zusanli acu-points;
2) Acu-point: Formula assessments resulted in a significant decrease of P300 amplitudes during the acupuncture and post-acupuncture periods. However, there was significant difference in P300 amplitudes in the non-acupoint assessment.

Acupuncture stimulation of both Zusanli acu-points resulted in a decrease of P300 amplitudes, suggesting the involvement of the cerebral cortex in sensory interaction when simultaneous sensations of the two types are received. No similar changes were observed in the non-acu-point assessment, which have been suggested to be related to so-called acu-point specificity. Results obtained using the acu-points formula were not significantly different from those using acu-points alone. These findings suggested those neuropsychological effects from stimulation of the cerebral cortex resulted from stimulation via the Zusanli acu-points (Hsieh *et al.* 1998)

Acupuncture for the regeneration of nerves: The regeneration distance of sensory nerve, twitch tension & tetanic tension, sciatic nerve functional index (SFI), and motor nerve conduction velocity (MNCV) were monitored in 2, 4, 6, 10 weeks of operative intervals respectively. After treatment with electro-acupuncture (EA), they were significantly higher than in control. EA had the effect of promoting regeneration of injured peripheral nerve (Chen, *et al.* 1998).

Acupuncture on the MPTP-induced Parkinsonism in Mice: In order to evaluate the effect of acupuncture and Chinese medicine treatment on the effects of 1-methyl-4-phenyl-1,2,3,6-tetrahydropyridine (MPTP) induced-Parkinson's disease, MPTP-lesioned C57BL mice were investigated. The result showed that MPTP significantly decreased caudate nucleus (CN) dopamine (DA) and dihydroxyphenylacetic acid (DOPAC) levels and midbrain DA levels. The ratio of DOPAC/DA increased in CN. After treatment, the CN and midbrain DA levels increased in acupuncture. The results showed that acupuncture, Chinese medicine and conventional levodopa therapy can increase the decreased DA levels in MPTP mice, and DOPAC/DA ratio in CN of acupuncture. These observations suggested that acupuncture and Chinese medicine therapy may have protection effect on neuron that is different from the replacement therapy of levodopa (Zhu *et al.* 1996).

Auricular Acupuncture Stimulates the Sympathetic Nervous System: The stimulation of the auricular sympathetic via the auricular acupuncture (AA) point would affect the sympathetic nervous system. Stimulation of the sympathetic AA point significantly decreased the stimulus-evoked electrodermal response (EDR) when compared with an AA stimulation to a non-sympathetic nervous system (placebo) point (Young, *et al.* 1998).

Acupuncture Moderates the Immune System: During the investigation of the role of acupuncture in the regulation of cellular immune function, the changes of T lymphocyte subsets (CD3+, CD4+, CD8+), soluble interleukin-2 receptor (SIL-2 R) and beta-endorphine (beta-EP) in the peripheral blood of patients with malignant tumors before and after acupuncture were observed with double blind protocol. Forty patients were divided randomly into two groups of 20 each. One group was treated with acupuncture and the other one without as the control. Results showed that acupuncture has the effect of enhancing the cellular immunity of patients with malignant tumors. Acupuncture treatment could increase the percentage of T lymphocyte subsets CD3+, CD4+ and the CD4+/CD8+ ratio ($P < 0.01$) and the level of beta-EP, as well as decrease the level of SIL-2 R ($P < 0.01$). The correlation analysis of the three criteria showed there was a positive correlation between beta-EP and T lymphocyte subsets. Based on these results, a discussion on the acupuncture immunomodulation network was conducted in this article in order to explore the possible mechanism of acupuncture on immunomodulation. (Wu *et al.* 1996)

Acupuncture in the Treatment of Drug Abuse: Morphine dependence was induced in Wistar rats using an 8-day-morphine-injection regime. Heart rate and blood pressure of the rats were recorded after 18–24 h of morphine abstinence, and 100 Hz EA stimulation was then given.

The result was: Tachycardia of the rats was ameliorated by 100Hz EA, those effects were reversed by injecting opioid-receptor antagonist naloxone, or by administrating selective K-opioid receptor antagonist nor-BNI. The conclusion was that the effect of 100 EA in ameliorating tachycardia during morphine abstinence was mediated by K-opioid receptors in CNS. (Yu *et al.* 1999)

Acupuncture in the Reduction of Drug-induced Side Effects: Acupuncture can be used for drug detoxification or alleviating the side-effect of chemical (synthetic) drugs. To observe the effect of electro-acupuncture (EA) on succinate dehydrogenase (SDH) of gentamycin (GE) induced ototoxic cochlear hair cells, Preyer's reflex normal guinea pigs were selected and divided randomly into three groups: GE group, EA group, control group. Brainstem auditory evoked potentials (BAEP) and SDH levels in the cochlear hair cells were taken as indexes. In the GE group BAEP reaction threshold rose markedly, while that rose slightly in EA group. The difference was significant between two groups ($P<0.05$). The change of SDH within cochlear hair cells and degree of hair cells injury in the EA group were lower than those in GE group. EA therapy could relieve GE ototoxicity, protect SDH in cochlear hair cells and might be a possible mechanism of action of EA. (Kang, 1998)

Acupuncture Protects Body's Anti-oxidant System against Radicals: Cyclophosphamide (CTX) can damage the anti-oxidation system of the body, by causing the damage of hyperlipoxide. Acupuncture can protect the anti-oxidase system of body by improving the activity of super oxide dismutase (SOD), decreasing the accumulation of metabolites of lipid, lowering the side effects of CTX. SOD acts as scavenger of reactive oxygen radicals generated from drug molecules. But the effects are co-ordinated with the points (Zusanli is better than Duzue), stimulated duration (5 minutes is better than 10 minutes) and method (acupuncture is better than moxibustion (Shang, *et al.* 1998).

Electro-acupunture on Pressor Response: The effects of electro-acupuncture (EA) on the pressor response and reversible myocardial dysfunction induced by application of bradykinin (BK) on the gallbladder were studied in cats anesthetized with a-chloralose. The cardiovascular responses evoked by application of BK included a pressor response, an increase of LVP and its dP/dtmax, tachycardia and a decrease of local wall motion of the left ventricle with a supplying branch of the left anterior descending coronary artery ligated beforehand. Following EA of bilateral Neiguan acupionts, the pressor response of BK was inhibited, while the regional left ventricle myocardial dysfunction was alleviated significantly. The effects of EA were reversed by intravenous injection of naloxone (0.4 mg/kg). The observations indicated that EA had an inhibitory effect on the BK-induced pressor and ischemic dysfunction, which may be related with endogenous opioid peptide (Chao, *et al.* 1999).

Electro-Acupunture on Apoptotic Neuronal Death: The effect of Electroacupuncture (EA) on apoptotic neuronal death induced by focal cerebral ischemic in rats was evaluated. In the cerebral ischemic +EA treated group, the number of apoptotic neuronal cells in the infarcted area reduced significantly. The result suggested that EA inhibited apoptotic neuronal death induced by focal cerebral ischemia (Yan, *et al.* 1998).

Acupuncture-Moxibustion (AM) on Neurotransmitter Levels in Experimental Parkinsonism: Changes of three monoamine transmitters such as dopamine (DA), nor-adrenaline (NA) and 5-hydroxytriptamine (5-HT) in the striatum corpus of Parkinson's disease rat model induced by 6-hydroxydopamine (6-OHDA) before and after administration of acupuncture-moxibustion (AM) were compared. The results showed that the levels of three transmitters were significantly elevated after AM treatment. AM can raise monoamine transmitter levels in experimentally induced Parkinson's disease (He *et al.* 1998).

Acupuncture on Cerebral Ischemia: The model of reversible middle cerebral artery occlusion (MCAO) was used to study the effect of EA on SEP, the volume of cerebral lesion and the atrophy of thalamus. The result is: The volume of cerebral ischemic lesion in EA+MCAO group are smaller than that in MCAO group ($p<0.05$), the atrophy of thalamus in MCAO group was much serious than EA+MCAO group (p,0.05). EA has a cerebroprotective effect on the lesion by cerebral ischemia.(Si, *et al.* 1998)

Acupuncture on Hypophrenosi: Hypophrenosis is a difficult disorder to cure, but the clinical research of acupuncture appear to produce some effects. The author used filiform needle to treat 37 children of hypophrenosis, comparing with 15 cases of control group. Clinical symptoms were improved much better than the control group. Cortisol and growth hormone levels in blood were much higher after acupuncture (Ma, *et al.* 1998).

Concluding Remarks

As acupuncture becomes more and more popular over the world, paying attention to the adverse effects of acupuncture is necessary.

Examining the records in the Medline database for the years 1981–1994 one could find out that a total of 125 papers was localised by the keywords "Acupuncture adverse effects". Excluding the articles without case reports, 78 reports formed part of the basis for the present paper. A total of 193 patients were reported with adverse effects of acupuncture in 14 years. Pneumothorax is the most common mechanical organ injury, while hepatitis dominates among infections involved in the acupuncture procedures. Acupuncture treatment is claimed to be responsible in the death of three patients. One patient died from bilateral pneumothorax, another received endocarditis, and died of complications. The third patient died of severe asthma while under acupuncture treatment. Most adverse effects of acupuncture seem to be linked to insufficient basic medical knowledge, low hygienic standard, and inadequate acupuncture education. Serious adverse effects, however, are few, and acupuncture can generally be considered as a safe treatment and a useful medical procedure in healthcare for the public.

References

Bai Bo, Wang Hong, Liu Wenyan, Song Chaogu (1999) Effect of anti-opioid peptide sera on the enhancement of electroacupuncture analgesia induced by neurotensin in pag of rats. *Acta Physiologica Sinic* 4(2), 2.

Bian Xueping, Zhang Zhihong, Liu Yongda, Wang Lijun. (1998) He-Ne Laser Acupuncture in Treatment of Cholelithiasis-A Report of 310 Cases. *Chinese Journal of Laser Medicine*, 11(4), 15, 8.

Chan, K. (1996) Critical assessment of traditional Chinese medicine: *A Fellowship Report* submitted to the Winston Churchill Memorial Trust, London, April 1996.

Chao Dongman, Shen Linlin, Cao Yinxiang, Li Peng: (1999) Inhibitory effect of electroacupuncture on the cardiovascular response evoked by applying Bradykinin on the gallbladder *Acta Physiologica Sinica*, 4(2), 1.

Chen Xiaodong, Gu Yundong, Xu Jianguang, Chen Liang, Shen Liying (1998) Electroacupuncture (EA) promote sciatic nerve regeneration. *Journal Chinese Hand Surgery* 6(2), 10.

Cheng, P.T., Wong, M.K., Chang, P.C. (1998) A therapeutic trial of acupuncture in neurogenic bladder of spinal cord injured patients. *Spinal Cord*, 36(7), 476.

Cheung, L. and Chan, K. (2000) Examples of interactions between Chinese herbal medicinal products and orthodox drugs. *In: Interactions between*

Chinese Herbal Medicinal Products and Orthodox Drugs, Chapter 7 57–98, Harwood Academic Publishers, Amsterdam, 2000.

CTHM (1994) China National Corporation of Traditional and Herbal Medicine, The Resource of Traditional Chinese Medicine, Science Press, Beijing, China, 1994

Gan, S.-S., Li, Z.-J. and Zou J-Q. (1998) The Development Strategy Plan of Modernization of the Practice and Use of CMM. The Publisher of Science and Technological Documents, Beijing, China 1998

He Chong, Wang Linlin, Dong Hongtao, Wang Junmei, Ma Pin. (1998) Effects of Acupuncture—Moxibustion on the contents of monoamine transmitters in the striation of rats in Parkinson's disease. *Acupuncture Research*, **23**(1), 44, 24.

Hsieh, C.L., Li, T.C., Lin, C.Y., Tang, N.Y., Chang, Q.Y. and Lin, J.G. (1998) Cerebral cortex participation in the physiological mechanisms of acupuncture stimulation: a study by auditory endogenous potentials. *American Journal of Chinese Medicine*, **26**(3–4), 265–274.

Hsu, D.T. (1996) Acupuncture: A review. *Regional Anesthesia*, **21**(4), 361.

IMPLAD (1979, 1982, 1985, 1988, 1994, 1998) Institute of Medicinal Plant Development *Chinese Materia Medica (Zhongyaozhi)*, Vol. I–VI. People's Health Publisher, Beijing, China.

IMPLAD (1991) Institute of Medicinal Plant Development's publication on "The Agronomy of Chinese Medicinal Plants". China Agriculture Press, Beijing, China

Kang Songjian. (1998) Effect of Electroacupuncture on Succinate Dehydrogenase of Gentamycin Induced Ototoxic Cochlear Hair Cells in Guinea Pigs. *Chinese Journal of Integrated Traditional and Western Medicine.* **6**(6), 20.

Liu Chang-Xiao and Xiao Pei-Gen. (1993) An Introduction to Chinese Materia Medica. Peking Union Medical College & Beijing Medical University Press, Beijing, China.

Liu, X.-M., Xiao, P.-G. and Chen, S.-A. (1997) The Way of CMM Forward to 21 century. In: the Proceedings of TCM-Doctoral Symposium on Modernization about CM, p42–43, Beijing, China.

Ma Xiaoping, Gao Guangzhong, Xia Zhiping, Zhang Zhongyu, Gao Liqun. (1998) Acupuncture infleuence of blood serum cortisol and growth hormone on children of hypophrenosis. *Shanghai Journal of Acupuncture and Moxibustion.* **17**(3), 4.

MOH (1988). Ministry of Health Guidelines for Good Manufacturing Practice, Beijing, China

MST (1993). Ministry of Science and Technology Guidelines for Good Laboratory Practice (GLP) for Non-Clinical Laboratory Studies. Beijing, China.

Peng Yong and Xiao Pei-Gen. (1993) A review on the Resource Utilization of Chinese Medicinal Plants. *Journal of Plant Resources and Environment*, **2**(1), 49–55.

SDA (1999). At *http://www.sda.gov.cn*

SATCM (1999). At *http://www.satcm.gov.cn*

Shang Minghun and Sun Yisong. (1998) Influence of acupuncture and moxibustion on the damage of hyperlipoxide mice with CTX chemotherapy. *Shanghai Journal of Acupuncture and Moxibustion*, **17**(1), 40.

Si Quanming, Wu Genchen and Cao Xiaoding. (1998) Protective effect of electro-acupuncture in cerebral ischemia. *Shanghai Journal of Acupuncture and Moxibustion*. **17**,(4), 40.

Sun Dongxin, Ding Caiying. (1999) Effect of He-Ne Laser Acupoint Irradiation on T Lymphocyte Subpopulations in Patients with Herpes Zoster. *Chinese Journal of Laser Medicine* **2**(1), 1.

Wang Chuanduo, Lon xing, Zhu Xiaozhen, Li Cuilan, Deng Zhenmin. (1998). A study on the clinical curative effect by acupuncture for myofascial pain dysfunction syndrome. *Chinese Journal of Stomatology* **9**(5), 25.

Wang Junfu, Peng Huanrong. (1998) Ultrashort wave combined with acupuncture therapy for suprapatellar bursitis: *Chinese Journal of Physical Therapy* **8**(4), 20.

Wyon, Y., Hammar, M., Theodorsson, and Lundeberg, T. (1998) Effects of physical activity and acupuncture on calcitonin gene-related peptide immunoreactivity in different parts of the rat brain and in CSF, serum and urine. *Acta Physiologica Scand*, **162**(4), 517

Wu, B., Zhou, R.X. and Zhou, M.S. (1996) Effect of acupuncture on immunomodulation in patients with malignant tumors. *Chung Kuo Chung His 1 Chieh Ho Tsa Chih*, **6**(3), 139.

Xiao Pei-Gen. (1988–1997) Chief-editor of the series on "A Pictorial Encyclopaedia of Chinese Medicinal Herbs" (Vol. I–XII). The Commercial Press (H.K.) Ltd. and People's Health Publisher, Hong Kong.

Xiao Pei-Gen. (1992) Traditional Medicine and New Drug Development. Herba Polonica, Vol. XXXVIII No 3.

Xiao Pei-Gen and Chen Ke-Ji. (1987) Recent advances in clinical studies of Chinese medicinal herbs, I. Drugs effecting the cardiovascular system. *Phytotherapy Research* **1** No. 2.

Xiao Pei-Gen and Fu Shan-Lin. (1987) Pharmacologically Active Substances of Chinese Traditional and Herbal Medicines. *Herb, Spices, and Medicinal Plants*, **2**, 1–55.

Xiao Pei-Gen and Peng Yong. (1992) Product Development of Medicinal Plants, Spices and other Natural Products in China. In: Proceeding of Seventh Asian Symposium on Medicinal Plants, Spices and other Natural Products. Manila, The Phillipines. 151–163.

Xiao Pei-Gen and Peng Yong. (1994) A Review on Research of Chinese Materia Medica. *Chinese Pharmaceutical Journal.* **29**(10): 584–586.

Xiao Pei-Gen and Peng Yong. (1998) Ethnopharmacology and research on medicinal plants in China. *Plants for Food and Medicine* (Chief in Editor by N.L. Etkin), 31–39.

Xiao Pei-Gen, Wang Li-wei and Chou Gui-Sheng. (1986) Statistical analysis of ethnopharmacologic data on Chinese medicinal plants using an electronic computer I. Magnoliidae. *Chinese Journal of Integrated Traditional and Western Medicine.* **6**(4), 253–256.

Xiao Pei-Gen, Wang Li-wei and Chou Gui-Sheng. (1989) Statistical analysis of ethnopharmacologic data based on Chinese medicinal plants using a computer (II) Hamamelidae and Caryophyllidae. *Chinese Journal of Integrated Traditional and Western Medicine.* **9**(7), 429–432.

Xu Liufeng, He Chenna, Wu Qun, and Tian, F. (1996) Evaluation of Therapeutic Effects of 50 Patients with Postpartum Breast Stasis with Acupuncture. *Shanxi Journal of Nursing.* **6**(3) 28.

YYJM (1999) At *http://www.yyjm.net.cn*

Yan Huichang (1998) Clinical Application of combined Acupuncture-Drug Anesthesia in Cerebral Function Area Operation. *Chinese Journal of integrated Traditional and Western Medicine*, 3(3), 20.

Yan Yi-ping and Sun Fengyan. (1998) Effect of Electro-acupuncture on neuronal death induced by focal cerebral ischemia in rats. *Acupuncture Research*, **23**(1), 33.

Young, M.F. and McCarthy, P.W. (1998) Effect of Acupuncture stimulation of the auricular sympathetic point on evoked sub-motor response. *Journal of Alternative & Complementary Medicine*, **4**(1), 29.

Yu Changqin, Zhao Shuhua, Zhao Xueliang, Guo Jun, Qi Shan, Fang Meishan, and Gai Xueliang. (1998) Treatment of Simple Obesity in Children with Photo-Acupuncture. *Chinese Journal of Integrated Traditional and Western Medicine*, **6**(6), 20.

YU Yun-Guo, Chui Cailian, Yu Jiren and Han Jisheng. (1999) 100 Hz electroacupuncture amelioration of tachycardia of morphine withdrawal rats mediated by K-opioid receptor in central nervous system *Journal of Beijing Medical University* 18(2), 1.

Zhu, W. and Xu, Z. (1996) Alterations of plasma beta-EP and cortisol contents in thyroidectomy under acupuncture anesthesia and acupuncture anesthesia combined with tetrahydropalmatine. *Chen Tzu Yen Chiu*, **21**(1), 15–17.

Zhang Dong, Wang Shuyou, and Fu weixing (1998) A preliminary Study on Evaluation of Electro-Acupunctural Effect by Using Cortical Infrared Thermography. *Chinese Journal of Integrated Traditional and Western Medicine* 12(4), 1.

Zhang, S., Tang, Z., Wu, Z., Li, L. and Zhang, R. (1996) Research of clinic and laboratory of face acupuncture effect and the exploration of their afferent pathways. *Chen Tzu Yen Chiu*, **21**(1), 39–44.

Zhu, W., Xi, G., Ju, J. (1996) Effect of acupuncture and Chinese medicine treatment on brain dopamine level of MPTP-lesioned C57BL mice. *Chen Tzu Yen Chiu*, **21**(4), 46–49.

Zou Jun (1999) The experimental investigation about regulating function of acupuncture at inverse rhythm of mitotic index of digestive epithelium *Chinese Journal of Basic Chinese Medicine*, **2**(2), 28.

12 THE PROGRESS OF CHINESE MEDICINE IN SOME COUNTRIES IN EUROPE: BELGIUM, GERMANY & HOLLAND

Christoph Kunkel
Jan Nauta
Pierre Sterckx
You-ping Zhu

Historical Introduction

The earliest records for introducing acupuncture, one of the aspects of Chinese medicine, to Europe as a medical discipline are those due to Wilhelm Ten Rhyne (1647–1700) and Engelbert Kaempfer (1651–1716). They spent two years in the enclave of Nagasaki, where the Dutch-East-Indian Trade Company had a registered office. Their publications formed the foundation for European acupuncture. The Dutch surgeon, Ten Rhyne, published his experiences and observations in 1683 in London and Kaempfer followed these with "Curatio Colicae Per Acupuncturam Japonicus Unitata". Later on the French Jesuit Priests brought their knowledge to Europe, and Du Halde published the "Description de l'Empire de la Chine" in 1753.

The first pioneers of acupuncture in Europe were the French who led the philosophical leadership of Chinese medicine. One particular Frenchman, Soulié de Mourant, together with his students and followers spread the teaching of acupuncture. Some of the first Belgian, Dutch and German acupuncturists had also studied under the tutelage of these persons. French authors such as Cloquet who, in 1826 published the "Traite de l'Acupuncture" and later on in the same year Dabry, published "La Medicine Chez Les Chinoises".

In Germany at the beginning of the 20th Century, as a result of the colonial relationship between the "Kaiserreich" and the "Qing Dynasty" there was a significant rise of interest in acupuncture. The famous sinologist Richard Wilhelm, who practised as a priest in Tsingdao, translated several very important Chinese classic text books such as Yi Jing, and those written by Kongfuzi and Laozi. These publications placed an image in the minds of the German people of China.

Early Development of Chinese Medicine in Belgium, Germany & Holland

EARLY DEVELOPMENT OF CHINESE MEDICINE IN BELGIUM

Although Belgium is relatively small country compared with other European countries, she is the Capital of the European Union. She is a unique nation made up of two ethnic groups, French and Flemish and is one of the best producers of chocolates and French/Belgian fries! In Belgium, no written historical account is available on the origin and the development of Chinese medicine. The present description is therefore based on verbal accounts and personal experiences. Readers are asked to accept these accounts as the author was told them. The author has tried to authenticate these accounts but was unsuccessful. It was generally accepted that Belgium's first experience of acupuncture was in the early fifties. Then in 1960s professional or scientific organizations started to emerge.

As in many western countries, the first encounter with traditional Chinese medicine is usually acupuncture. The introduction of acupuncture into Belgium was very much due to individual rather than organised efforts. Many of them had personally experienced the benefits of Chinese medicine. These persons' backgrounds were diverse and colourful. In the absence of any records, it is impossible to evaluate their achievements. They have however, made important contributions to the development of Chinese medicine in Belgium.

Some of the first Belgian acupuncturists had studied under the tutelage of Soulié de Mourant and his students. Later on, some went to the UK to study under Gill and Rose-Neal and some went to Hong Kong, China and Japan. Consequently, many acupuncture styles were being and are still practised according to the schools where these practitioners originally studied. When Westerners, including Belgians, were able to study at the acupuncture centres for foreigners in Beijing, Chengdu, Guangzhou, Nanjing, and Shanghai a true and unique TCM-style of acupuncture emerged. This new style was then adopted but with modifications, by most of the European schools of acupuncture. These courses are simplified to three or six-month long. Despite the acupuncture's diverse development, the practitioners of acupuncture were already assigned to three distinctive groups whose membership is today still operating. These are the Western or orthodox medicine qualified acupuncturists (medical doctors with acupuncture training), physiotherapist-acupuncturists (physio-therapists who also study acupuncture) and non-classified acupuncturists (individuals who have neither medical nor physiotherapy background).

The first personal account of Chinese medicine development in Belgium

Jean Basens, an orthodox medical practitioner, is practising acupuncture as acupuncturist MD according to the above mentioned classification. Dr. Basens was stricken by a debiltating disease which orthodox medicine could not treat. The disorder was eventually treated and resolved by one single acupuncture session. Subsequently, Dr Basens went to study acupuncture in France in 1951 under Dr. Delafuye. He came back to practise in 1954. In 1964, he created the first Belgian association of acupuncture with other colleagues. He became its first president. He was also the first Vice-president and former professor of the Association of Belgian Acupuncturists Medical Doctors (ABAMD); the Belgian representative of the French International Association of Acupuncture of Dr. Delafuye; and the Vice-president of the International College of Chinese Medicine. According to Dr Basens the association was set up with about ten acupuncturists in Belgium, led by Dr. Willy Gerniers, a former student of Soulié de Mourant. However, that attempt to organize acupuncture properly was aborted one year later. In 1972 Doctors De Fymovsky, Beyens and other colleagues formed another association known as Association Belge des Medecins Acupuncteurs (ABMA). The objectives of that association were to:

- Establish a constructive relation between MD acupuncturists and non-MD acupuncturists;
- Defend acupuncture and its practice
- Promote a scientific knowledge of acupuncture; conduct scientific research into the mechanisms of acupuncture and its application in medical practice;
- Set up an acupuncture course for MDs in Belgium;
- Create relations with acupuncture societies of other countries;
- Collect all documentation and articles published about acupuncture.

Since then tremendous efforts were put into compiling a complete dossier with scientific evidence of the effectiveness of acupuncture, in order to obtain recognition from both the medical and the political authorities. Unfortunately, the Academy of Medicine refused. Later on, the Association Belge des Medecins Acupuncteurs incorporated Chinese herbal medicine as part of its activities after inviting Dr. Chen Kai Yan from Hong Kong to teach this new Chinese herbal medicine subject.

The second personal account of Chinese medicine development in Belgium

The second account was given by Mr. Jos Struelens, an acupuncturist belonging to the group of non classified acupuncturists. He too had personal experience of acupuncture in a similar manner as Dr. Basens. His affection for judo was threatened when he received a severe trauma to his shoulder at the beginning of the sixties. Fortunately, a Japanese Judo expert and acupuncturist was teaching at that time in his father's dojo. This "sensei" treated him with acupuncture and he was able to resume his regular judo training. Jos Struelens left Belgium for Japan where he devoted four years to studying acupuncture, first mastering the Japanese language. On his return to Belgium in 1969 he started to practise acupuncture. In 1973, he was invited by the St. Francis Hospital of Amsterdam (Netherlands) to use acupuncture anaesthesia to perform a complete hysterectomy. This attempt in the Netherlands appeared to have been convincing enough as he was later invited by the Holy Family Hospital at Reet (Belgium) to participate in a research program on acupuncture anaesthesia. At this hospital, he had apparently performed more than a hundred anaesthesia for a variety of surgical operations including dental surgery, kidney stones, gallbladder removal, vasectomy, laparoscopy, sterilization, appendectomy, etc. Jos Struelens also wrote a report to illustrate the economic advantages of using acupuncture in the general medical care.

Later, with W. Boermeester (MD), E. Vandeperck (physiotherapist) and P. Rausenberger (osteopath), Struelens opened an acupuncture school called Eastern Healing Arts (Opleiding Oosterse Geneeswijzen). The curricular contents consisted of the teaching of Dr. Kespi in France and Gill and Rose-Neal in Great Britain. Unfortunately, not long afterwards, the partners split and went their separate ways to work with other organisations like the European University of Traditional Chinese Medicine, Jing Ming, etc.

EARLY DEVELOPMENT OF CHINESE MEDICINE IN GERMANY

Influence of the work by Franz Hubottter on development of CM in Germany

Based on the data from early publications, Franz Hübotter (1929) developed the foundation for German acupuncture. Hübotter, a western doctor of orthodox medicine (OM) and a Sinologist, was the genius and chief instigator of Chinese medicine in Germany. His works on Chinese medicine, Tibetan herbal materials and obstetrics were for many decades unique. With his publications he researched the Chinese classics and commented on their practical application. He spent most of his time living in Asia, which gave him very little chance to teach Acupuncture to the European students.

Before World War II Hubotter taught very few acupuncturists; according to an informed source from a famous acupuncturist, G. Bachmann who was, perhaps, the only student taught by Hubotter. Thus, the teaching of the acupuncture aspect of CM probably started after World War II in Germany. In 1953 Hubotter was deported from "Red China" and subsequently taught in West Berlin until his death in 1967. Unfortunately, due to the Cold War and his past links with China, Hubboter and his method (perceived as an Eastern method), were strongly disapproved of by his colleagues in West Berlin.

The German doctors were inspired by the translations and speeches of the author Georges Soulier de Mourant from Paris who, together, with P. Ferreyrolles and R. Dela Fuye helped to create modern European acupuncture. The famous World Congress of Acupuncturists held in Paris in 1956 was the first great meeting of German and French Doctors and pointed the way forward. Since then, G. Bachmann, E. Stiefvater (and Hubotter), are now considered as the sages of this new knowledge. Gerhard Bachmann, who then was teaching in Munich, published his book "Akupunktur-eine Ordnungstherapie". His work has helped the spreading of acupuncture and his own style of acupuncture is still in practice. Erich Stiefvater on the other hand taught in Freiburg.

In Bremerhaven a doctor named Mrs. Roeder has practised acupuncture since 1952. She first became interested in acupuncture through her husband, whom she met in Prague in 1943 during an exchange with doctors from Tibet. Those therapists were accepted by their patients but experienced rejection from their colleagues. However, because of the free choice of therapists and methods of treatment in Germany, none of these critics could really attack them.

Another pioneer of acupuncture was Ernst Kluger who, in 1979, published a book, which became very popular among the practitioners. The book highlighted a strong link with the Francophone era before the "Opening of China" by Guido Fisch in Lausanne and Nguyen van Nghi in Marseilles inter alia.

Other famous names include Heribert Schmidt and R. Dela Fuye, who published a handy and unique Vademecum (1952), in which they demonstrated the technique of choosing acupuncture-points in order to inject homeopathic dilutions into them. Every point had its own dilution. The method is called homoeo-siniatrie. This was at a time when ordinary acupuncture needles were rare and gold and silver needles were the standards. It was a period characterised by needling "sedative", "tonification" and "master" points. When taking pulses therapists focused on "Mother and Son" or "Noon and Midnight" rules etc. Another famous name at this time was Elisabeth Finckh, who left behind three precious books about Tibetan medicine (1990).

These men and women provided the mental stimuli that lead the German practitioners out of the paralysis caused by the destruction of World War II. In this context, the works of Stephan Palos, a Sinologist born in Hungary, were important. He first lectured in Budapest and then came to Germany in 1964. Above all, he worked on *Qi Gong* exercises and published extensive sinological research concerning Chinese medicine (1980). In 1966, in Munich, he published "Chinese Herbs", his most important dissertation. For a time he edited the "Comsilium Acupuncturae", Cedip. Vlg.. With the death of Bachmann and Hubotter, acupuncture in Germany lost its leaders and obtained little further academic stimulus.

Influence of the cultural revolution in China on CM in Germany

During the "Great Cultural Revolution" of the People's Republic of China, the German public became aware of a dramatic, new change in China. The "Great Cultural Revolution" forced acupuncture to modernise itself. The acupuncture analgesia was emphasised as being the anaesthetic procedure in the People's Republic of China. Many doctors in Germany saw a link between acupuncture analgesia and the neurophysiological basis of their own cellular pathological medicine and could, thus, accept the effects of acupuncture in this aspect. But, they ignored the underpinning philosophy of acupuncture. Also, the approach of Chinese doctors who dedicated themselves to their own traditional medicine was viewed in a narrow scientific manner. In addition to these innovations, China also produced much written work incorporating the classics. With the visit of Nixon in 1972, China was able, once again, to open its doors to the outside world. In German operating rooms acupuncture was used for minor operations such as curettage and dental extractions. New in this field were electric current and steel acupuncture needles.

Aided by neighbouring countries such as Austria, Belgium, Switzerland and France the old, traditional connections remained the same in spite of this superficial declaration of acupuncture according to neurological basis. In Austria, it was mainly Johannes Bischko who quickly integrated acupuncture into routine hospital medicine and he created a standard by publishing papers and books (1971). It was mainly the Vietnamese Nguyen Van Nghi (1974) and Chamfrault (1957) who had an effect on the German "slumber" during the 1960's via Switzerland and France. At the beginning of the 1970's it was, to a great extent, Guido Fisch (1973) in Lausanne who gathered Belgian, French, German and Italian acupuncturists around him.

The search for a method of acupuncture analgesia in China as well as in Canada and Europe brought forward interesting scientific bases such as the Control-gate, the Serotonin and the Endomorphin-theory. Chinese discussions on the mechanisms of acupuncture also examined whether there is a connection between the transportation via blood or via the effective nerve system for the transmission of an acupuncture effect. Acupuncture points can now be objectively measured by instruments. All acupuncture points have similar characteristics including the finding that the resistance of the skin decreases exponentially on the points. On this basis, a completely new acupuncture principle was developed in the People's Republic of China. Hundreds of new points were discovered, not only in China. Paul Nogier (1969), a French doctor, developed his own system of ear acupuncture. It was empirically developed out of ancient Indian philosophical bases and suggested that there were two important theories in ear acupuncture and this had important affects on the field of medicine, mainly in Germany.

With the end of the "Great Cultural Revolution" it has to be stated that the successes of acupuncture analgesia among the enthusiastic Chinese masses shrank to a realistic 15–25% of all cases. The study of the ancient texts was once again possible in China as well as in other parts of the world. The famous German Sinologist, Manfred Porkert (1973) of Munich University acted as a translator bringing the original Chinese texts to the European doctors, lost in a Babylonian confusion of languages. He created a standard nomenclature, which however drove medical doctors into a permanent dilemma because of its placid clumsiness due to the fact that the terminology is Latin and requires either an extended education or the permanent use of a dictionary. Nevertheless it has to be mentioned that M. Porkert is nowadays considered as the academic leader of the modern TCM in Germany. His edited or published works and lectures and also his federation Societas Medicinae Sinesis, SMS, Fran-Joseph-Str. 38, D-80801, Munchen) that publishes "Chinesische Medizin" quarterly have reached international standard.

EARLY DEVELOPMENT CHINESE MEDICINE IN HOLLAND

Varying views on success and failure of orthodox medical treatments

The medical doctors of early days in western society earned respect from their patients for their skills, their knowledge and their care for people. This is especially true at the countryside, together with the priest and the teacher, they were considered by many as providers of care and help in the community. In those days the relationship between a patient asking for help and the professional healthcare was a personal one. Nowadays, this relationship is often characterised by technology, by glossy technical equipment and hard-to-understand mysterious figures and numbers. Advanced technology has not only made its way to the hospitals and the doctor's office, but also into our daily lives. With modern technology we can organise our lives. With a remote control in our hands we witness bombardments with astonishing precision. We expect the same results from our medical technology with "magic bullets".

From a scientific point of view medical science and technology may have reached new heights in other domains of science affecting mankind. Most people, however, have their doubts when they or their loved ones fall victims to incurable diseases. Western medicine cannot fulfil their hope and dreams of a happy and healthy undisturbed life. So modern medicine lacks something. For doctors, therapists and patients it is hard to accept the shortcomings of modern medicine as a "part of life". The doctor wants to cure. The patient wants to be cured. Instead of accepting the facts of life they try to find another way out. Traditional medicine thus fulfils a "void", which orthodox medicine has failed.

Other health care systems that have survived hundreds or thousands of years may give a solution. Especially health care systems far away from our academic medicine become attractive. It is remarkable that in discussions with adherents of alternative medicine, the application of modern scientific analysis of the clinical results of an therapeutic method in traditional Chinese medicine (TCM) and other systems is considered invalid. In the same discussions people demonstrate their anger towards academic medicine as the result of a conspiracy of doctors and industries. People feel threatened by the scientific-technological complex. In their experience modern medicine is beyond the human scale.

Reasons for turning towards Chinese medicine

Traditional Chinese Medicine (TCM) is not included in the official programmes of the Dutch medical faculties or paramedical colleges. TCM is therefore considered as alternative or complementary medicine. Nevertheless, TCM, in particular Chinese acupuncture, is widely accepted by the public. While TCM education is not included in officially approved and controlled educational programs, private organisations offer teaching-programs for a wide variety of students, students with a professional medical or paramedical background (doctors, physiotherapists, nurses) and students without any medical or even biological knowledge. To evaluate these private-courses, it is necessary to analyse the different views that exist on Chinese acupuncture, Chinese herbal medicine and physio-therapeutical techniques like *Tuina* or *Qigong*.

For several reasons TCM forms the solution for the above-mentioned threat. First of all, a health care system with a history of continuing use of 2000–3000 years would not have survived the test of time if it were not effective at all.

Secondly, the therapeutic methods used in TCM are simple, visible and understandable without complex technological tricks. The same applies for the diagnostic procedures. Furthermore the procedures of observation, palpation, smelling and questioning in diagnostics enables TCM practitioners to give a "personal touch". No blood samples and no sophisticated machines degrade the patient from a human being to a block of tissue. The use of natural substances, by definition in harmony with nature, in TCM instead of synthesised drugs with their side-effects are very appealing to people; they come to the conclusion that modern society with its technology does not realise the health and happiness they expect.

Present Progress of Chinese Medicine

THE PRESENT SITUATION OF CHINESE MEDICINE IN BELGIUM

The practice of acupuncture in Belgium

There are three kinds of acupuncturists: medical doctors (MD), physio-therapists (PT), and others (including graduates from China, CMD). There are two main professional organizations, one for MD, one for PT. According to the statistics from NVA—the Dutch Association of Acupuncturists, there are about 400 MDs to 100 PT (on paper). Realistically, there could be about 30 MD and 15 PT, practising acupuncture as their main activity, i.e. those who treat more than 10 patients per week. There are five CMDs (or OMD) who were trained in the traditional method in China (four of Chinese nationality and one of Belgian nationality). Most acupuncturists are in private practice and a few in the pain clinic of a regular hospital.

The training and education of acupuncture are only available on a part time basis from private schools. The courses are usually about eight weekends per year for two to three years. The best curriculum covers 200 to 300 hours of theory plus 100 to 200 hours of clinical practice. There are also some crash-courses of one to two weekends. They are referred to as scientific acupuncture without the traditional philosophy. The main MD-organization considers that a minimum of 200 hours is necessary in order to educate an acupuncturist properly. PT-organizations on the other hand propose at this moment 500 hours to attain the same target. CMD (OMD) had a full-time university cur-riculum of about 3500 hours.

Acupuncture is considered as a non-conventional medicine (or therapeutic technique). It is not legally recognized. Medical colleges prefer to ignore it. The academy of medicine rejects it. Legally, it is non-existent, but it is actually practised. There are two legal facts: Firstly, acupuncture practised by non-MD or non-PT is subjected to VAT. Secondly, piercing the skin with a needle, based on a medical examination and diagnosis and using a therapeutic objective, is considered a medical act; and this activity is reserved to MD. Similarly, little research is conducted into the use and effectiveness of acupuncture.

Despite this anomaly, acupuncture is much sought after by the public. It is also the most popular non-conventional medicine after homeopathy and chiropractice (and osteopathy). The public is quite oblivious of the "warring" that is going among the acupuncturists of different background and does not really differentiate between MD-acupuncturists and non-MD acupuncturists as revealed by a research conducted by the country's most important consumers' organization (Test Aankroop, 1991).

Based on the European Lannoye-report on non-conventional medicines, the Belgian government decided to regulate acupuncture. The basic principles are as follows:

- The practice of acupuncture will be limited to licensed MD and PT (plus the existing practising few graduates from China, four Chinese residents and 1 Belgian)
- The license will be granted by the Minister of Health upon advice of a commission (to be created), which will define all the necessary conditions to obtain the license.
- The Commission will be composed of 7 MD (proposed by the faculties of regular medicine) and seven practitioners of the non-conventional medicines.
- The Commission will determine the licensing criteria and define the medical conditions allowed in each non-conventional medicine
- Within the Commission there will be one professional Chamber per non-conventional medicine and composed of 3 MD (representing the medical faculties) and six practitioners of the non-conventional medicine.
- The advice of the Commission will always originate from the Chambers.
- The Chambers are responsible for producing the guidelines on good medical practice, registration, a deontology and a tarification system. They will also determine the transitory rules for all practitioners who are already active in the field and who do not yet respond to the licensing criteria.
- All licensed practitioners will always report their treatments to the regular MD of the patients they have treated.
- In the first instance it will just be a new article in the law on the practice of medicine, mentioning the existence of non-conventional medicines. Later on different Commissions will have to determine all aspects of medical practices.
- At present the conditions to be a licensed acupuncturists are either (which can still be changed) be a MD-acupuncturist or Physiotherapist-acupuncturist with a complementary education in acupuncture of 1,000 hours (including theory, clinical practice and training). The education programme will be proposed by the professional and scientific organizations and the universities and finally defined by the Minister of Health.

From this we can conclude that all measures are being taken to maintain acupuncture within the bounds of the regular orthodox medicine. It is felt that there is no need to organize education and research on a controlled basis; orthodox medicine remains the basis of an acupuncture curriculum, which has to be completed by a self-limited specific education program of 1000 hours. Finally the aim of this law is to control acupuncture as a medical act without real respect for or understanding of the philosophy of the Chinese medicine. Nevertheless, this law will officially recognize acupuncture, which can be considered a real progress. There are still discussions on the definitions of the indications and acupuncture techniques to be finally accepted, and the proper terminology to be used. At this juncture everything is possible, the best and the worst.

The practice of Chinese herbal medicine in Belgium

Chinese herbal medicine is generally practised by acupuncturists as a supplement in their practice. Those practitioners may have only studied for between 50 and 100 hours inclusively. In most cases, this training is supported by the importers and distributors of Chinese herbs and herbal preparations. The education is also partly based on a mixture of Japanese kampo-yaku, orthodox medicine and TCM principles.

The genuine Chinese herbal products are not usually prescribed and used in the traditional principles. They are formulated powder, liquid extracts and herbs. These are mainly produced in Taiwan for the local and the Japanese, European and American markets which represent 80% of the market. Ready–made (Proprietary) medicines have about 15% of the market with 5% for the regular Chinese herbs used in decoctions. The dosages that are recommended for these products when compared with those prescribed in China show a marked variation (see Table 12.1)

Table 12.1 A comparison of a dosage for herbs, formulated powdered and liquid extracts prescribed in Belgium and in China

Belgium		China
Powdered extracts	3–6 g/day	3 × 5 g/day
Proprietary (readymade) medicine (pills)	2–4 pill/day	20–40 pills/day
Regular herbs	20–40 g/day	60–120 g/day and often more

Only a few practitioners who have a Chinese medicine degree are prescribing normal dosages. There is a suggestion that Western patients prefer not to prepare decoctions because of their smell and their taste, and therefore practitioners are compelled to prescribe extracts and pills. However, this does not seem to be borne out with the patients who are under the care of China-graduated practitioners. They accept the traditional prescriptions.

Bad publicity of Chinese herbal medicinal materials

In Belgium, Chinese herbs had received very bad publicity as a result of several scandals both outside and inside Belgium. There were regular articles about Chinese ready-made (proprietary) medicines being adulterated with orthodox drugs (paracetamol, corticosteroids, etc.). In addition, the World Wildlife organization has been highlighting the traffickers of endangered species and other animals and is also very critical of the use of endangered animals in Chinese medicine. In the early 1990s, Chinese herbs were used in slimming cocktails mixed with orthodox medicines and about 100 patients got irreversible kidney damage. After four years of research into this tragedy, two reports indicated that the Chinese herbs were not until now found responsible for this damage. More recently, Chinese herbs were used in smart-drugs (e.g. mahuang-ephedra). As a result, the Belgian government legislated against Chinese herbs in December 1997.

Initially, there were only laws on regulating registration of pharmaceutical products. These laws require medicines (including herbs which claimed to be medicines), to be registered as in most countries. Before there was no clear ruling on the selling of herbs as medicines or as food supplements. The new law implemented categorizes the herbs and places under a different list. **List 1** herbs are considered lethal for the human consumption and are banned from sale as food products. **List 2** cites all the mushrooms that are allowed to be sold as food for humans. Any mushroom not on the list is forbidden. **List 3** comprises all herbs sold in pre-dosed forms (ready-made or proprietary medicines, granules, powders, and other extracts) that must be registered before being sold commercially.

From the point of view of Chinese Medicine, List 1 includes Baizhu (*Rhizoma Atractylodis Macrocephalae*), all kinds of *Paeonia* (Baishao, Chishao, Mudanpi), Yanhusuo (*Rhizoma Corydalis*), Mahuang (Herba Ephedrae), Houpo (Cortex Magnoliae Officinalis), Gouqizi (Fructus Lycii), Buguzhi (*Fructus Psoraleae*), Huangqin (*Radix Scutellariae*), etc. Fuling and Poria are not on the permitted List 2. This means that some of the major herbs used in Chinese medicine are also forbidden. This makes the practice of Chinese herbs very uncomfortable (not to say impossible). On List 3, there are about 70 herbs and all their combinations that should be registered when sold in pre-dosed forms. To gain registration there must be adequate scientific (bibliographic) proof that these herbs are safe in their prescribed form and dosage. Each herb is then registered at the cost of £100. Consequently, a company which sells all these 70 herbs plus 100 mixed formulas comprising one or more of these herbs, may add to these 170 products, and has to register. The companies are given six months to comply. In addition each company has to register these herbs.

There were, of course, some reactions against this law. At first, there was no concerted effort to remonstrate owing to the fierce rivalry against each other among the herbal companies. At this moment, the Ministry of Health has activated the Commission installed by this law in order to revise a part of the list of forbidden herbs. If the herbal companies can give sufficient scientific evidence that the herbs in List 1 are safe, these items will be transferred to List 3. But this could take some time. Not much animal toxicological research, as those performed for orthodox drugs, has been conducted on these herbs which had been safe for human use for centuries. Looking at the other side of the same coin, it is also a surprise that so many safe Chinese herbs are on the forbidden list of dangerous herbs. These lists were drawn by one professor in pharmacology, one member of the botanical garden at Meise, the Ministry of Agriculture, organisation of producers, distributors and shops of dietetic and western herbal products and the Food Inspection Service of the Ministry of Health without consulting any experts of Chinese medicinal herbs. As a result it is now legally impossible in Belgium to prescribe 80% of the most used Chinese formulas. As this chapter is being written, some critical reactions about this law were noted in the overseas specialist journals.

It is interesting to note the following statements in the Dutch Journal of Phytotherapy (1998)—"*Certain herbs on the forbidden list are well chosen, but some are disputable. It is difficult to comprehend it really, as these lists are made up without reference to any scientific criteria, which could be, e.g. the presence of certain toxic products in the herbs. Also concerning the registration, no clear references to the trustworthy bibliographic sources were given. ...*"

Cynics may say that this is the Belgian way of doing things, that is first rush in a law and never mind the quality in order to satisfy a minority of powerful lobbyists and afterwards ask a Commission to correct it, in order to satisfy the majority of powerless victims. In the meantime three herbal companies have already left the country rather than face the official hassles, likened to inquisitory prosecution. Some others are setting up agencies in the neighbouring countries to ease the escape should the need arise. What a strange European country is Belgium! What was perfectly innocent and legal in most European countries became terribly toxic and criminal overnight in Belgium.

Fortunately bad laws do not live long in one way or another. The incriminated herbs will be rehabilitated. In the mean time, the official recognition of Chinese medicine is impossible. Instead the ever-resourceful ordinary Belgians, accustomed to this kind of behaviour from their successive governments will purchase medicine and health products from abroad that they know will work for them and which they can trust.

CURRENT VIEW ON HEALTH CARE SYSTEMS IN HOLLAND

Recent difference of opinions on acceptance of types of healthcare from the public has created problems for the government. Other health care systems that have survived hundreds or thousands of years may give a solution, in particular health care systems far away from our academic medicine that have become attractive recently. It is remarkable that in discussions on alternative medicine the application of modern scientific analysis of clinical results and therapeutic method in TCM and other systems is considered invalid. In the same discussions people demonstrate their anger towards academic medicine being the result of a conspiracy of doctors and industries. People feel threatened by the scientific-technological complex. In their experience modern medicine is beyond the human scale.

Regulatory views on Chinese medicine and Chinese herbal products in Holland

The above mentioned arguments make it understandable that TCM education and research never found a place in official universities and academic training programs in developed countries, even when it was known that thousands of patients visited the TCM-practices. Until the beginning of the nineties, administering medical care was the exclusive responsibility of orthodox medical doctors. Acupuncturists, as well as all other alternative therapists, were considered as illegal practitioners. Although "de jure" illegal, or "de facto" the health authorities did not pay any attention to this "illegal" and by law unlicensed practising of medicine. Health authorities will only become involved after a patient has lodged a complaint.

Nowadays a new law is being implemented. This law defines the conditions, under which individuals may practise medicine and other alternative forms of health care including alternative medicine. The administration of these individuals is handed over to their respective professional unions. All health care workers will be entered into a register controlled by the health-professional unions. Enrolment in such a register can only take place when the applicant has fulfilled certain criteria with regard to his education, hygienic measures in his practice, patient administration and postgraduate education, etc. The unions themselves will define the criteria.

There are several organisations, which are very active in the education of TCM. There are two organisations admitting only medical doctors and dentists. Another organisation accepts physiotherapists and medical doctors. Several others accept everyone, eventually, after an introductory course in basic physiology and anatomy. All of these organisations offer their own training programs based on their own views on TCM and modern medicine. Attempts to certify these different programs so far have been unsuccessful, not only because of the incompatibility of their different views on TCM, but also on economic grounds. The organisations offering TCM-courses badly need their students for survival! In the University of Groningen, an introductory optional course on acupuncture is being offered to medical students.

In contrast to the academic medical education programs, the courses in the different forms of alternative medicine, including TCM, are only subjected to the rules of their own organisations and thus, not to any other independent quality control system. The old saying, "TCM is a costly pearl in the treasure-house of Chinese tradition" is undoubtedly true, but people who do not know how such a pearl looks like can not find the real pearl. The worth of TCM cannot be found without a thorough knowledge and understanding of history of Chinese language, philosophy, educational system and science. That understanding cannot be reached by reading the Dutch translation of an English or German translation of an old Chinese manuscript.

Chinese herbal products are also not subject to legislation in The Netherlands. The quality assurance of TCM practice and Chinese herbal products is a matter for self-control. There are very competent TCM doctors and self-claimed TCM doctors, who are providing TCM treatment without sufficient professional monitoring. The quality of imported Chinese herbs and herbal products also vary dramatically from one supplier to another, especially concerning crude herbs.

In 1996, several Chinese herbal preparations sold in the Dutch market were found containing high level of heavy metals, and were forced to be withdrawn from the market. In the same incident, a large number of preparations made from animals and plants listed in the protected biological species were detained. It was later revealed that these animal and plant ingredients were not from the wild origins but from domestically bred sources or artificial substitutes.

A patient developed a severe chorea while taking Taiwan-made Chien Pu Wan pills. Investigation later showed that a high level of (3 times the normal value) heavy metal was found. Chemical analysis of these pills showed that each pill contained 14 mg of manganese. By taking 3 to 5 pills a day, the patient was receiving 42 to 70 mg of manganese over and above the normal absorbed quantity of 60–90 mg daily. Because the chorea developed during the use of these pills and resolved when the blood levels of manganese went down, and because the high manganese blood levels were the only abnormality found, it was assumed the Chien Pu Wan pills and the subsequent manganese intoxication to be the cause of chorea (De Krom *et al.*, 1994). Acute hepatitis in a patient using Chinese herbal remedy was also reported (Levi *et al.*, 1998).

In addition, adulteration of Chinese herbs under similar commercial names largely goes unnoticed in the Netherlands due to lack of expertise and regulations. The author encountered several Chinese herbs with multiple plant sources. Misuse one for another, particularly at large doses, may cause serious consequences. These herbs include "Fang Ji" which is produced from the roots of Stephania tetrandra or Aristolochia fanchi, "Mu Xiang" whose source plants range from *Aucklandia lappa* to *Aristolochia debilis* and several *Vladimiria* species, and "Mu Tong" which often comes from the stems of *Aristolochia manshuriensis* but sometimes declared as the stems of *Clematis armandii* or *C. montana* (Zhu, 1998). Overdose of *Aristolochia* species have been reported causing acute renal failure (Wu, 1964, Hong *et al.*, 1965).

Adulteration is reported to be the cause of an incident in Belgium involving the Chinese herb "Fang Ji" (Vanherweghem *et al.*, 1993). Although the cause of this incidence has been challenged (Malak, 1998), the fact that the misidentified herb was being used unchecked is enough to ring a bell. This incidence shows that how neglected in the education of TCM in the West is. In Chinese herbal medicine, adulteration of herbs due to multiple sources or name similarity is not uncommon and need to be dealt with seriously if TCM is to be taken seriously by the authorities and medical professionals in the Netherlands.

CHINESE MEDICINE IN TODAY'S GERMANY

The dominating position of acupuncture in Chinese medicine

Chinese medicine today is still fundamentally acupuncture in the perception of the public in Germany. Only hesitatingly was it accepted that Chinese herbal therapy was an essential part of the practice of CM as are the energy meditation therapies *Qi Gong* and *Taijiquan*, diet and *Tuina* massage. As a result, there is no standardised education and all the different branches are not understood to be part of the whole CM. There are hostilities between the different medical boards and, thus, there is no overlapping help. Professional access to the associations and the motivation to learn all the methods of CM are so different that mutual acceptance cannot be easily produced. An educational order among the associations is lacking. In the first instance, it is difficult to classify the parts of the conventional CM in Germany. For many years, CM herbs were difficult to obtain; this is, however, no longer a problem nowadays. This explains the extreme overemphasis of acupuncture among German practitioners and doctors. It is also true that several doctors only practise acupuncture as second job as they are reluctant to learn the more complex body-acupuncture: many, therefore, turn to the much easier ear-acupuncture which exists as the combined Chinese and the French style of acupuncture, developed by P. Nogier. In "The Deutsche Akademie fur Akupunktur und Aurikulomedizin", Feinhals-Str. 8, D-81247 Munchen, the Nogier-system is characterised by a sort of technical mystification. For example, the use of pulse quality changes for finding the right ear points is not well defined. Beside ear-acupuncture, there are other special techniques like scalp needling or hand-acupuncture. Doctors who apply these methods are not members of the "Deutsche Arztegesellschaft für Akupunktur" which can be called the most important and traditional medical association since 1952. With the journal "Akupunktur in Theorie und Praxis", (Medizinisch Literarische Verglagsges. Uelzen, Potsfach 1151, D-29501) it has, for decades, been the catalyst, responsible for much correspondence and feed back among professionals. These include official and obstinate matters, brilliant and minor ideas out of the spirit of European medicine permeated into the Chinese world of thought and vice versa. However, nowadays the journal publishes largely uninspired considerations of the statistical relevance of acupuncture methods. Slowly, however, this important and professional group has begun to realise that the use of CM herbal therapy is much more the pillar of Chinese medicine.

The emergence of Qi Gong and related aspects of Chinese medicine
At the end of the "Cultural Revolution" in China, during the 1970's, a new mass movement has developed. In public and in large circles in China, people practised *Taijiquan* and *Qi Gong* in the parks. It became an official subject in the universities and schools. This mass movement also met with a response among the German public. From this time on, *Qi Gong* has been offered by different societies and is also taught at adult education centres and propagated by the health insurance companies as a prophylactic measure. There was also a programme on television, going out once a week, in which the viewer can simultaneously take part. Apart from the usual mystery of everything coming from the Far East there were serious theoretical reports on the television programmes, explaining Taijiquan and Qi Gong from the Chinese culture. It was, to a large extent, the Bonn Society (Medizinische Gesellschaft für Qi Gong Yangsheng, Herwarth-Str.21, D-53115 Bonn) influenced by Professor Jiao Guorui (1992) who, unfortunately killed in an accident in 1997, did much to enlighten the public introducing some essential terms relating to energy meditation to the public.

There is presently, a large circle of practitioners, psychotherapists, doctors, physiotherapists, and non-medical practitioners, teachers and nurses who work with either *Qi Gong* or *Taijiquan*. Long before this time, however, Stephan Palos and another forerunner of Chinese medicine in Germany, Erich Stiefvater, had referred to breathe and energy meditation. Many will remember Josephine Zoller who, for many years, had worked alone in this field (1991). Further academic influences came to Germany via Sri Lanka. Many young researchers went to a Clinic in Colombo, Sri Lanka, in order to study the practice of acupuncture there. The Indian lady, Radha Thambirajah, who was teaching there and is living in England presently, introduced many generations of young German students to Chinese medicine at her Academy of Clinic Acupuncture (The Willow Clinic, 105 Short Heath Road, Erdington, Birmingham, B23 6LH, England). Andreus Noll (Arbeitsgemeinschaft fur Klassische Akupunktur und TCM, in D-12205 Berlin) also contributed much, especially to homeopaths. He succeeded mainly in engaging English-speaking therapists, such as J. Ross, G. Maciocia, B. Flaws and B. Kirschbaum, as experts.

Thus, English literature also found its way into therapeutic everyday life. It was mainly the standard works of Maciocia, the acupuncture works of J. Ross and "The Formulas and Strategies" of Berolet and Bensky that outstripped the classics dominating in this field. Above all, they are characterised by their integration of the psychosomatic of J. Ross into acupuncture, making possible a colloquial access to the Chinese original literature. In comparison, the immensely diligent and broadly constructed work of Porkert seems monolithically accepted in the field of acupuncture, medicinal herbs, diagnostic or fundamental research.

Meanwhile, CM has also developed further in other directions. The "pressure or pushing massage", *Tuina*, is increasingly used therapeutically. It is mainly Dr. A. Meng (1991) from Vienna who spread therapeutic standards in this field. In order to have original and direct access to the knowledge of the People's Republic of China, different societies organise study trips to major cities in China. Under the good cultural and political conditions that existed in the 1980's several important institutions were founded. Based on the Munich model, the "Erste deutsche Klinik für TCM", Ludwigstr. 2, D-92444 Kötzting" was founded in 1989. This is the TCM Klinic in Kötzting which is the very first Chinese medicine hospital founded in Germany. This project has enabled the Chinese scientists and practitioners to travel to Germany much more easily. Thus through the extension of trading relations, the possibilities of CM therapy were improved. (A fuller account of the TCM Klinic in Kötzting is given is Chapter 5).

The position of Chinese herbal medicine
Gradually, Chinese herbs have become available in pharmacies in Germany. The official Pharmacist Chambers have to fix purity regulations regarding the issue of a Quality Control Certificate of limiting pesticides and heavy metal pollution on the crude materials imported to Germany according to the Commission E guidelines. Besides treatment with the crude herbal materials, (these are the classically prepared, Chinese medicinal plant parts, minerals and animal parts), granules of these are also used. These are mainly imported from Taiwanese herbal manufacturers as medicinal herbal decoction extracted granules. These are ready-made herbal combination of herbal ingredients boiled according to Pharmacopoeia guidelines; the extract is then granulated and drawn up with a thickening agent and then sold as an easily drinkable powder to the United States of America and Europe. Some of the Taiwanese manufacturers also supply granules of decoction combinations of the Japanese Kampo medicinal herbal products. (Chapter 14 gives further details of Kampo medicine that is a modified Chinese medicine practised in Japan.). There was massive ideological discussion in Germany, especially concerning the use of Chinese medicinal herbs and

their composite formulae or prescriptions. For instance, the Societas Medicinae Sinensis under the leadership of Porkert very frequently accepted the original CHM composite formula or recipes as the basis for treatment of diseases. Their theoretical transactions have been based on long history of use and recorded in the Chinese Pharmacopoeia. However another group under the leadership of Fritz Friedl, a TCM doctor from Wasserburg-Reithmering, has begun to break loose of this rigid concept and have developed their own combinations based on the old recipes. A mailbox network of therapists, called DECA, has developed steadily using the Internet as the medium of discussions over such development.

The use of Chinese medicinal herbs as dietetics
Apart from medicinal herb therapy, dietetics is also slowly finding its way into the therapeutic standards of the TCM doctors. In the beginning, there was only a rough idea of how dietetics could be used for prevention and treatment of diseases. However, the original Chinese literature quoted in the ancient medical works has been sifted through and worked out that practical translations of functional food from CHM sources were made. The voluminous textbook on this area by Engelhardt und Hempen (1997) was published. However, this book lacks practical application. Subsequently the use of CHM materials as functional food for the practical side of traditional cooking for every day needs of working people was published (Kunkel, 1997). Chapter 3 of this book gives an account on this topic.

The standard and qualification of Chinese medicine practitioners in Germany and their training
The teaching of CM in Germany varies immensely in regard to quality and its main focuses. Whereas the "Deutsche Ärztegesellschaft für Akupunktur" mainly teaches acupuncture and lately, as a side-subject, also offers courses in Chinese Herbalism. Recently an important non-medical practitioners' association, the "Arbeitsgemeinschaft für Klassische Akupunktur und TCM" has probably become the most complete academic base in Germany. The elitist association the "Societas Medicinae Sinensis" offers its extensive education only to OM doctors. The members, having passed the examination, are sparsely spread throughout Germany. The Kötzting TCM Klinic near Munich has offered training courses for CM to OM practitioners too.

The German public has to tolerate and face the difficulty of choosing which CM practitioners would be "properly" qualified or trained. This is due to the confusion consequential to the lack of an official designation of CM therapists whom should be able to offer various aspects of CM treatments such as acupuncture, CM herbalism, CM nutritional regime, *Qi Gong*, and *Tuina* etc. As the associations do not recognise each other, or agree to a basic standard of practice, it is, obviously, impossible have a rational control over professionalism, in spite of all the professional competence that has been acquired. Each association is trying hard to be accepted by the therapists as the only official institution for representation of their welfare and professionalism. A co-operation with the non-medical practitioners and other therapists by the OM doctors with CM therapy skill is out of the question at present in Germany. This results in a colourful, but, not uninteresting, patchwork of herbalists or acupuncturists. In general Germany is far from a licence system in this aspect, as is found positively acted on in the United States of America. Personal qualifications are achieved through self-education and during weekend seminars. A knowledge of the Chinese culture and the language or, even, of the country, is not absolutely necessary. One major handicap for spreading CM in Germany is that the discipline is not taught at university institutes. The only hospital with a clinical TCM education in Germany is the Anthroposophic Clinic Witten-Herdecke 25l.

Presently various Chairs of nature healing have been appointed in universities in Germany. Of these professorships of TCM should also be considered. Unfortunately if these are offered they may be put up with the not very experienced, young and unsecured disciplines such as the homoeopathy or, the anthroposophic medicine, as well as modern phytotherapy. There are also the non-medically qualified Sinologists who lecture privately and disseminate their knowledge. Therefore, such training and education system of TCM can hardly be conveyed to a German OM doctor as a desirable professional course, simply because of the confused education that is offered at the present time.

The ideological difference between the orthodox medicine and so-called alternative therapies has become even more emphasised during the past few years. The hardening of attitudes has become so strong that an agreement seems impossible. Apart from the massive economic interests of in some of the OM practices, it is also the pharmaceutical industry to a large extent, that wants to prevent changes in therapeutic strategies within the German health service. As most illnesses are treated with the help of chemically produced medicines, specifically in Germany, other medicines using natural remedies would be considered as dangerous competition for the pharmaceutical industry. Thus, it is understandable that the OM doctors restrict themselves to their scientific knowledge and deny TCM a separate scientific character.

As a result, there is very little communication opportunity between the practitioners of OM and CM. The medical insurance companies take pleasure in coming to the conclusion that they do not, or, only exceptionally, bear the costs of the TCM therapies. There is, however, a Supreme Court decision concerning the possibility of reimbursement for unconventional cures being fulfilled, if there is no therapeutic approach of orthodox medicine or if all the possibilities of orthodox medicine have been exhausted in an individual case. Again and again, medical insurance companies succeed in refusing their financial support in individual cases. The fact that therapists are not organised and do not have a uniform standard of education in this respect comes in very useful on the side of the conventional OM doctors and medical insurance companies as well as for the pharmaceutical industry.

Future Directions for Progress of Chinese Medicine in Europe

FROM BELGIUM: AN APOCALYPSE NOW OR LATER?

Is there a future for Chinese medicine (CM) in Belgium? Could it happen to other European partners? Will the future happen before or after an apocalypse? In China, CM is making tremendous advances in the treatment of chronic and recalcitrant diseases because there is mutual integration of orthodox medicine into the Chinese medicine. She is preparing the road to a new medicine of the future.

Unfortunately, this positive reputation for the Chinese medicine refound to China's credit is being rapidly tarnished by some unscrupulous organisations. They are collaborating for personal gains to offer dubious diplomas and certificates of acupuncture and Chinese herbal medicine to Westerners and Chinese alike who have had inadequate Chinese medicine education. For whatever reasons these certificates or diplomas are sold, and CM will suffer most from long lasting damage, if and when the public is harmed from receiving treatments from these inadequately prepared persons. Today, many such agencies are set up overseas.

There is a gap growing between Western practitioners of Chinese medicine and Chinese medicine in China. Westerners find it difficult to study true Chinese medicine for a variety of reasons such as hasty fashions and inadequate course design and language difficulties. Given this perception, China is taking the simplistic and economic solution to resolve the growing demands for the Chinese medicine beyond her shores.

It is the author's belief that this growing gulf will affect the future of Chinese medicine in Belgium. Even though it is only a wish on the author's part, it is not too much to hope that:

- The future of the Chinese medicine is rooted in and informed by its traditions;
- The confrontation of knowledge of these old traditions with a modern spirit of scientific creativity could be a powerful catalyst of development and progress;
- Intercultural, inter-professional and inter-personal respects are an essential conditions for a profitable and peaceful dialogue in order to help both Chinese medicine and orthodox medicine to coexist and complement each other to benefit the patients;
- Those who have the power could lead the way and leave a legacy for future generations to remember that their health was secured beyond any price.

FROM GERMANY: CAN CHINESE MEDICINE BE ACCEPTED?

It is against a sceptical and believing background that the private disputes between Prof. M. Porkert and Prof. P. Unschuld have to be considered. Unschuld (1980), a former pharmacologist, who later devoted himself to Sinologist research claims that what is nowadays called "TCM" cannot be a homogeneous field at all. He is also of the opinion that there is no comprehensible, uniform TCM at all, but, that it is historically an extremely varied and incoherent creation calling itself "Chinese Medicine" with a changing focusing. Unschuld claims that this historical incoherence is not a reliable indication for a scientifically unanimous creation for any European scientific standards. Porkert objects to this assertion. He considers, with undisputed and unanimous opinion among other experts, that Chinese medicine has the background and recorded historical knowledge and experience, supported by the classical Chinese texts. These are available to us for consideration and assessment, from whatever different epoch they may date. They, at least, show so much uniformity on the basis that we may fall back upon them as uniform ideas. Porkert produced his textbooks from tireless translations of the classics. Rightly, he points out that the theoretical bases of TCM over the centuries remained homogeneous in the core, in spite of so many influential changes in China politically, socially and economically. The sustaining practice of Chinese medicine along side with orthodox medicine in China since 1950s can be seen as an historically valid basis for the various theoretical and practical approaches for looking after the healthcare of her people in the most populous country of the world.

Thus, it can be stated that the Chinese medicine has been handed down in writing for more than 2000 years, complete and like no other medicine of this world. However, Unschuld's opinion is likely to attract extreme support from official sources. It helps the OM professional associations in Germany with their arguments that Chinese medicine can only be certified as a practice with a lack of scientific character and incoherence. Generally, Chinese medicine in Germany is considered as a medical care evolved from "the colourful picture of a non-standardised education" which is supplemented with increasing qualification of the therapists via improved knowledge, standard and supply of education from translation. An acceptance of the public develops mainly against the background of the economic measures within the health service.

As the medical insurance companies no longer accept various costs anyway, one turns to a solid, but the useful treatment given by private doctors. The media increasingly report about various branches of the Chinese medicine. Furthermore, the great economic connections with the People's Republic of China facilitate a larger exchange of professional personnel. In spite of all the provincial principals there is a future perspective for the Chinese medicine in Germany. The German Sinology has made a serious, fundamental contribution to the dissemination of Chinese medicine outside of China. This cannot be appreciated enough against the background of an Anglophone dominated world public.

FROM HOLLAND: IS THE CHALLENGE TOO BIG?

By and large the scientific community in the Netherlands is still sceptical about TCM even the interest is high, particularly with certain effective Chinese herbs. In the University of Groningen, a research project to produce artemisinin (qinghaosu), a potent anti-malarial agent against anti-multi-resistant malaria parasites isolated from the Chinese herb "Qing Hao" or Artemisia annua, through plant tissue culture and through this technique to select high artemisinin yielding plants with the aim of reaching optimal artemisinin contents in *A. annua* plants for an economically feasible production of artemisinin-related anti-malarial is under way. Sterilised seeds of *A. annua* were germinated on agar plates in the laboratory and subsequently the small plant-lets were analysed for their artemisinin content. Plant-lets (young shoots) with an artemisinin content higher than 0.2% were transferred to the open, in an experimental field in The Netherlands. The artemisinin content of the individual plants was followed during their development. It was found to be maximal just before flowering, in mid-September. More than 50% of the plants that were selected on a high artemisinin content in the laboratory, also yielded plants with a high content in the field. Some individual plants contained three times more artemisinin as compared with plants that were grown in the open without selection (Woerdenbag *et al.*, 1994).

Another Chinese herb, "Feng Wei Cao" or *Pteris multifida*, has also been investigated in the same laboratory for anti-neoplastic activities. Two diterpenes, ent-kaurane-2b, 16a-diol and ent-kaur-16-ene-2b, 15a-diol, have been isolated. Both compounds showed a moderate cytotoxicity to Ehrlich ascites tumour cells (Woerdenbag *et al.*, 1996).

The effect of Chinese herbal medicine against atopic eczema also attracted attention from dermatologists of the Groningen University Hospital. They evaluated the effectiveness of Chinese herbal remedy against constitutional eczema (Stam-Westerveld and Coenraads, 1995).

To promote TCM, as a valuable tool in modern healthcare requires a close co-operation between Western physiological and medical scientists and scientifically trained experts who are knowledgeable about Chinese medicine and related fields. And even then, there will be many great challenges to be faced in various aspects such as cultural, philosophical, linguistic, and psychological gap between the two.

Comments from the Editors

One of the Editors has combined 3 contributions from our colleagues in Europe into one chapter using the Editors' privilege. However the authors' original intention and ideas have not been altered at all. All their efforts have been grouped together in a coherent way such that readers would find the text more fluent and easy to follow. During the editing stage we have discovered so much similarities for the development of CM in Europe. Together with the picture in UK (please refer to Chapter 16) a similar picture can be painted:

- The historical introduction of CM has been amazingly but not surprisingly similar. The introduction of acupuncture, one part of Chinese medicine, dominated the scene since the 16 century when European exploration started towards the East. The gradual modification and specialisation of regional acupuncture have actually altered the traditional concepts of CM. The biomedical and physiological changes measurable by OM technology helped to convince OM practice that acupuncture actually works. However those who do not have a OM-medically qualified degree are not accepted as professionals to practise acupuncture. Hence there are 3 different types of acupuncturists in almost of these 4 countries in Europe.

- An identical problem has been pointing towards the training and education systems of the CM practitioners and acupuncturists in these 4 countries. On the one hand there are "cowboy" practitioners whose practice actually damaged the name and practice of CM as well as the patients' health. This does not help to gain confidence from the OM colleagues. The length and extent of training and education is also varied as can be observed from the part-time courses run in all 4 contributions. Some practitioners travelled to China to do short-courses that may not be truly helpful as some institutes in China are not offering proper training but charging fee as a business. Such acts have been recently eliminated and sanctioned in the future by the order of the State Administration of TCM in China.

- It is also interestingly, worryingly and annoyingly to observe that the poor quality of Chinese herbal medicinal (CHM) products appearing in the European market does not help to give confidence to Chinese herbal treatment. Regulation is indeed needed to stamp out "cowboy" practice. Unfortunately due to the lack of expertise even good CHM herbs are banned for use as reported in Belgium. The safety of patients is of paramount importance. All OM drugs are poisonous and dangerous if not controlled or prescribed by people who know their jobs. The information pointed out in Chapter 4 on poisonous CHM products have been substantiated by information from the European colleagues of this chapter. Proper regulations for the use and prescribing of CM herbal products are needed and should be drafted together with inputs from CM professionals.

- An open-mind is needed for all professionals who work in the healthcare systems of all countries where the use of complementary medicine is increasing. Patients are more informed than most doctors nowadays due to the Internet. They also have the right to choose. Enough evidence had shown that some diseases that are resistant to OM treatment can be helped by Chinese medicine (See data at the TCM Klinic Kotzting, Chapter 5). An ideal situation will be that OM and CM practitioners, scientists and professionals should work together for the benefit of the patients.

References

Bachmann, G. (1980) "Die Akupunktur-eine Ordnungstherapie", Haug Vlg., Heidelberg, 3. Aufl.

Bensky, D. and Gamble, A. (1986) Chinese herbal medicine-materia medica, Eastland Press, Seattle.

Bischko, J. (1971) "Akupunktür für Anfénger", Haug Vlg., Heidelberg

Chamfrault, A. (1957) "Traitä de Medicine Chinoise", Angoulême

De Kram, M.C.T.F.M., Roreas, A.M.H.P., Hardy, E.L.M. (1994) Mangaanintoxicatie door het gebruik van Chien Pu Wan tabletten. *Nederlands Tijdschrift voor Geneeskunde*, **138**, 2010–2012.

Dela Fuye, R. and Schmidt, H. (1952) "Die moderne Akupunktur" Hippokrates Vlg., Stuttgart

Engelhardt/Hempen (1997) "Chinesische Diatetik" Urban & Schwarzenberg, Munchen

Ernst Kluger (1979) "Die traditionelle klassische Akupunktur in der täglichen Praxis", Druckerei Thierbach, Muhlheim a.d. Ruhr

Fratkin (1986): Chinese herbal formula—a practical guide, Institute for TCM and Preventive Health Care, Portland.

Finckh, E., "Grundlagen tibetischer Heilkunde, Vol. I+II, (1975/1986) "Der tibetische Medizin-Baum", 1990; all Vol. at Medizinisch Literarische Verlagsges., Uelzen

Fisch, G. (1973) "Akupunktur", DVA, Stuttgart

Goldmann, H.R. (1991) 1991 "Franz Hübotter, ein Berliner Arzt zwischen Ost und West", Dissertation v, FU Berlin

Hong, Y.S., Huang, Y.L., Wang, Y.J. (1965) Overdose of Mutong caused a death due to renal failure. *Zhejiang Journal of Traditional Chinese Medicine*, **8**, 415.

Hübotter Franz (1929) "Die Chinesische Medizin zu Beginn des XX. Jahrh. und ihr historischer Entwicklungsgang" Asia Major-Vlg., Leipzig

Jiao Guorui (1992) "Das Spiel der 5 Tiere", Medizinisch Literarische Verlagsges. Uelzen

Kunkel, Ch (1997) "Die chinesische 5-Elemente-Ernahrung", Falken Vlg.

Levi, M., Guchelaar, H.-J., Woerdenbag, H.J., Zhu, Y.-P. (1998) Acute hepatitis in a patient using a Chinese herbal tea—a case report. *Pharmacy World & Science*, **20**, 43–44.

Malak, J. (1998) Chinese herb nephropathy is not a (dex-)fenfluramine nephropathy but a serotonin nephropathy. *The Journal of Alternative and Complementary Medicine*, **4**, 131–135.

Meng, A. (1991) "Lehrbuch der traditionellen chinesischen Massage, Tuina-Therapie", Haug Vlg, Heidelberg, 3. Aufl

Nguyen Van Nghi (1974) "Pathogenese und Pathologie der Energie in der chinesischen Medizin" 2 Vol., 1974, Medizinisch Literarische Verlagsges., Uelzen

Nogier, P. (1969) "Introduction practique a l'auriculotherapie", Maisonneuve

Noll, A. Arbeitsgemeinschaft für Klassische Akupunktur und TCM; D-12205 Berlin.

Palos, S. (1980) "Atem und Meditation", Barth Vlg., 2. Aufl

Porkert, M. (1973) "Die theoretischen Grundlagen der Chinesischen Medizin" F. Steiner Vlg. Wiesbaden

Porkert, M. "Chinesische Medizin", 4 Vol p.a., Urban & Vogel, Lindwurmstr. 95, D-80337 Munchen

Stam-Westerveld, E.B., Coenraads, P.J. (1995) Constitutioneel eczema: behandeling met traditional Chinese medicine. Wetenschappelijk Deel van de 272e Vergadering van de Nederlandse Vereniging voor Dermatologie en Venereologie, 20–22.

Test Anskoop (1991) Survey on alternative complementary medicine in Belgium, No. 336, September 1991.

The Belgian law on production and the commerce of food products containing or made of plants or plant preparations, 29 August 1997.

Unschuld, P. (1980) "Medizinin in China", BeckVlg., München

Vanherweghem, J.-L., Depierreux, M., Tielemans, C., Abramowicz, D., Dratwa, M., Jadoul, M., Richard, C., *et al.* (1993) Rapidly progressive interstitial renal fibrosis in young women: association with slimming regimen including Chinese herbs. *The Lancet*, **341**, 387–391.

Woerdenbag, H.J., Lutke, L.R., Bos, R., Stevens, J.F., Hulst, R., Kruizinga, W.H., Zhu, Y.-P., *et al.* (1996) Isolation of two cytotoxic diterpenes from the fern Pteris multifida. *Zeitschrift fur Naturforschung*, **51c**, 635–638.

Woerdenbag, H.J., Pras, N., van Uden, W., Wallaart, E., Beekman, A.C., Lugt, C.B. (1994) Progress in the research of artemisinin-related antimalarials: an update. *Pharmcy World & Science*, **16**, 169–180.

Wu, S.H. (1964) Two cases of acute renal failure due to ingestion of large doses of Mu Tong. *Jiangsu Journal of Traditional Chinese Medicine*, **10**, 12–13.

Zhu, Y.P. (1998) Chinese Materia Medica: Chemistry, Pharmacology and Applications, pp. 256–262, 325–327, 379–383. Amsterdam: Harwood Academic Publishers.

Zoller, J. (1991) "Das Tao der Selbstheilung", Ullstein Vlg. Berlin, 4. Aufl.

13 THE PROGRESS OF CHINESE MEDICINE IN HONG KONG SAR, CHINA

Kelvin Chan
Hin-Wing Yeung

Historical Development of Chinese Medicine in Hong Kong SAR

GENERAL INTRODUCTION

Hong Kong Special Administrative Region (SAR) had been a British colony for more than one and a half centuries until July 1997. Over 90% of Hong Kong residents are of Chinese origin and have maintained very close economic and cultural relations with Mainland China throughout her colonial history. In the past decades, Hong Kong has been one of the three most influential regional communities in terms of economical and technological development and growth (the other two are Mainland China and Taiwan) in the world.

Chinese medicine (CM) as an integral part of the Chinese culture has been widely used within the Hong Kong Chinese community for a long time despite the fact that western orthodox medicine (OM) is the main stream in use. Hong Kong is also an important trade centre of Chinese herbal medicinal (CHM) materials due to her close economic relationship with China and Chinese communities overseas. China is the main producer and exporter of CMM and Hong Kong is the most important first destination of this export trade. The open policy of Mainland China since the 1980s has created many new trading channels. Direct export of CMM to Hong Kong in terms of weight, though declining, makes up around 30% of Chinese medicinal products (including both CMM and ready-made CM products (See Table 13.1).

Early British government policy makers in Hong Kong did not consider the practice of Chinese medicine as part of the healthcare provided to the public. Although CM has been widely used by the public in Hong Kong on an unofficial basis, regulating departments disregard the profession and the industry. CM practitioners, including CM physicians (Zhong Yi Shi), bonesetters and acupuncturists etc. were not

Table 13.1 Chinese Materia Medica (CMM) exported to Hong Kong (Jia Qian, 1998)

	CMM To HK in tonnes	Total CMM in tonnes	%	CM products To HK In US$mill.	Total CMM In US$mill.	%
1991	55.9	111.6	50	13.1	36.8	36
1992	48.7	123.4	39	14.0	41.1	34
1993	51.3	128.7	40	11.2	39.0	29
1994	47.4	261.5	18	20.3	65.1	31
1995	41.9	228.9	18	19.8	65.5	30

required to register as health care professionals. A business registration was good enough for anybody to practise CM in Hong Kong. Trading of CMM and related medicinal products were not regulated; only those ready-made CM products in conventional dosage forms similar to OM pharmaceutical products are regulated. However, the control was limited to merely screening for adulteration with OM drugs.

CHANGES OF GOVERNMENT POLICY

In general, traditional medicine is widely practised by various ethnic groups all over the world. The World Health Organisation (WHO) has long supported its development. In May 1977, a resolution of the 30th World Health Assembly was adopted urging "Interested governments to give adequate importance to the utilisation their traditional systems of medicine and to incorporate them into their own national health systems" (WHO, 1985). However, the progress of development of CM in Hong Kong (compared with that in Mainland China and Taiwan, see appropriate chapters for comparison) has been slow and without government participation throughout the 70's and 80's.

There was a drastic change in government policies upon the signing of the "Joint Declaration" between the UK and China. Article 138 of Basic Law states that the Government of the Hong Kong Special Administration Region shall, on its own, formulate policies to develop western and traditional Chinese medicine and to improve medical and health services for the population in Hong Kong.

The Hong Kong government started to review the situation 5 years after the beginning of the transition period. In August 1989, the

Secretary for Health and Welfare of Hong Kong appointed the "Working Party on Chinese Medicine" (WPCM), chaired by Deputy Secretary for Health and Welfare, to review and make recommendations on the use and practice of traditional Chinese medicine (TCM) in Hong Kong. A report was published on Oct 1994 recommending that the government should set up a preparatory committee consisting principally of members of the CM profession. This committee, the Preparatory Committee on Chinese Medicine, would advise on future legislation for the promotion, development and regulation of CM.

The "Preparatory Committee on Chinese Medicine" was then established in April 1995 and a report was published in March 1997. The committee proposed to establish the "Traditional Chinese Medicine Council" to administer CM practitioner and Chinese medicinal products

The government published a "Consultation Document on Development of Traditional Chinese Medicine" in November 1997. It proposed that registration of both CM practitioners and CM products be started by 2000.

THE CHINESE MEDICINE PROFESSION

Over 60% of the Hong Kong population have, at least once, consulted a CM practitioner (CMMRC, 1991). An even higher proportion of Hong Kong people regularly include herbal soup with CMM (see Chapter 17 for more information on the topic), herbal tea and herbal tonic food in their normal diet. Popular newspapers and magazines usually have columns inviting CM practitioners to answer questions posted by readers. CM prescription formulae are easily given solely based on the written information provided by readers.

There has been no reliable information about the size of CM profession until the Preparatory Committee on Chinese Medicine recorded that 6890 (of which 66% working full-time) were active CM practitioners in 1996. Among which, 63% are predominantly general practitioners (Zhong Yi Shi), 23% bonesetters (Gu Shang Ke Yi Shi), 7% acupuncturists (Zhen Jiu Yi Shi) and 7% do not take CM practice as their principal occupation. This list will be the basis of subsequent registration as proposed by the Committee. About 60% of all the practitioners work in clinics and 19% are hired by CMM shops. The conditions are usually unsatisfactory for CM practice in CMM shops. Space is limited and the surrounding is noisy.

In general, local residents seldom regard bonesetters as "Chinese Medicine Practitioners", however patients take their service as an alternative to OM osteopathy in treating even serious bone fracture. Resistance does exist among OM orthropaedic surgeons and CM bonesetters.

About 50% of the 4315 Chinese medicine-general practitioners (CM-GPs) recorded that they had received post-secondary education; 48% were trained in CM schools (full-time or part-time) and 43% via apprenticeship.

As compared with CM-GP's, bonesetters received less educational training and the majority of them were trained through apprenticeship (77%). Only 19% had post-secondary education.

About 60% of the 473 acupuncturists had received post-secondary education; some 46% were trained in CM schools and 33% by apprenticeship. The rest of the 20% received some other form of training including self-learning.

In Hong Kong the CM-GPs use primarily Fu Fang (composite formulae of CMM) and crude CMM as the mainstream of their practice, though most of them had received training in acupuncture. (Ko, 2000)

STATUS OF ACUPUNCTURE (*ZHEN JIU*) WITHIN CHINESE MEDICINE IN HONG KONG: A COMPARISON WITH WESTERN CONCEPTS

In the west, practice of acupuncture is better received than that of Chinese herbal medicine (CHM). A survey in Australia (Bensoussan, Myers, 1996) showed that 54% of CM practitioners practise predominately acupuncture, while only 3% practice predominately used CHM (while 28% combined both CHM and acupuncture). Over half of the Australian CM practitioners surveyed seldom used crude/prepared Chinese medicine to treat patients. In the west, consumers and academics are in general not familiar with CM theory. Since practice of acupuncture to treat certain symptoms may not require the application of holistic approach of CM, patients and consumers in the west often regard acupuncture as a physiotherapeutic technique and demonstrate much greater acceptance towards acupuncture. Several other chapters, describing CM in other countries and regions, in this section make similar observations.

In Hong Kong the CM-GPs use primarily Fu Fang (composite formulae of CMM) and crude CMM as the mainstream of their practice, though most of them had received training in acupuncture. *Zhen Jiu* (though commonly referred to as acupuncture, consisting of *Zhen* that is the act of acupuncture and *Jiu* is moxibustion) is not as often practised by CM-GPs in Hong Kong.

As CM is an integral part of Chinese culture, knowledge and belief from generation to generation are deep-rooted in Chinese communities. Coupling with own personal experiences, the publics in Chinese communities accept CM theory and practice more readily and are not as skeptical to Fu-fang as their counterpart in the west. In Hong Kong, *Zhen Jiu* is merely a supplement to Fu-fang treatment.

OTHER RELATED CHINESE MEDICINE TRADES

The majority of the Hong Kong Chinese come from the Guangdong province. With respect to culture of food and beverage, Cantonese style always prevails. Various kinds of soups with CMM (functional food, see Chapter 17) form an important part of the local Cantonese menu, many households may prepare these in their meals on a weekly basis. Local residents frequently intake CMM tonic soups (cold-resistant type, *Qi* nourishing type, and "blood" nourishing type etc.) in autumn and winter. A variety of packaged compound CMM formula for soups are available in the market.

Hong Kong is situated in the sub-tropical zone and climate is hot and humid. Therefore, "*Damp*" relieving soups and "*Heat*" relieving herbal teas are popular beverages all through the year. Some of the varieties are packed in aluminium cans and tetra-pack exactly the same way as ordinary soft drinks. There are lots of herbal teashops in Hong Kong selling herbal tea for curing and preventing common flu.

With some knowledge (whether correct or not) of CM, it is quite common for many Hong Kong residents purchasing over-the-counter ready made or proprietary CM products and CMM without CM practitioners' prescriptions and/or consultation. Most local CMM processors and proprietary CM manufacturers operate on small scale and relatively primitive techniques. Imported or locally manufactured proprietary or ready-made CM products are available from most pharmacies, drugstores and CMM shops.

There are approximately 1600 retail CMM shops in Hong Kong (WPCM, 1994). Experienced dispensers are short in supply. Dispensers have usually received little formal education or training and their working conditions are unsound, with long working hours, low salary and great responsibilities. Unlike pharmaceutical professionals of OM, CMM dispensers are responsible for identifying CMM, since the labelling of toxic/potent crude CMM is not regulated.

The Public Concerns of Chinese Medicine in Hong Kong

When comparing the rapid progress of CM in Hong Kong the progress of CM in other developed communities will help to focus how Hong Kong should respond to various concerns in terms of internationalisation and modernisation of CM. As Hong Kong has been developed over the past 150 years under British influence many of the public are still skeptical about the practice of CM, and all healthcare has been run by the OM system.

In the West the use of Chinese herbal medicines (CHM) is one of the most rapidly growing in popularity of the complementary and alternative medical disciplines of the English speaking western world (Sino-British, 1998). It is particularly utilised as the second tier of CM treatment by western acupuncturists who have learned how closely CHM and acupuncture are integrated into clinical practice of CM and with orthodox medicine in China. It is interested to observe, in the 1993 British Medical Association Report, that it is recommended more vigorous professionalism and regulation would be placed upon acupuncture and herbalism (being among the top 5 disciplines singled out from the report) in order to safe-guard patients' interests (BMA, 1993).

Apart from popularity, problems relating to the practice of CM become more apparent when this discipline is being utilised more by the public in the west. Adverse effects, ready-made CHM products containing undeclared orthodox drugs, poor standard of acupuncture procedures, supply of fake herbal substitutes and herbs not properly processed or detoxified were noted over the past decade. More appropriately, apart from quality issues of these mainly imported products, the issues on efficacy and safety of CM have not been addressed collectively.

The followings are general comments brought about by the public and healthcare professionals in the west, which are similar from some of the public in Hong Kong:

- What is known about the quality, safety and efficacy of the CMM used?
- Do CHM products have to pass through the same strict legislative procedures as pharmaceuticals?
- What is the level of education of practitioners of CM who diagnose and prescribe CM treatments?
- What do pharmacists and medical practitioners in the west know about acupuncture and CMM products and are they aware that their patients may be using a dual approach to health-care by indulging in OM and CM at the same time?
- Why are composite mixtures prescribed in CM prescriptions?
- How to obtain guaranteed good quality with efficacy-proven herbs and ready-made CHM products?

The public and OM healthcare professionals in Hong Kong who are either skeptical or not familiar with the practice of CM also commonly pose these questions to the authorities. In order to provide evidence-based services attention should be paid towards development of these services with approaches measurable by scientific protocols that are recognised by modern concepts. CM has been an experience-based practice utilised by our ancestors over 3 to 4 thousand years. Thus safety and efficacy of CM through experience rather than modern-scientific measurements have been observed. Re-assurance is needed to convince and give confidence to the evidence-based demands.

Training and Education of Chinese Medicine in Hong Kong

Hong Kong Government did not include CM education into her public education system until the late 90's and has not recognised CM training as any kind of professional qualification. Since there is no registration system for the CM practitioners and no regulation of CM practice, it is a natural consequence that there is no system of accrediting CM courses or schools at all.

TRAINING OF CHINESE MEDICINE IN THE 1950s

Private schools have been offering part-time (mainly evening and/or week-end) courses of very different formats, ranging from short interest courses to better structured under-graduate and post-graduate courses (qualifications not recognised by government) that last for several years. Qualified CM professionals from Mainland China set up some of these private schools since the early 1950s. Both the authors were invited as honoured quests on separate occasions to preside at the graduate ceremonies of a well-known private school in Hong Kong Island. Students attending there also include OM graduates and practitioners. Some of these graduates are well qualified to train future professionals in the integrated practice of OM and CM. More than half of the active CM practitioners recorded recently (PCCM, 1996) claimed that they had received their training in Hong Kong. Representatives of CM profession recognised these courses as "making a valuable contribution to training of practitioners" (WPCM, 1994).

THE TRAINING OF CHINESE MEDICINE IN THE 1990s

Public funded tertiary institutions did not involve themselves in CM education or training until the early 90's. Currently 3 universities are offering part-time certificate type short courses, some of which are refreshing courses for practitioners.

The Chinese University of Hong Kong (CUHK)

In the early 1990s the Extramural School of the university offering continuous education to the public at large has been responsible for setting up part-time programmes on Chinese Medicine. The university has scheduled to open a 4-year degree course of Bachelor of Chinese Medicine in the coming 1999/2000 academic year with first intake of 15 students. The course will involve service teaching from academics in universities of Chinese medicine.

The Hong Kong Baptist University (HKBU)

The university has developed a full-time Bachelor of Science (Honours) in Chinese Medicine programmes and admitted the first batch of 30 students since September 1998. It is the first recognised degree programme in Chinese medicine in Hong Kong by the funding organisation, University Grant Council. The programme, originally consists of 170 credit units amounting to 4214 contact hours (including clinical practice and internship), will be restructured to a dual degree programme of Bachelor of Chinese Medicine; and Bachelor of Science (Honours) in Biomedical Science (consists of 202 credit units). A full time degree course of 4 year duration on Chinese Medicines (BScCMS) will be launched in

September 2001 to provide future pharmacists in Chinese Medicinal materials.

The School of Continuing Education of HKBU has offered a 4-years part time Professional Diploma of Chinese Medicine course (1872 contact hours) since 1997. Upon completion, holder of the Professional Diploma may transfer to the degree course of Bachelor of Health Science (Chinese Medicine) offered by Royal Melbourne Institute of Technology in Australia (additional 117 contact hours). This course will be moved to the newly built School of Chinese Medicine in the very near future. The new school will house all the units of teaching and research. The research and development arm is the Institute for the Advancement of Chinese Medicine. This Institute, apart from the current R & D for the modernisation and industrialisation of CM, has also established post-graduate M. Phil and Ph.D. research degree programmes since Sept 1997.

The Hong Kong Jockey Club has arranged to donate HK$100 million to the HKBU for establishing a building to house the School of Chinese Medicine and all related units.

The University of Hong Kong

Since 1991 the university has been offering part-time programmes on Chinese Medicine. Currently, her School of Professional and Continuing Education (SPACE) offers a wide range of part-time courses covering the following areas: Chinese Medicine, Chinese Medicine Pharmaceutics, Acupuncture and Moxibustion, Chinese Medicine and Acupuncture (for western medicine practitioners), Continuing and Professional Development Courses for Chinese Medicine Practitioners, and Acupuncturists and Bonesetters. A 4-year Diploma of Traditional Chinese Medicine course was offered in 1997/98. The course was then changed to run by credit unit system and expandable to a 6-year Bachelor of Traditional Chinese Medicine degree course in 1998/99. Students may enroll either course depending on own qualifications and choice. Over 300 students have been enrolled on these two programmes.

On Chinese Medicine Pharmaceutics, a 3-year Diploma in Pharmaceutical Management in Chinese Medicine course and a 4.5-year Bachelor of Pharmacy in Chinese Medicine degree course have also been established. Two diploma course on acupuncture, namely, Diploma in Clinical Acupuncture (designed for western medicine practitioners) and Diploma in Acupuncture and Moxibustion (designed for existing CM practitioners) are available. A 2.5-year

Master of Traditional Chinese Medicine (Acupuncture and Moxibustion) course will be launched for degree holders of either Chinese medicine or orthodox medicine, or practitioners with recognized qualifications.

There is also a Diploma in TCM Orthopaedics and Traumatology course designed for practitioners.

Courses offered by SPACE of HKU are normally instructed in Chinese language while those primarily designed for orthodox medical practitioners may be taught in English.

It will be interesting and useful to compare the Degree Courses in Chinese Medicine offered in the 3 different universities. (Table 13.2).

It is encouraging that the present government has fully supported and recognised that the training and research development of CM are important procedures for the future modernisation and inter-nationalisation of CM along side with the promotion of the CM industry.

Research of Chinese Medicine in Hong Kong

The Hong Kong Government is now well prepared to take a more active role in the promotion and development of research programmes in various aspects of CM. The Government Laboratories which were previously only concerned with the screening of herbal medicinal products that contain OM drugs have been allocated resources to conduct research in CM for later regulation and registration of CMM and proprietary CM products.

Table 13.2 Comparison of general CM courses offered by the three universities

	CUHK	HKBU	HKU
Theory of Biomedical Science	32	65	42
Theory of Chinese Medicine	77	121	102
Clinical practice & Internship	40	40	46
General Subjects (non-medical)	17	16	0
Total Credit Unit	166	202	190
Course Duration (years)	4	5	6–9

The Preparatory Committee on Chinese Medicine proposed that at the present stage, research activities would be focused on ensuring the safety, quality and efficacy of the use of crude CMM and CM products. Priority of obtaining methodology and analytical assays will be given to areas such as identification of CMM to avoid adulteration, toxic ingredients in CMM, contents of heavy metal, residual pesticides and toxicity of proprietary. Others of equal importance will include quality assurance of proprietary CM products, their stability analysis and clinical research on the efficacy of CM products and research and development (R&D) of new formulations of proprietary CM.

The Committee also urges local pharmaceutical industry to collaborate and support CM research projects in tertiary institutes. The Hong Kong Government Industry Department has implemented several schemes for R & D of new technology. Research funds have been granted to 12 projects related to CM from 1995–1997, amounting to nearly HK$50m (Ip, 1998). Individual academics have started scientific researches on CM since the 1970's. Some of the units and centres have been established in various universities and institutes in Hong Kong.

THE CHINESE MEDICINAL MATERIAL RESEARCH CENTRE (CMMRC)

This centre is located at the Chinese University of Hong Kong (CUHK) and was established in 1979 to promote and facilitate multidisciplinary and interdisciplinary research on CM. The Centre aims to document and evaluate the efficacy of CM and to explore better application of TCM and upgrade the scientific contents of CM. Currently the Centre focuses on four major areas of research in the development of new products for diseases involved in the central nervous system, cardiovascular system, immunodulation, and on birth control. There are also researches working on cures for controlling AIDS, cancer and hepatitis.

THE BIOTECHNOLOGY RESEARCH INSTITUTE (BRI)

This Institute is situated at the Hong Kong University of Science and Technology (HKUST) was founded in 1990 with the mission to develop and train specialists in biotechnology for Hong Kong. One of the current major research areas is Chinese Medicine. The Institute has established a TCM Centre for Drug Development, Safety, Standardisation, and Reformulation to provide high-technology services to the industry, establish collaborative efforts between in Hong Kong and China.

THE INSTITUTE FOR THE ADVANCEMENT OF CHINESE MEDICINE (IACM)

The IACM at the Hong Kong Baptist University (HKBU) was established in 1997. The mission of the institute has been to:

- conduct scientific and industry/trade-related research on CM
- offer research-orientated postgraduate program to train high level personnel of CM
- establish links with relevant institutions all over the world for the advancement of CM
- promote public education on CM as a scientific and effective health care system, and
- provide support to undergraduate CM degree program of the university.

Other researches currently conducted include diseases of the aged population, socio-economic aspects of CM and application of scientific and strategic management in CM. The Quality Research Laboratory (QRL) of IACM focuses on Quality Assurance, Quality Control and Standardisation of CM products. One of the major techniques heavily utilised is LC/MS/MS (Liquid Chromatography/Mass Spectrometer/ Mass Spectrometer) for identification and authentication purposes. The QRL also performs contract R&D and testing services for private manufacturing and trading enterprises of CM. The Chinese Medicine Informatics Centre (CMIC) at the IACM was established to develop new techniques and application of information technology for CM researches. The Centre works on information base, pattern/finger-printing discovery, and data mining of CM and has already completed a Bibliographic Search System of CMM, an Information System for Toxic CMM.

RECENT REGIONAL ACTIVITIES INVOLVING CHINESE MEDICINE IN HONG KONG

The geographic position, established networks with China and bilingual capability of Hong Kong make her an excellent meeting point of CM experts for dialogue and sharing of research experiences and information. Several key activities along this line could be identified over the recent past years.

Department of Health of the Hong Kong Government hosted, with cosponsor, the World Health Organisation, a 3 day workshop on "Regional Workshop on Traditional Medicine" in November 1995. Over 60 health administrators, public health physicians, Chinese Medicine practitioners and traders, academics, researchers and pharmacists had presented papers. Discussion groups recommended that the role of traditional medicine should be recognised with policies and regulations for supported training of practitioners, research and development.

Two Workshops were co-organised, on 13 December 1995, by the Hong Kong Society for Traditional Medicine & Natural Products Research and Hong Kong Caritas (Ming-Ai) Centre, on "Quality Control & Legislation of TCM Products" and "The Practice and Use of TCM in the United Kingdom. The meeting actually began the launching of the first ever 5-year full-time degree course in TCM taught in English in Europe, offered by the Middlesex University in October 1997 (see Chapter 12).

A three-day Symposium on "Quality Assessment and Assurance of Chinese Herbal Medicines" was held at the Baptist University of Hong Kong on 27 to 29 June 1996.

A two-day International Symposium on "Chinese Medicine & Public Health" was held at the University of Hong Kong on 23 to 24 November 1996.

In Mar. 1998, the IACM of Hong Kong Baptist University hosted a 1-day conference on "Challenges of Quality Assurance/Quality Control (QA/QC) of Chinese Medicine in the 21st Century". Ten speakers including CMM Traders, Chinese and overseas academics, representatives from Consumer's Council delivered speeches reflecting concerns of QA/QC of CM from the perspective of CM personnel, regulating scientists and consumers.

An International Symposium on "The Worldwide Herbal Industry: Present And Future" was held in CUHK on July 1998. More than 30 academics, manufacturers, government officers of regulatory bodies, academics presented on topics such as development of herbal medicines and dietary supplements, relevant regulation and legal aspects, manufacture and marketing, quality controls and clinical researches.

The IACM of HKBU hosted a 3-day's conference on research of CM for their tripartite collaborative program with Tsinghua University and

Beijing University of Chinese Medicine and Pharmacology on Dec 1998.

A one-day International Symposium on "Hong Kong Can Be a Centre for the Continuing Development of Chinese Medicine" was co-sponsored by the Hong Kong Society for Traditional Medicine and Natural Products Research and Hong Kong Federation for Industry, on 23 January 1999.

On 17 to 19 May 1999, the IACM of HKBU and United States-China Intellectual Property Institute (USCIPI) organised a 3 day workshop on "Intellectual Properties and the Internationalization of Chinese Medicinal Products" with Federation of Hong Kong Industries. The Industrial Department of HKSAR Government supported the running of the workshop.

A 3-day duration of International Conference on "Chinese Medicine and Successful Aging" was recently held in June 2000 with collaboration of several CM institutions of China, Stanford University of USA and HKBU.

Regulations for Registrations of Practitioners and CHM Products

BEFORE SITUATIONS 1997

Hong Kong government, before 1997, exercised very limited control on the trade of crude Chinese herbal medicinal (CHM) and proprietary (ready-made) CHM products as compared with their counterpart in orthodox medicines. Related ordinances of Hong Kong can be summarised as follows:

Public health and municipal services ordinance (cap 132)

If any proprietary CM were found to be unfit for human consumption whether externally or internally or falsely labelled, traders involved would be prosecuted. The ordinance also empowered the Department of Health to seize those relevant drugs. There is no general exemption for CMM under this ordinance.

Pharmacy & poison ordinance (cap 138)

Traditional CMM are expressly exempted from registration under this ordinance. Pharmaceutical products of orthodox western medicine must register with the Pharmacy and Poisons Board before they can be sold in Hong Kong. However CMM listed in the *Ben Cao Gang Mu*; (本草岡目) and those CMM herbs customarily used by the CM from the open market are exempted from registration. The sale, manufacturing, dispensing or compounding of these CMM is not regulated by the ordinance. Department of Health officials conduct analyses to ensure that proprietary CM are not adulterated with components of western drugs or content other toxic ingredients such as unacceptable amount of heavy metal. This practice does not apply to raw or processed CMM.

Undesirable medical advertisements ordinance (cap 231)
The ordinance prohibits advertisement about any medicine, surgical appliance, treatment or prevention of a list of diseases specified. The restrictions apply to all medicines, whether Chinese or western. Such a control aims at protecting the public from being induced by such advertisements to seek treatment from unqualified persons or to resort to improper self-medication. CM practice itself is not bound by any legal commitment. Undesirable Medical Advertisements Ordinance is the only ordinance regulates certain CM practice.

Animal and plants (protection of endangered species) ordinance (cap 187)
Certain CMM traditionally used are of part of endangered species, such as bones of tigers and horn of rhinoceroses. Manufactured products of these species are strictly prohibited to trade. Use of some other endangered species for CMM requires license and registration.

Import and export ordinance (cap 60)
Proprietary CM products are currently subjected to licensing control for both import and export. License of a particular proprietary CM would be issued if there were no adulteration with any ingredients of western medicine found. Although CMM is not exempted in proprietary form, trading of raw or processed CMM do not need any license under this ordinance. Most CMM (properly processed) are mild in nature, however, some commonly used CMM are toxic or at least potent in their unprocessed raw form. These toxic/potent CMMs may require appropriate preparation and/or compound into CMM formula to neutralise their toxicity for human consumption.

Trade descriptions ordinance (cap 362)

Traders counterfeiting CMM may be prosecuted, this ordinance only treats CM products as other ordinary commodities and does not regulate them in the sense of pharmaceuticals.

PROPOSED FRAMEWORK FOR REGULATION OF CM PRACTITIONERS

Sharing with the experience from development of CM in China and current modes of regulation of other health service profession in Hong Kong, the government plans to set up a statutory administrative body tentatively called "Chinese Medicine Council". The Council will be responsible for promoting, developing and regulating CM, and to take up the overall administration of CM practitioners and CM products. Two committees, "CM Practitioners Committee" and "Chinese Medicine Committee" under the Council, will regulate the profession and the medicine industry respectively.

A list for active CM general practitioners was drawn up in 1996, which would be the basis for eventual registration. In the long run, all CM practitioners must register before being permitted to practise in the same way as other health service professions do. From 2000 onwards, to register as CM practitioner, applicants must have completed a degree course in CM (or equivalent qualification) recognised by Council and pass registration examination. However, there will be transitional arrangements for existing practitioners. Those practitioners who have practised CM for 15 years or more will be exempted from any registration examinations or assessments. With less than 15 years of practice, applicants may be exempted from registration examinations assessment if they have continuously practised for a certain period and pass a vetting assessment.

A disciplinary system will be set up to ensure professional conduct. The Council will draw up a Professional Code and Conduct. Those practitioners breach the Code will be subject to disciplinary action.

PROPOSED FRAMEWORK FOR REGULATION OF CM PRODUCTS

Regulation of a list of toxic/potent CMM is the starting point for controlling CMM products. Sale of toxic/potent CMM will be restricted to those patients having prescriptions from registered CM practitioners.

Processors, manufacturers and importers of CM products will be required to register under new licensing system. Registered premises will be regularly inspected by law enforcing departments for sanitary and health standards of premises, fittings and machinery and random sampling test of CM products. Registration of proprietary CM will be based on certificate of registration from place of origin, and/or guarantee of quality and safety from manufacturer or importer. Government will conduct test on samples submitted by traders and will also regulate labelling, adulteration and advertisement of CMM and CM product.

Government officials have estimated that it will take 2 years to register the entire 3200 proprietary CM currently on the local market, starting with those entering the market after Mar. 1999.

IMPLEMENTATION SCHEDULE

Regulation and registration will be implemented on a step by step basis, expected timetable for legislation and subsequent regulations are as follows:

- Legislation for establishment of TCM Council   1998/1999
- Legislation for regulation of CMM and
  registration of CM traders   1999/2000
- Registration of CM and regulation of CM trades   2000 onwards

When regulatory system is in operations, ways of regulation and registration of CM dispensers will then be examined.

Future Developments of Chinese Medicine in Hong Kong

THE INTENTION OF THE HONG KONG SAR GOVERNMENT

Orthodox medicine has been the mainstream of national health care service all over the world in the 20th century. However, acceptance of traditional medicine as an alternative choice to patients is growing. USA, the largest market for pharmaceutical products in the world, established the Office of Alternative Medicine in 1991 and introduced the Dietary Supplement Health and Education Act (DSHEA) in

1994. A booming market for alternative medicine has and will further be developed in a big way. The principles of CM stress on preventive measures and many common and popular CHM products are used as food (See Chapter 3). CHM products from the Chinese communities in Asia may take this golden opportunity to take a share of this blooming dietary supplement market, provided that manufacturers can cope with demand of quality products from the consumers overseas.

Past performance has demonstrated that the Hong Kong industry possesses good abilities to understand, interpret and satisfy the needs and preferences of very diversified national markets and customers. However, Hong Kong has to produce new generations of high-value-added goods to face the economic challenge of the 21st century. Consumers in both the developed countries and emerging economies seek assurance of quality, purity, reliability and brand reputation of the products they buy.

The potential and prospect of Hong Kong to manufacture service-enhanced CM products to meet the increasing acceptance of CM all over the world is attractive and encouraging. A MIT research team recently recommended the Hong Kong SAR government to develop a new CM industry (Berger, Lester, 1997), which aims at using CM as a base for new drug discovery leading to patent-protected products that will compete with orthodox drugs. The team concluded that Hong Kong has greater advantages to develop this new CM industry than other economies.

The MIT researchers suggested the Hong Kong SAR government should establish some form of regulatory agency similar to the US Food and Drug Administration. This agency could provide guarantees for CHM products handled or produced in Hong Kong. With a monitoring and assurance system to meet consumer demands, consumers all over the world are prepared to pay a premium price for this new breed of nutraceuticals and natural products.

To advance and develop the existing CM industry, the government, the industry, the profession and academic institutions should work closely together to strengthen technological capabilities of government. Scientific research, systematic standardisation, stringent quality assurance, public education, data mining and clinical testing are major areas to be tackled.

The Chief Executive of Hong Kong SAR had shown positive support to develop Hong Kong into an international centre of Chinese medicine in both practice and products (Tung, 1997 and

Tung 1998). He also disclosed that the government is considering establishing an Institute for Chinese Medicine that will focus on applied research to strengthen the scientific and technological base of Hong Kong and facilitate commercialization of medicinal products made by Hong Kong.

FOCUSES FOR FUTURE DEVELOPMENT OF CHINESE MEDICINE IN HONG KONG

In the recent Hospital Authority Convention-2000 hosted by the Hong Kong Hospital Authority, the first ever Special Plenary Session of Chinese Medicine was focused on how Chinese Medicine should be developed in Hong Kong (Chan, 2000). Some of the views can be sum-mariesd here for discussion:

Open-mindedness in the training and practice of OM and CM for better healthcare

Over 95% of the population of Hong Kong are of Chinese origin yet their ways of life have been under British influence over the past 150 years to such as extent that they are quite different from those in the Mainland.

For example, the well established degree in orthodox medicine (OM) that was established in early 1911 in a private medical school, that later became part of the University of Hong Kong, has trained many OM prac-titioners to serve the public in Hong Kong. However the launching of official training courses for CM in Hong Kong by the government is occurring nearly 80 years later. Inevitably there is skepticism and concern from OM practitioners in Hong Kong in accepting CM practice into medical care. The situation of CM practice in the Mainland and other regions such as that in Taiwan and Japan is quite different where the integrated or parallel practice of CM and OM has been officially implemented since the early 1950s. Concerns, misunderstanding, protect-ionism, skepticism, and suspicions, though in existence, have been put aside by co-practice experience or via regulatory means throughout the past 50 years. In Hong Kong the government's decision of regulating the qualification of CM practitioners and quality of treatment products has helped towards the right direction for the progress of CM. Nevertheless there is a need for open-mindedness in achieving the aims and objectives set up by the government's 10 year plan in launching CM as part of the healthcare and future industrial development. The followings can be discussed as possible steps to achieve open-mindedness and respectable CM practice.

- Once the competence, quality and evidence-based outcomes of CM treatments have been demonstrated and recognised professionally and legally there should be enough opportunity to work towards the common goal of quality service for patient care.
- Apart from the common Chinese cultural background shared between most of the OM and CM practitioners in Hong Kong initial understanding between the two different aspects of medical practice, can best be achieved by launching joint seminars, academic and professional meetings in order to build up the learning curves for collaboration.
- Educating the public on general healthcare issues should include both CM and OM aspects towards guidance on effects and safety of dual treatments. This will eliminate the misunderstanding and blame of either treatment when adverse effects arise during the treatment period.
- Academic and professional discussions can be focused on integrating advantages and avoiding disadvantages of medical treatment and prevention of certain themes of illnesses as a mission for giving the best possible patient care. Such examples can be found from the well-known Kotzting Chinese Medicine Hospital in Munich, Germany (See Chapter 5)
- With the common goal of assessing the efficacy of CM treatment, whether through acupuncture or using CHM products, the setting up of evidence-based clinical studies and control on quality, safety and efficacy of CM treatment is a good opportunity for encouraging open-mindedness.
- To achieve such evidence-based treatment studies, other scientific professionals related to both CM and OM practices will be needed to support various aspects involving patients monitoring, outcome measurements. These professionals may include biomedical scientists who are familiar with both disciplines, other paramedical supporting staff such as special nursing staff and pharmacists who can recognised CM terminology as well as medications, experts who can authenticate, identify and quantitate crude CM materials. There is a lack of such expertise not only in Hong Kong but also in other developed countries. Mainland China can provide some in-puts; however, their professionals may need to be re-orientated towards competitive overseas markets.

- Both CM and OM practice have their own documentation system for patient diagnosis and treatment. It will be most valuable for future actions that if and when integrated medicine is being practised a generalised reporting and documenting system can be derived such that progress of treatment and adverse reactions or interactions can be recorded.

- In desperate situations for the benefit of patient care and progress of medical science a concerted effort should be made towards targeting chronic diseases that are resistant to OM with either integrated CM and OM approaches or using CM to complement OM treatment. Several areas can be identified. Treatment of certain types of cancer can use CM composite herbal prescriptions to relieve side effects of cytotoxic drugs and help to improve the immuno-system that is weakened by cytotoxic drug treatment. In the prevention of bacterial resistance when orthodox antibiotics are compromised CM decoction can be co-administered. For myocardial infarction acupuncture, or CM decoctions with microcirculation activities are used in conjunction with orthodox beta-blocking agents. All these and other examples are cited (Chan & Cheung, 2000).

RESEARCH AND DEVELOPMENT ASPECTS

The need for modernisation in Chinese medicine

The practice of Chinese medicine, co-existing with orthodox medicine introduced in the early 1900s, in China has never been stopped throughout the history of the development of healthcare in China. However the improvement of this form of healthcare has not been keeping pace with the advance in science and technology and that of orthodox medicine. The recent increase of interests and concerns of CM practice in the west has indirectly hastened and induced the already planned national decision to implement the "Plan of Modernisation of Chinese medicine". Such decision has helped to cope with the increasing demand of good quality crude materials and finished products. The recent "Plan" proposed in general by 15 ministries in China, was led by the Ministry of Science and Technology, jointly with the Ministry of Health, the State Administration of Traditional Chinese Medicine (SATCM), the State Drug Administration (SDA), National Foundation Committee of Nature Science and so on.

The aims of the Plan have mainly been to modernise and internationalise various aspects of Chinese medicine based on inheriting and carrying forward the advantages and distinguishing features of the traditional system of healthcare. The Plan will fully utilise the methodology and measures of modern sciences, draw lessons and experiences from international standards and regulations on materia medica, in order to develop Chinese herbal products that can compete and enter the international medicinal markets. The Plan started in 1995 and aims to increase the share of the world market from the then 3% to 15% in 10 to 15 years' time. (See Chapter 20 for details).

A complete new approach in R & D is needed

Two levels of R & D on the progress of development of medicinal products from Chinese herbal materials can be identified.

Firstly, the local needs—To address local needs on herbal and other natural products that are used in CM treatment, it is our duty to ensure quality, efficacy and safety (QES) of these materials. We need to address the sources of CHM materials (Good Sourcing Practice, GSP) with guaranteed reference to the collection, identification and authentication of these medicinal materials that are prescribed by CM practitioners.

In order to safeguard the QES of these medicinal products from natural sources and avoid accidental poisoning by the public due to supply of wrong herbs and adulteration, commonly prescribed Fu-Fang and individual herbs can be supplied by reputable CM herbal manufacturers, as dried extracts or granules of the decoctions. R & D on the procedures for manufacturing these products are needed urgently to produce acceptable dosage forms for use in CM practice. This approach of using CHM products will help the development of regulation for registration of medications or health food manufactured from CHM crude materials.

There are several advantages of this approach.

- The granules produced can be QA-guaranteed with acceptable monographic details for identification and standardisation purposes.
- Such quality medicinal products can then be used for clinical trials with confidence comparable to those for OM pharmaceutical.
- Patients will no longer worry about preparing the decoction themselves. Their preparations may not give consistent products; thus efficacy may be compromised.
- Patients will find carrying of new CHM dosage forms, comparable to those OM medications, is convenient.

- Such medicinal products, though with complicated chemical compositions, can be regulated according to nationally and internationally agreed monographs complied by expertise groups consisting of government health authorities, CM herbal manufacturers, and appropriate academicians.

Secondly, a higher level of Biomedical Research—research staff from different universities and institutes can use their own expertise to develop up-market medicinal healthcare products or medications from their research programmes of CM natural products that have been used for centuries. These will involve up-to-date/cutting edge biotechnology. Apart from general pharmacological/toxicological screening models that we have developed, there is now the available expertise to develop advanced biomedical testing using in vitro systems, such as tissue cultures containing cell-lines that are useful: phage lysins, anti-cytokines, novel immuno-pharmacological screening and rapid biotechnological and microbial diagnostic tests. These technologies can be utilised for the preliminary screening of crude, and subsequently refined extracts from natural products. Such technology can generate future patents for the benefit of the country in the areas of Natural Products Research and Clean Environment Research.

Several areas can be shown to be benefited from these approaches:

- Infectious diseases—rapid diagnostic tests, new antibiotics, antiviral,
- Immunology related disorders.
- Rapid screening test for environmental contamination
- Phage display technologies

Develop SOP for control on quality, safety & efficacy of CHM products; (university, industry, government)

Without quality products the success of any clinical investigations or trials of CHM products will be compromised. Here several disciplines of expertise will be required to set up guidelines on GAP, GSP, GLP, GMP, and GCTP. Thus herbal manufacturers of CHM products, government regulatory body, and legal expertise on natural products should make sure standard operation procedures (SOP) have been included in the industrial monographs for all products to be registered as prescription only CM medications, or OTC products

Streamline basic and applied research programmes for CHM products; (Mainland, university, industry)

With respect to the general industrialisation of CM the national plan for modernisation can be used as a guideline. The universities and academic institutes in Hong Kong should make a joint-venture to identify and research into niche marketable areas of health and treatment needs with local manufacturing industries of CM products.

Input biomedical science measurements on acupuncture & CHM treatment (university, clinics)

These areas of clinical research into the mechanism of how acupuncture works have attracted a lot of interest in developed countries. Other areas of CM treatments including Qi-Gong, Tai chi and acumassage should also be looked into as part of their evidence-base studies. The joint effort should come from academic departments in universities and hospitals and clinics.

SETTING UP THE INTERNATIONAL INSTITUTE FOR CHINESE MEDICINE IN HONG KONG—THE MISSION POSSIBLE

We have previously proposed (Chan *et al.*, 1999) and it has been recently announced (Local newspapers 30 June 2000) by the Chief Executive of the Hong Kong SAR that the setting up of an International Institute for Development of Chinese Medicines has become more possible due to the financial support offered by the Hong Kong Jockey Club.

In line with the actions for national modernisation of Chinese medicine our proposed model aims to provide a co-ordination role in close contact with institutes in Mainland China. The ultimate common goal has been to create one of the national Centres of Excellency for promoting Chinese medicine globally in the right directions. National efforts in several areas should be addressed towards an assurance of quality of clinical and professional practice in CM, the launching of CM herbs and herbal products with good quality safety and efficacy, the promotion of a workable regulatory system to cope with international demand on quality, safety, and efficacy of crude CM herbs and manufactured products.

The Model Organisation (See Figure 13.1 modified from ref. Chan *et al.*, 1999) should be responsible with complete accountability to an independent Board of Trustees, which is formed to oversee that public

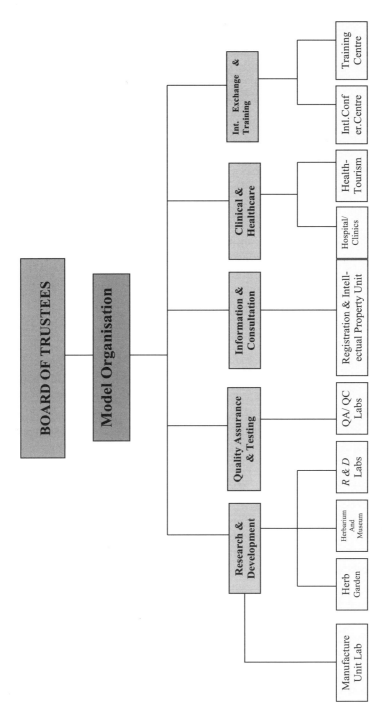

Figure 13.1 Organisation chart for development of CM based institute (adopted from Ref. Chan *et al.*, 1999)

funding for the execution of duties by the Organisation is used appropriately. After initial support from public funding over a definite period, subsequent development should be self-supporting. Apart from generating capital via manufacturing CM products, joint venture projects and consultation income should be the logical sources of revenues. A successful model to promote the co-ordination roles for the development of a Chinese medicine based industry should be set up to achieve the following goals.

- To develop for Hong Kong a global Centre of Excellency with unique and stand-alone identity for Chinese medicine in order to counteract misconception that CM is a myth.
- To co-ordinate, incubate and realise ideas from various universities' units on CM in Hong Kong and Mainland into action for basic and applied research in all aspects of Chinese medicine.
- To create an international center for co-ordination of the harmonisation of regulations for registration of CM products with quality, safety and efficacy for treatment and prevention of diseases; development for registration of intellectual properties on CM product manufacturing.
- To set up trouble-shooting facilities for Hong Kong's CM manufacturing companies or small or medium sized industries, which cannot afford such facilities, with due regard for the confidentiality of their products.
- To set up training facilities for Hong Kong's, perhaps global, need of professionals, technicians, dispensers specifically required by the CM industries that other university institutes cannot offer.
- To incubate and realise environment for R & D programmes in conjunction with experts in various local university research departments and institutes as well as those in Mainland China on new formulation, novel composite prescription products, manufacturing procedure with GMP guidelines.
- To provide facilities for small scale pre-manufacturing R & D production for small and medium size industries.
- To set up functionally viable CM hospitals or clinics, similar to the one set up in Kotzting in Munich, Germany, complementing existing OM hospitals such that the public can have a choice for their treatment.
- The future development of healthcare tourism based on CM treatment and prevention of diseases can help to promote Hong Kong's

economy and culture as well as improve the quality of life for the public when the know more about the use of CM information.

- Taking a role of international link for CM the Institute can start organising ICH regulations to clamp down supplying adulterated and fake CHM Products
- Working with Mainland on encouraging GAP for producing raw materials is a very much-needed direction in order to replenish shortage of CHM materials. Indirectly, this approach will help preventing unnecessary exploitation and is positively environmental friendly to prevent extinction of natural materials.

Concluding Remarks

THE NEED OF MODERNISATION AND PROFESSIONALISM OF CHINESE MEDICINE

Modernisation and improvement will be needed to make better use of this traditional medical practice for complementing and co-existing with well-advanced orthodox medicine. Implementing and maintaining of existing regulations for both practitioners and product-related treatment is also important to safeguard the quality of CM for providing and improving healthcare of the population.

In Hong Kong and developed countries in the west, in order to be recognised and accepted into practice in healthcare as part of the medical and health professional team, the CM practitioners have to be able to demonstrate their competence of practice and level of their training. The demonstration of professionalism requires a concerted effort of those who are practising various roles of Chinese medicine. Professional organisations apart from self-regulating their membership should be able to demonstrate their working ethics and professionalism in order to obtain national and international recognition by aiming at:

- Maintaining and developing educational standards
- Continuing professional development and modernisation
- Being familiar with healthcare affairs (improving linking via various OM and CM professionals)
- Keeping with development of ethics and safety issues
- Being aware of research & development in Chinese medicine as well as those in orthodox practice

- Liaisoning with government regulation agency for better service
- Helping to develop monographs or formulary of CHM products for local use

THE LINKING ROLE OF HONG KONG

Hong Kong has the right "environment" to take up the role for building up links between east and west for future development of Chinese medicine. This is because in Hong Kong various ingredients, such as the global reliable infrastructures for business, monetary, trading and technology for local and international development, are available to provide presently a unique advantage over the Mainland cities for the promotion and expansion of Chinese medicine.

The way forward to make better use of Chinese medicine for healthcare of the public in a global situation will require tremendous efforts from professionals and health officials in China where Chinese medicine originated and those from countries where Chinese medicine is practised. Both east and west have to work closely together to get the right approach for professionalism, regulatory issues for control of quality of practitioners, Chinese herbal medicines and other treatment related therapies. It is not the responsibility of one country to see to the implementation of efficacy, safety and quality of Chinese medicine. The areas for building bridges can be summarised as follows:

- International development for regulation on authentication of Chinese medicinal plants
- Dialogue between regulatory bodies from Chinese regulatory authorities and those from other countries
- Control of quality of import and export of CHM substances
- Co-ordination of GAP and GSP of CHM materials to avoid extinction of endangered species
- Development of methodology for assessment of efficacy of CHM products
- Development of regulatory issues for the international harmonisation of setting monographs for CHM materials and products.

As indicated in the early section of this Chapter, the delayed development of CM in Hong Kong has given Hong Kong an opportunity to contribute the right approach for future development. We sincerely wish those healthcare professionals, researchers, administrators and academics from institutes, universities, health authorities and other related government departments in Hong Kong can come together and work towards a common good course for development of Chinese medicine as soon as possible.

References

Bensoussan, A. and Myers, S.P. (1996) Towards a Safer Choice: The Practice of Traditional Chinese Medicine in Australia, University of Western Sydney, Macarthur, 1996.

Berger, S. and Lester, K. (1997) Made by Hong Kong, 1997.

BMA (1993) British Medical Association Report on Complementary Medicine: new approaches to good practice. Oxford University Press: Oxford, 1993.

Chan, K. (2000). How should Chinese medicine be developed in Hong Kong? In: The Proceedings of the Hospital Authority Convention-2000, 7–9 May 2000.

Chan, K. and Cheung, L. (2000) Interactions between Chinese Herbal Medicinal Products and Orthodox Drugs, Harwood Academic Publishers, 2000.

Chan, K., Chia, D., Yeung, H.W. (1999). Development of a Chinese Medicine based Industry in Hong Kong. In: Biotechnology in Hong Kong, A.W-K Chan (Ed), United States-China Intellectual Property Institute, New York, Chapter 3, P61–81, 1999.

Chinese Medicinal Material Research Centre (CMMRC), Chinese University of Hong Kong (1991) Report on the Utilisation of Traditional Chinese Medicine in Hong Kong, Hong Kong, 1991.

Health and Welfare Bureau, Government Secretariat HKSAR (1997), Consultative Document on the Development of Traditional Chinese Medicine in the Hong Kong Special Administrative Region, Hong Kong SAR, 1997.

Ip, Nancy, Y. (1999) Traditional Chinese Medicine in Hong Kong, In: Biotechnology in Hong Kong, A.W-K Chan (Ed), United States-China Intellectual Property Institute, New York, Chapter 2, p30–58, 1999.

Jia Qian (1998) Analysis on Situation of TCD Export in Recent Years, *Chinese Journal of Information on Traditional Chinese Medicine, Beijing*, Vol 5, No. 6, 1998.

Ko, W.M. (2000) Status and Trends of Traditional Chinese Medicine in Hong Kong. In Abstracts of the Conference of the Development of Chinese Medicine in the 21st Century. Hong Kong Convention & Exhibition Centre, 27 to 30 January 2000 (in Chinese).

Sino-British Co-operation (1998) Traditional Chinese Medicine in Britain: Report of a Seminar. *Pharmaceutical Journal*, 261: 641.

The Preparatory Committee on Chinese Medicine (PCCM) (1996) Report on Record Project of CM Practitioners in Hong Kong, Hong Kong, 1996.

Tung Chee Hwa (1997) Building Hong Kong for a New Era, the 1997 Policy Address by the Chief Executive, Hong Kong Special Administrative Region, 1997

Tung Chee Hwa (1998) From Adversity to Opportunity, the 1997 Policy Address by the Chief Executive, Hong Kong Special Administrative Region, 1998

The Working Party Chinese Medicine (WPCM) (1994) Report of The Working Party Chinese Medicine, Hong Kong, 1994.

World Health Organization. (1985) World Health Organization Handbook of Resolutions and Decisions of the World Health Assembly and the Executive Board. Vol 11, 1973–84, Geneva, 1985, p. 136–137.

14 THE PROGRESS OF KAMPO MEDICINE IN JAPAN

Katsutoshi Terasawa

Introduction

Because of the recent remarkable progress of modern medicine, it has become possible to recognise pathological evidence even at the molecular level. Accordingly, diagnostic and treatment procedures have made considerable progress in Japan. Nevertheless, the number of patients who request treatment with Kampo medicine has increased rapidly in the past 20 years. In the present paper, attempts are made to explain the reasons for this paradoxical phenomenon in Japan by means of a review of the historical background and an analysis of the characteristics of Kampo medicine, and then to discuss the problems of Kampo medicine that should be resolved for its universal development.

Historical Review

Buddhist monks by way of Korea introduced traditional Chinese medicine into Japan in the 6th century. Later, in the 7th century, Japanese envoys went to China to study Chinese culture that was subsequently introduced into Japan. This included the Chinese system of medicine, which for about one thousand years after that played an essential role in medical care in Japan. Then, by the mid-18th century, this system of medicine became more identified with Japan as a result of a renaissance of Japanese culture, in which ancient ideas of simplicity and naturalness were revived. From this interaction, Japanese Oriental (Kampo) medicine was developed.

When in 1858 Japan opened its doors to the West, it began to take in Western ideas and culture. In 1874, the government discarded Kampo medicine and accepted modern German medicine, which at that time was the most developed in the West. Since then, new doctors were not trained in Kampo medicine, but only in the Western style, and the art of practising Kampo medicine almost died out. Thus by

1920 there were less than 100 doctors practising Kampo medicine. This system of medicine, however, has survived because of the efforts of a few farsighted medical leaders who recognised the potential of Kampo medicine and kept the system alive, so it could be passed on to subsequent generations.

Present Situation of Kampo Medicine in Japan

During the last 25 years, Kampo medicine has gradually been making a reappearance for the reason set out below. Since the World War II, the Japanese people have increasingly come to respect the dignity of the individual. The growing idea in Japan that medical care should be adapted to the individual is closely related to this change in thinking. Therefore, Kampo medicine, which gives the patients individualised treatment, has come to be regarded by many Japanese as the most appropriate for our modern times.

The development of public health services, and the development of excellent antibiotics, has almost eradicated fatal infectious diseases from Japan. Now non-specific, constitutional, or psycho-somatic diseases have become the most pressing medical problems, as for example, arteriosclerotic diseases, autoimmune disorders, allergic diseases, malignant neoplasms, and degenerative diseases of the central nervous system. These diseases are often caused by an interaction of factors, some of which are unknown. They therefore present pressing problems for modern medicine, which has been based on the hypothesis that each disease is caused by one specific factor.

Disillusion with modern medicine has on occasion been brought about by severe adverse effects from synthetic medicines such as thalidomide, or by unexpected death caused by clinical examinations. The policies of the National Health Insurance Plan have also brought about discouragement with current medical practice. Because charges for medical treatment are defrayed on a formula based upon the indications applied to each patient, the physician's income depends on the margin of profit provided by the administered drugs, a scenario that can easily lead to excessive drug dispensation.

A general desire for the maintenance of healthy conditions has increased among the populace, but the system of modern medicine is not based on any concrete concepts for individual well being. Kampo medicine, however, is able to present some basis for the concept of "Ki" as vital energy. In other words, Western medicine is based solely upon a negative idea of health; that is, the absence of apparent sickness. Kampo medicine, however, recognises health as a positive condition, which can be maintained or achieved by a correct life style, and by the use of appropriate natural medicine.

Kampo medicine considers each person as a small universe, and signs and symptoms shown by the patient are integrated and interrelated by the "Yin" and "Yo" concept. The Yin and Yo are the two fundamental principles or factors in the universe, ever opposing and complementing each other, an ancient philosophical concept used in traditional Chinese medicine to refer to various antitheses in anatomy, physiology, pathology, diagnosis, and treatment; e.g., feminine, interior, cold, and hypofunction being Yin, while masculine, exterior, heat, and hyperfunction are Yo.

The system of Kampo medicine allows the doctor to be able to adapt the treatment according to the specific conditions and needs of each patient. In other words, the prescription for each patient is made up by the physician in accordance with the specific condition of the patient. The Kampo doctor also modifies the treatment according to the progress of the patient's illness or recovery. Therefore, Kampo medicine is both creative and individualised.

As a result of the philosophical changes in regard to the medical field and its applicability, the Ministry of Health and Welfare of Japan has entered Kampo prescriptions into the National Health Insurance Plan. Since 1976, about 150 Kampo formulations, which are extracted preparations from combinations of several herbs are available in our country. The medicinal plants that comprise such ethical Kampo prescriptions are also allowed to be covered by the Insurance Plan, so that it is possible to make up any kind of prescription as a decoction. As a matter of course, this official approval of Kampo medicine has also, concomitantly, stimulated more research in the field of Kampo medicine.

With the progress in chemistry and pharmacology in the last 20 years, the activities of components of the plants included in Kampo medicine have also been defined. These activities have made Kampo medicine more acceptable to many physicians who had previously felt somewhat suspicious and uneasy about the system of Kampo medicine.

At the Department of Japanese Oriental (Kampo) Medicine, Toyama Medical and Pharmaceutical University, there is an average daily attendance of 100 patients, almost all of whom received modern medicine prior to visiting the clinic. These patients can be classified into two groups.

1. No effective modern treatment available because of:
   (a) Difficulties in establishing a diagnosis, e.g., pyrexia of unknown origin, unexplained weight loss, lassitude of unknown origin;
   (b) Lack of effective treatment, e.g., neurodegenerative disorders, liver cirrhosis, chronic renal failure, and chronic obstructive lung disease.
2. Difficulty in application of modern medicine because of:
   (a) Drug hypersensitivity, side effects;
   (b) Multifoods or multisystem disorder in which treatment for one organ exacerbated others;
   (c) patient's distrust of modern medicines or preference for traditional Kampo medicine.

In the field of primary health care in Japan, Kampo medicine also plays an important role, especially in Groups 1(a) and 2. In addition, Kampo prescriptions are applied in a supportive role for diseases such as hypertension, common cold, headache, arthritis, neuralgia, bronchial asthma, collagenous diseases, chronic hepatitis, diabetes mellitus, chronic glomerulonephritis, and so on.

There are about 230,000 medical doctors in Japan, of whom about 300 doctors mainly use Kampo medicine in their daily practice. In addition, some other physicians use Kampo prescriptions, but only for extremely restricted cases such as chronic hepatitis. According to a recent report, about 65% of the physicians of Japan make use of Kampo prescriptions as a part of their daily practice in some manner.

In Japan, the license to practice medicine is given only to those who graduated from a Western style medical college, but there are no restrictions about adopting different kinds of medical procedures including acupuncture. It follows that the combined use of synthetic drugs and Kampo prescriptions is possible within the guidelines of the Medical Insurance Plan. As mentioned above, the present situation of traditional Kampo medicine in Japan is different from that of China and Korea, where two separate educational systems for medical doctors of the Western and traditional systems exist. On the other hand, in Japan, the license to practice acupuncture is given to those who graduated from a acupuncture school. There are about 100,000 acupuncturists in Japan.

Problems to be Resolved in the Future

Although Kampo medicine has been revived and is playing an important role in medical care in Japan, several critical problems remain. In respect to the efficacy of Kampo medicine there are four problems to be resolved:

1. Methods of pharmacological or biological assessment of the efficacy of the medicinal plants contained in Kampo prescriptions;
2. Pharmacological assessment of the efficacy of Kampo prescriptions as a whole, because Kampo formulations usually contain a combination of several plants;
3. Clinical assessment of the efficacy of Kampo medicine by using the procedures of modern medicine;
4. Clinical evaluation of the efficacy of Kampo medicine by way of controlled studies or similar substituted methods.

The active substances that can be obtained from medicinal plants have been detailed as a result of a tremendous amount of scientific research. As a result, however, of the lack of suitable assay systems, the various effects of the drugs of Kampo medicine have not yet been completely identified. Furthermore, from the viewpoint of Kampo medicine, each drug possesses a pharmacological vector that corrects a person from a shifted condition back to normal. The efficacy of Kampo medicine is traditionally assessed by the extent to which it is able to redirect a patient back to a state of normalcy. It is therefore necessary to include this characteristic concept in the assessment of the effects of Kampo drugs.

The next problem to be solved is the assessment of the Kampo prescription as a whole. The ancient textbooks of Chinese medicine describe the indicative condition for each formulation, which consists of several kinds of plants. For example, Kakkon-to (Ge-Gen-Tang in Chinese), one of the most popular formulations, consists of 7 kinds of plants; namely, Pueraria, Ephedra, Cinnamon, Ginger, Liquorice, Paeonia, and Jujube. The indication for this prescription is described in the textbook (Terasawa, 1990) as the first stage of the Yo state in which there is a sensation of stiffness and heaviness in the neck and back, mild chills, fever with tense and rapid pulse, but no perspiration. Viewed from the side of Western medicine, Kakkon-to can be recognised as a kind of anti-pyretic. The expected effect by Kampo medicine, however, is the regulation of circulatory vital energy on the surface of the body, improvement of blood circulation, and the increased production of vital energy in the digestive system. Therefore, Kakkon-to is widely adopted not only for the common cold but also for enteritis, tension headache, depression, and even for autoimmune disorders. As mentioned above, there are fundamental differences between the two systems of medicine, a situation that indicates the need for the development of new assessment procedures for the efficacy of Kampo prescriptions.

The third problem needing to be solved is a clinical assessment of the efficacy of Kampo medicine using the procedures of Western medicine. Actually, this problem does not seem particularly difficult. In our daily practice, we assess the efficacy of Kampo medicine by using laboratory data that we obtain before and after the treatment. In the strict sense, however, it is very difficult to estimate the efficacy of this medicine, because it considers every human as a small universe, and as part of the system of this medicine, spirit/mind and body are unable to be separated. Consequently, the parameters depended upon by Western medicine are not enough fully to estimate Kampo medicine's effectiveness.

The fourth problem, which needs to be resolved, is how to adapt a controlled study system to Kampo medicine. To succeed in such an approach, we first have to make clear the concept of "Sholl of Kampo medicine. Sho is the condition of the displacement from a state of normal health, and is shown by the interrelation of various signs and symptoms, according to the principle of Yin and Yo. As mentioned above, it is characteristic in Kampo medicine that the signs and symptoms presented by a patient consist of both subjective complaints and objective expressions. The indicative condition of the Kampo prescription is expressed as Sho. In other words, as shown in Figure 14.1, Sho represents the degree and type of shift from a normal condition, and each Sho has a corresponding Kampo prescription that will restore it to a normal state. In other words, it can be considered that the relationship between a Sho and its indicative prescription can be compared to a lock and a key. Therefore, the term Sho also has a meaning from the point of view of the Kampo prescription itself. The concept of Sho is completely independent of Western medicine. As shown in Figure 14.2, different methods of Kampo treatment can be applied to the same kind of disease in the light of different physical conditions and clinical manifestations.

For example, in the treatment of chronic hepatitis different methods such as cooling heat around the liver, tonifying the digestive system,

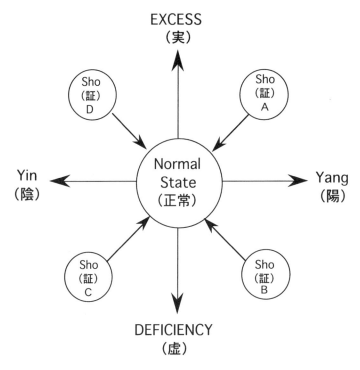

Figure 14.1 Two-dimensional display of "Sho", which recognises a patient as the displacement from a state of normal healthy by using "Yin"/"Yo" and deficient/excessive vital energy. The corresponding Kampo prescription for each Sho is applied to correct the shifted condition towards a normal state.

restoring the normal functioning of the liver, etc. should be used, dependent on whether liver dysfunction is due to heat in the liver, deficiency of vital energy or stagnancy of vital energy in the liver. Therefore, it is necessary to make clear the indicative condition, i.e., Sho, for a prescription to be tested. In other words, prior to adopting a controlled study of Kampo formulations, we have to be able to present a large number of readily understandable indicative criteria for the prescription under study. That is, a prescription can be assessed only in terms of its effects on its corresponding Sho. As described above, Kampo medicine diagnoses and treats illness along different dimensions from Western medicine; therefore, it depends on different (or additional) criteria of assessment.

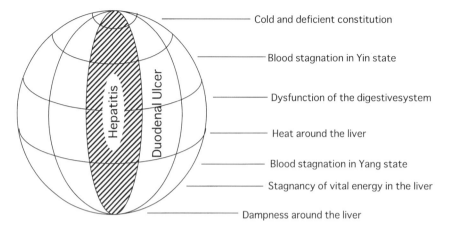

Figure 14.2 Treatment of chronic hepatitis by Kampo medicine. Different methods of treatment are applied to the same kind of diseases in the light of different physical conditions.

The Ministry of Health and Welfare of Japan is now reassessing Kampo prescriptions that are accepted in the National Health Insurance Plan. So far as I understand, the Ministry recognises the significance of Sho in Kampo medicine and proposes to perform the reassessment program under the direction of the Sho concept by using a double-blind controlled study. As the first step. the Ministry intends to re-evaluate the efficacy of Shosaiko-to (Xiao-Chai-Hu-Tang in Chinese) in the restricted indication as a drug for hepatic diseases. The Sho of Shosaiko-to consists of Yo (febrile and hyperreactive) state with thoracocostal distress, nausea, vomiting, and abdominal distress. Therefore, in initiating a controlled study the patient should be selected from the view point of Sho. In the program of the ministry, the Sho concept will be applied to the indicative hepatitis patients under treatment of Shosaiko-to excluding those displaying Yin symptoms who are deemed unsuitable for the study; e.g., a patient who has cold intolerance, severe lethargy, and diarrhoea with indigestion is excluded from the controlled study, because Shosaiko-to therapy is aggravative of patients with Yin symptoms. This kind of double-blind controlled study is essential for the universalization of Kampo medicine, although it may be possible to perform such controlled studies only with certain limited Kampo prescriptions. Based on this concept, the double-blind controlled studies were carried out, and the efficacies of Shosaiko-to on chronic hepatitis (Hiyamama *et al.*, 1989), Shoseiryu-to on allergic rhinitis (Baba *et al.*, 1995) and Daio-kanzo-to on constipation (Miyoshi, *et al.*, 1994) were reported. Further, We demonstrated by a double-blind study that Choto-san was effective in treating vascular dementia (Terasawa *et al.*, 1997).

Teaching System of Kampo Medicine

As already mentioned, not a few physicians take Kampo medicine into their daily practice in our country. However, no systematic educational system for Kampo medicine is available in Japan except at Toyama Medical and Pharmaceutical University. Therefore, almost all such physicians have learned Kampo medicine through their own efforts, by attending lectures held by Kampo drug companies, or by attending some private school of an expert in Kampo medicine who inherited knowledge of the system from his master. It is really critical, however, that this system of medicine be taught to both postgraduate doctors and medical students systematically, because Kampo medicine exhibits its full power only through a thorough recognition of its fundamental concepts.

Concerning the teaching system for postgraduate doctors, the Society of Japanese Oriental medicine started a registration system of specialists in Kampo medicine in 1990. This new system requests all registered specialists to attend the authorised meetings of the society and present any papers or medical journals at the meeting. Through this postgraduate educational system, it is expected that the understanding of Kampo medicine will be dramatically improved among the doctors of Japan.

In our concern with undergraduate education, we have been teaching the system of Kampo medicine for about 15 years at Toyama Medical and Pharmaceutical University. Lectures are given to fourth-year medical students, and fifth-year students undergo clinical training. In total about 30 lecture hours and 32 hours of clinical training are in the curriculum (Table 14.1).

This course in our university, however, is the only one dealing with Kampo medicine in our country. I hope that Kampo medicine will be

Table 14.1 The undergraduate curriculum of Kampo Medicine in Toyama Medical and Pharmaceutical University

---

1. Histories of Japanese and Chinese medicine (2h.)
2. The role of traditional Kampo medicine in contemporary health care in Japan (2h.)
3. On the concept of "Ki"/vital energy (4h.)
4. On the concept of "Yin" and "Yo" principles (6h.)
5. An outline of acupuncture and moxibustion (4h.)
6. Constitution of Kampo prescriptions (4h.)
7. Diagnostic procedures of Kampo medicine (8h.)
8. Clinical training (32h.)

---

taught to all undergraduate students, but for the following reasons, it has yet to be adopted in the curriculum of medical education in other medical colleges.

1. The planning of the curriculum is under the control of the faculty council of each college. But almost no members of these planning councils recognise the potential of Kampo medicine.
2. As a natural consequence of the aforementioned lack of educational Kampo programs in medical colleges, there are very few qualified teachers of Kampo medicine.
3. The Ministry of Science, Education and Culture of Japan has yet to take a fully positive attitude towards promoting the education of Kampo medicine.

These three factors, therefore, constitute a vicious circle, which, if left to continue in its present form, can hardly be expected to break out of its self-restrictive pattern. Some extra effort must be made, and aggressive steps taken, change the form of this circle into a series of progressive developmental stages.

For the universalization of Kampo medicine to succeed, good textbooks and qualified teachers are a necessity. Toward this goal, I have issued a textbook (Terawasa, 1990) in which the diagnostic criteria of fundamental pathological concepts are presented by clear definition. Since then, the textbook was translated into English (Terasawa, 1993) German (Terasawa, 1994) and Chinese. I believe this kind of effort is one concrete way to achieve universal understanding of Kampo medicine.

Conclusion

In this paper, I have attempted to describe the present situation of Kampo medicine in Japan, and I have discussed the problems that need to be resolved in the future to promote Kampo medicine.

In conclusion, it seems of the utmost importance to develop a system correctly to estimate the potential of Kampo medicine, so that a new style of medical care can be established, incorporating both western and traditional Kampo medicine.

References

Baba, S., *et al.* (1995) Double-blind clinical trial of Shoseiryu-to (TJ-19) for perennial nasal allergy. *Jibirinsho*, **88**, 389–405. (in Japanese)

Hirayama, C., *et al.* (1989) A multicenter randomised controlled clinical trial of Shosaiko-to in chronic active hepatitis. *Gastroenterologia Japonica*, **24**, 715–719.

Miyoshi, A., *et al.* (1994) The clinical effect of Tsumura Daio-Kanzo-To extract granules for ethical use (TJ-84) by double blind test against the constipation. *Gastroenterology (Tokyo)*, **18**, 299–312. (in Japanese)

Terasawa, K. (1990) *Case-oriented Japanese Oriental (Kampo) Medicine*, Igaku-shoin, Tokyo. (in Japanese)

Terasawa, K. (1993) *Kampo, Japanese-Oriental medicine, Insights from clinical cases*, Translated by Bacowsky. H. and Gerz, A. Standard McIntyre, Tokyo.

Terasawa, K. (1994) *Kampo, Prexis czer t:raditionallen ferndstlichen Phytotherapie anhand von klinischen Fallbeispielen*, Translated by Bacowsky, H. Karl F. Haug Verlag, Heidelberg. (In German)

Terasawa, K. (1997) Choto-san in the treatment of vascular dementia. a double-blind, placebo-controlled study. *Phytomedicine*, **4**, 15–22.

15 THE PROGRESS OF CHINESE MEDICINE IN TAIWAN

Chieh Fu Chen
Yau Chik Shum
Ming Tsuen Hsieh

Introduction

Owing to political turmoil, Japanese occupation and early economic hardship, the long envisioned organized educational and research programs in traditional Chinese medicine (TCM) in Taiwan did not take root until the 195Os. The development programmes started several years after Taipei became the site of the Nationalist government even though traditional Chinese medicine had long been an integral part of the rich heritage of the Chinese culture. In Taiwan its practice was officially recognised in March 1956 with the passing of the Chinese Medicine Education Act. The Act established educational and research institutions for the development of TCM to be an integral part of the overall modernisation of Taiwan's medical care. It is given the same status, support and fair share of available resources as orthodox medicine. Nonetheless, the path to respectability and acceptability among the general public, academic and healthcare professionals has been arduous. This chapter offers a brief history and major achievements in the history of TCM so far.

The Development of Education and Training of Chinese Medicine

THE DEVELOPMENT IN CHINA MEDICAL COLLEGE

The history of TCM development began with the creation of the China Medical College in Tai Chung in the early 1950s. The Ministry of Education formally recognised the College in June 1958. Subsequently, the pace of development quickened by 1973 when the Basic Medical Sciences department was built. In the same year, the Faculty of Public health was created to offer postgraduate programmes leading to

Master's degree for Pharmacy in the spring of 1974 and TCM in the following year. In 1977, orthodox medicine education and training was for the first time, offered to practitioners of TCM.

To accommodate the increasing demands for TCM, the College was moved in February 1983, to a more spacious campus in Pei-Kang. This lead to the establishment of a post-graduate programme in TCM and to the building of an affiliated hospital thereafter to support the clinical parts of the TCM programmes.

TCM continued to evolve satisfactorily with doctoral degree being offered in 1987. December 1991 marked the beginning of a new phase in the progress of TCM in Taiwan. An exhibition Hall for TCM was opened. This was quickly followed by the offer of doctoral degree at the Graduate Institute of Chinese Medicine and Chinese Pharmaceutics. Near the end of the twentieth century, TCM was gaining both stature and physical growth. The affiliated hospital built earlier in Taichung and mentioned above was designated a medical centre, an accolade befitting the continuing growth of TCM in Taiwan.

From the founding premises of the China Medical College to promote education and training of Chinese medicine till the present time, the modernization of traditional Chinese Medicine and the integration of East-West Medicines have been the unwavering guiding principle. From the early joint East-West medical and pharmacy curricula to today's 12 faculties, 6 graduate departments, 2 affiliated teaching hospitals the China Medical College has evolved to be a multidisciplinary all-round educational, research and health-care institution. The development of a healthy system permits the expansion and attainment of objectives. The Government and various business sectors have translated the high respectability commanded by Board Chairman Li-Fu Chen into strong and unwavering support. Soon after his appointment the Basic Medical Sciences Building was erected. Unprecedented loans from the Government and donations from the business sectors enabled the building of the affiliated hospital, elevating basic and clinical medical education to a World-caliber level. On July 1 1997 the affiliated hospital in Taichung gained candidate status for Medical Center designation.

To date, Taiwan has five major institutions offering undergraduate and post-graduate programmes and a range of exciting research projects such as pharmacokinetics, phytochemistry, toxicology, signal transduction, diabetes, cardiovascular and central nervous system pharmacology as well as receptor dynamics. These institutes were established:

THE DEVELOPMENT IN CHANG GANG UNIVERSITY

This University was founded in April 1987 as the Chang Gang Medical College. Adequate funding, good incentives and facilities allowed it to quickly become a leading teaching and research center in Taiwan. Following years of offering top-notch medical services largely in the orthodox medical mode by its affiliated hospitals, a Department of Traditional Chinese Medicine has been established in recent years in response to popular demand. Consequently the proper training of practitioners of traditional Chinese medicine attracted the attention of the policy-makers. Following lengthy research, discussions and preparations, the Faculty of Traditional Chinese Medicine was established in the fall of 1998

THE DEVELOPMENT IN NATIONAL YANG-MING UNIVERSITY IN TAIPEI

The National Yang-Ming University was founded in 1975 as the National Yang-Ming Medical College with the intention of training and eventually providing health care professionals for rural areas and the veterans' hospitals. According to the "Universities and Technical Colleges Act" post-secondary colleges enjoy the same statuses as universities. The granting of university status merely reflects the diversification in academic programmes. The National Yang-Ming Medical College quickly established a reputation as one of the leading medical colleges in Taiwan. The Department of Pharmacology was among the original academic departments which established and attracted the services of several renowned pharmacologists. Research projects on orthodox and Chinese medicinal aspects include pharmacokinetics, phytochemistry, toxicology, signal transduction, diabetes, and cardiovascular and central nervous system pharmacology and receptor dynamics.

THE DEVELOPMENT IN THE INSTITUTE OF TRADITIONAL CHINESE MEDICINE

Established in 1991, the Institute of Traditional Medicine at the National Yang-Ming University is the only institute devoted to the postgraduate teaching and research of traditional Chinese medicine (TCM) among national universities in Taiwan. Her main objectives include (1) training of teachers and researchers in TCM; (2) integration of TCM into mainstream health care and (3) modernization of TCM along the lines of standardization, systematization of the practice of TCM. Research activities in the Institute are based on a multidisciplinary approach. Through cooperation with faculty members in other departments in the National Yang-Ming University and clinical researchers at the Veterans' General Hospital, innovative approach to the research of TCM is fostered.

Research training is available in subjects including the theory and practice of acupuncture, biophysical properties of TCM meridians and points, purification and identification of biologically active compounds from Chinese medicinal herbs, cardiovascular effect of TCM and effects of medicinal herbs on sperm motility, lipid peroxidation, virus and cancer cells. Ph.D. programmes were offered since the fall of 1998.

THE DEVELOPMENT IN THE INSTITUTE OF BIOPHARMACEUTICAL SCIENCES

The Institute of Biopharmaceutical Sciences at Yang-Ming University was established in 1994. Although the scope of teaching and research are in theory very broad and flexible, in practice efforts are intensely focused on disorders for which modern orthodox medical treatments are not very successful and those with high local incidence. The approach is the employment of cutting-edge technology, including those in molecular and cellular biology, for the investigation of neoplastic disorders, vascular disorders and those related to aging and the immune system. The hope is of international attention that will be drawn to the involvement of biopharmaceutical sciences for the development of products from genetic engineering, traditional medicine, health foods and supplements. Cooperation and collaboration with other departments and institutes at the National Yang-Ming University permits the Institute to offer diversified programmes both in teaching and research. The approved Center for Drug Development, which is envisioned to coordinate actions required for the full development of active compounds to marketable drugs, began operation in the fall of 1998.

Thus all the five institutes offer various aspects in research and training in Chinese medicine. These include subjects such as theory and practice of acupuncture, biophysical properties of TCM meridians and points, purification and identification of biologically active components from Chinese herbs, cardiovascular effect of TCM and the effects of medicinal herbs on sperm motility, lipid peroxidation, virus and cancer cells. Some institutes possess cutting edge technology for the modernisation of Chinese medicine.

Accreditation of Qualification of Chinese Medicine

Throughout the development of TCM in Taiwan, practical experience has been handed down from generation to generation. The Central Government, through the Executive Yuen, has taken steps to rationalise the standards of education, training and practice for TCM practitioners. Individuals can now be qualified in TCM under several conditions as described below:

a) The person must have sat and passed the Qualifying Examination in TCM administered by the National Examination Board. The prescribed subjects are Chinese, Biology, Physiology, Diagnosis, Materia Medica, Prescriptions and Internal Medicine. The compulsory subjects and elective subjects for Special Examination of TCM are: Chinese constitution, Physiology, Materia Medica, Prescription, Diagnosis Internal Medicine, Acupuncture, and Obstetrics, paediatrics, Ophthalmology and Traumatology. The successful candidates for the Special Examination are required to undergo eight months (52 credits) of basic orthodox medical and Chinese medical sciences training and ten months (42 credits) of Chinese medicine clinical training in the China Medical College.

b) Orthodox medical graduates who have successfully completed 45 academic credits in Chinese medicine (13 credits of Chinese Internal medicine, 6 credits of Chinese Materia Medica, 4 credits of Chinese medicine, and any 3 credits of Chinese obstetrics, paediatrics, Ophthalmology, Surgery and Traumatology) can sit for the National Board Examination. The compulsory subjects for TCM are Chinese, Materia Medica, Prescription, Diagnosis, Internal Medicine and Acupuncture while the elective subjects are Obstetrics, Paediatrics, Ophthalmology, Traumatology and Surgery.

c) Graduates from an accredited Post-Baccalaureate 5 year Medical Programme in TCM, 7-year Medical Programme in TCM, 8 year combined TCM and Orthodox Medical Programme, or Orthodox Medical Graduates upon completion of a Master's Programme in TCM with a minimum of 27 credits in TCM are also allowed to sit for the National Board Examination for the TCM practitioners.

Taiwan has come a long way since it launched its first TCM programme in the early 1950s. Today, it boasts 4 public medical universities or colleges, 6 private medical colleges and two technical colleges of pharmacy. It has about 3430 licensed TCM doctors for its 21 million people. This nevertheless compares very unfavourably with 23150 licensed orthodox doctors.

Development of Research in Chinese Medicine

THE NATIONAL RESEARCH INSTITUTE OF CHINESE MEDICINE (NRICM)

The NRICM was created in 1957 through a government decree, under the direct auspices of the Ministry of Education (Chen, 1989; Chen, 1998). The institute is committed to the advancement of TCM through organisation, research, education, experimentation, development and other related activities. In 1996, two research buildings were added to the NRICM. The following year a 400-acre National Arboretum of Medicinal plants was established in Taipei County. The NRICM now boasts the following research sections:

a) Basic Chinese Medicine Unit consisting of Medicinal Plants and Pharmacognosy, Pharmaceutical Chemistry and Clinical Chinese Medicine.
b) Information Section consisting of National Arboretum of Medicinal Plants Museum, Library, and Computer Information Centre.
c) Archives of Chinese Pharmacopoeia and Department of Graphics and Medical Arts.
d) Medicinal Plants Quality Control Centre, and
e) Biological Activities Screening Centre

The research mission of the NRICM focuses on the isolation and identification of biologically active principles from natural products. These include those of marine origin, synthesis of purified compounds and their derivatives, testing of these compounds for potential use in the treatments of liver diseases including hepatitis, neurodegeneration, neoplastic diseases and other disorders related to ageing and the immune system. Modern techniques and tools such as NMR, IR, FT-IR, GC/MS, LL/MS, LL/MS/MS, preparative and analytical high performance liquid chromatography, tissue cultures, bio-molecular techniques, electro-physiology and flow cytometry are routinely employed.

In addition, the NRICM organises intramural, regional, national and international symposia, providing a forum for the exchange of ideas, coordinates research activities with collaborating institutions and between academia, industry and government. Its publishing arm organises, revises ancient pharmacopoeia and publishes them in modern language. It also publishes other books, newsletter and periodicals related to research in

TCM. The NRICM's information service branch establishes and constantly updates databases of research information and is usually dispensed free of charge to interested parties. In order to increase public awareness and retail handlers of Chinese medicinal products who may have already had many years of experience but had inadequate theoretical training, the NRICM organises continuing education programmes in modern pharmaceutical practices. Although not directly involved in policy making, the NRICM provides consultation to relevant government offices. The goal is to establish a centre for all activities related to the advancement of TCM complementary to orthodox medicine as part of the modern health care resources. The task is enormous and daunting but the NRICM, along with its colleagues in academia, industry and government, is steadfastly contributing towards that goal.

GENERAL STATUS OF RESEARCH IN CHINESE MEDICINE AND NATURAL PRODUCTS

The tradition of research in TCM in Taiwan dates back to the days of Japanese occupation. Today, Taiwan has an active research community of pioneers and research fellows. There are many eminent researchers whose contributions have helped to gain international recognition for Taiwan's TCM research portfolio. The scope of this chapter does not allow listing all these pioneers but wishes to acknowledge their invaluable contributions. Instead a representative selection of research projects will be highlighted to emphasize how TCM was enhanced. The names of individual researchers initially written by the authors were intentionally left out by the Editors to offer an objective perspective and to avoid any cause of offence.

Early efforts
An early review of research activities on natural products (Lee, 1982) indicated that many aspects were related to Chinese medicinal products.

- Some were performed at a well known privately owned establishment (Brion Research Institute), where research in pharmacognosy, phytochemistry and pharmacology and quality control of CM materials was carried out.
- Early work on TCM materials at the Faculty of Pharmacy of the China Medical College (CMC) included, anthelmintic, expectorant and antitussive effects of some the TCM. Other published works

were"Medicinal Botany", "Medicinal Plants of Taiwan", "Toxic Plants of Taiwan" and the therapeutic uses of Chinese Medicines in the treatments of cancers, poisonous snakebites and kidney diseases.

- At the Kaohsiung Medical College, 20 bioactive alkaloids from plants indigenous to Taiwan were isolated that had potential antibiotic and anti-neoplastic effects. Of these 7 had antibiotic effects and 9 cytotoxic among 70 alkaloids screened.

- The Institute of Botany at Academia Sinica worked on the isolation of antibiotic materials from Taiwanese soil.

- The Faculty of Medicine of Chung-Kung University studied the antipyretic effects of Chinese medicines and quantitation CM products using high-performance-liquid-chromatography and development of derivatives of glycerretinic acid.

- The Faculty of Pharmacy at the National Taipei University worked in steroids and terpenes, and studied the biological activities of anticancer principles from natural products as well as their syntheses. Work has also been aimed at the biological activities and synthesis of alkaloids from natural products and succeeded in the isolation and confirmation of the chemical structures of discretamine, stepholidine, and govadine. Others were on the isolation of alkaloids from *Uncarica hirsuta* Haviland for their anti-hypertensive mechanisms, anticancer activities of active principles from Chinese medicines and seaweed and characterisation of the anticancer protein isolated from *Absurd precatorius* L.

- At the National Yang-Ming Medical College, works were directed at the screening and confirming the anti-hypertensive, analgesic and antipyretic effects for a number of Chinese medicines and studied the diuretic effects of *Orthosiphonis Herba*, *Plantaginis Semen*, *Evodiae Fructus* and *Drabae Semen*.

- The Taipei Medical College pioneered the isolation of bioactive alkaloids from Taiwanese plants with more than 70 related articles, the antibacterial effects of 35 coumarins and the relaxant effects of butylidenephalide on smooth muscles.

Lee also pointed out (Lee, 1982) that the main obstacle in research in natural products in Taiwan lay in the lack of support from the pharmaceutical industry, financial support from the government and individuals and lack of interest on the part of doctoral students. In the last few years' research, Traditional Chinese Medicine in Taiwan has received a big boost from the fine efforts from various institutes. (Chen, 1988a, Chen 1988a and Chen 1989).

Recent progress in research of Chinese medicinal plants

In the 1970s The National Science Council in Taiwan initiated research programmes in anticancer potentials in Chinese medicines with core researchers recruited from the NDMC. In recent years under the auspices and support from the National Science Council and the Ministry of Health other experts from the NYMU, TMC, Kaohsiung Medical College, CMC and even the Tatung Technical College have helped to realize these goals. The pledging of substantial support from the Ministry of Education in 1988 breathed new life to research activities at the NRICM. Having enjoyed international recognition in its research in snake venom, the Research Institute of Pharmacology at the NTU has also branched into TCM research. At the same time the cross-Strait relationship between Taiwan and Mainland China has improved, allowing scholarly exchanges and fueling the pace of TCM research. Recently the Executive Yuan has assigned greater responsibilities to the NRICM in working closely with Taiwan's own National Health Research Institute (NHRI) and the National Science Council to expand TCM research in Taiwan with the development of new drugs as a designated goal.

Recent results were reported (Teng, 1991, Teng & Liu 1991) that in more than a hundred of Chinese medicinal herbs screened, approximately 10% were found to possess anti-hepatitis virus potentials. Others possessed central effects, some acted on the cardiovascular system, and some possessed anti-inflammatory actions. The following list summarises the names and actions of these plants.

- *Daphne odor* Thumb. var. *atrocaulis* Rehder (白花瑞香), *Caesalpinia sappan* L. (蘇木), *Syzygium tripinnatum* (Blanco) Merr. (大花赤楠), *Peucedanum japonicum* *Thunb.* (日本前胡), *Ganoderma lucidum* (Leyss ex Fr.) Karst. (fruiting body) (靈芝子實體), *Poria cocos* (Schw.) Wolf. (茯苓), *Salvia miltiorrhiza* Bunge (丹參), *Dysosma pleiantha* (Hance) Woodson possess anticancer effect. (八角蓮), *Bupleurum chinense* DC. (柴胡), *Lonicera japonica* Thunb. (金銀花), *Physalis angulata* L. (苦蘵),) *Cordyceps sinensis* (Fruiting body) (冬蟲夏草, *Psoralea corylifolia* L (若蘵)., *Magnolia officinalis* Rehd. & Wils. (原朴) possess immunological regulation and anti-inflammatory effects.
- *Lycopodium serratum* Thunb. var. *longipetiolatum* Spring (金不換), *Lycopodium casuarinoides* Spring (木賊葉石松), *Corydalis yanhusuo* W.T. Wang (延胡索), possess central effect. *Lithospermum*

erythrorhizon S. et Z. (紫草), *Litsea cubeba* (Lour.) Persoon (山胡椒), *Rhamnus formosana* Matsum. (台灣鼠李), *Wikstroemia indica* C.A.Mey. (南嶺蕘花), *Zanthoxylum schinifolium* S. et Z. (翼柄花椒), *Corydalis ochotensis* Turcz. (疏花黃堇), *Murraya euchrestifolia* Hay. (山黃皮, *Zingiberis officinale* Rosc. (薑), *Melastoma affinie* Don. (蘭嶼野牡丹), *Saposhnikovia divaricata* (Turcz.) Schischk. (防風), *Gentiana flavo-maculata* Hay. (黃花龍膽), *Epimedium sagittatum* (S. et Z.) Maxim. (淫羊藿), *Dendropanax pellucidopunctata* (Hay.) Merr. (台灣樹參),) *Acacia Polygonum cuspidatum* S. et Z (相思子)., possess antiplatelet aggregation effect.

- *Nymphaea tetragona* Georgi (睡蓮), *Aconitum carmichaeli* Debx. (烏頭), *Lindera megaphylla* Hemsl. (大香葉樹), *Dehaasia triandra* Merr. (腰果楠), *Cryptocarya chinensis* (Hance) Hemsl. (大香葉樹), *Evodia rutaecarpa* Hook. f. et Thom. (吳茱萸), *Melastoma candidum* D.don (野牡丹), *Fissistigma glaucescens* (Hance) Merr. (白葉瓜馥木), *Dictamnus dasycarpus* Turcz. (白鮮皮) had effects on the cardiovascular system and blood pressure.

A number of active principles have been isolated from these herbs and their chemical structures identified. These include dehydroevodiamine, evodiamine and rutaecarpine from *Evodiae Ruteacapae*. Their pharmacological profiles, mechanisms of actions as well as pharmacokinetics have been investigated. The development of the bioactive alkaloid aporphine is currently in progress. Not included in Teng's report are analyses by high performance liquid chromatography and capillary electrophoresis and pharmacokinetic studies, which have attracted international attention.

Reports on the progress between 1974 to 1991 (Chen, 1992; Chen, 1998c) described the work on steady advancements both in quantity and quality of studies on Chinese medicine in Taiwan, isolation and synthesis of bioactive compounds from medicinal plants, and procurement of four patents.

Since 1997 the screening of Chinese composite formulae (Fu Fang) for their inhibitory effects on inducible nitric oxide synthetase, amyloid beta-peptide secretion, amyloid beta-peptide binding to neurons, and PtdSer exposure on neurons, and antioxidant effects in the hope of finding potential neuro-protective agents has been a major research theme at NRICM (Chen, 1997). Examples of inter-institute collaboration has been started at the National Taipei University's School of Medicine on Chinese composite formulae (Fu Fang) for the treatment of asthma which attracted the participation of experts in basic and clinical fields from various institutions.

Conclusion

The credibility and popularity enjoyed by orthodox medicine has been helped largely by organized and integrated approaches in education, research and systematic documentation of observations. However, increasingly the orthodox medical profession is becoming aware of merits in other forms of medical practice in the treatment of diseases, particularly certain disorders for which orthodox medicine has not been very successful. For many such ailments, symptomatic relief is probably the only means of relief. However, due to lack of organization and accurate documentation, many of these other forms of alternative medical practice are shrouded in mystery, impeding their acceptability. Traditional Chinese Medicine has always been an integral part of the Chinese heritage. With thousands of years of experimentation and accumulated observations, it is a rich source of information and clinical wisdom waiting to be rediscovered. Regrettably "the art of healing" in traditional medicine had been passed on only on a personal basis, relying heavily on clinical experience rather than meticulous documentation. Many "secret recipes" are lost. Organized education and research so that the merits of traditional Chinese medicine can be verified and accepted are much warranted.

There has been an enormous effort in Taiwan to validate by orthodox and conventionally accepted methodology, the ancient Chinese medical recipes for the treatment of a range of diseases. It is widely recognised that much has been focused onto the characterisation of the principal natural products through isolation and identification of their active constituents and then to develop them as new medicinal products. The benefit of such an approach is difficult to dispute in the scientific world. However, it ignores the original reason for combining medical herbs together and there is no question that under certain conditions various herbal mixtures may interact and potentiate the efficacy. Therefore, alternative clinical effectiveness evaluation methodologies should be developed for assessing composite prescriptions, which contain multiple herbal mixtures, as is the case for TCM and many other traditional herbal medicines around the world. Thus, besides being used as health foods, partial purified natural products are now being seriously considered as medicinal products by the Food and Drug Administration (FDA) of the USA. Again, the clinical efficacy of well quality-controlled complete composite prescriptions containing multiple herbal mixture should be carefully evaluated (Way, Liu, & Chen, 1996).

In conclusion, there appears to be a long way to go for the right approach to confirm tradition by present day science. Both education and research are long term investments, the fruits of which are unlikely to be immediately achieved. It has been said that to cultivate a tree takes only 10 years but to cultivate a person would take 100 years.

References

Chen, C.F. (1988a) How to modernize Chinese herbal drugs, a viewpoint from the development of modern Materia Medica, *Chemistry*, **46**, 299–302.

Chen, C.F. (1988b) Past, present, and future of National Research Institute of Chinese Medicine [Chinese], National Research Institute of Chinese Medicine, Taipei, 1988.

Chen, C.F. (1998c) Abstracts of publications on Chinese medicine from Taiwan (1991–1996) [Chinese], National Research Institute of Chinese Medicine, Taipei, 1998.

Chen, C.F. (1998d) Brief introduction of the National Research Institute of Chinese Medicine, The National Research Institute of Chinese Medicine, Taipei, 1998.

Chen, C.F. (1989) Studies on traditional Chinese herbal drugs and natural products. *Science Monthly*, **20**, 413–418.

Chen, C.F. (1992) Abstracts of publications on Chinese medicines from Taiwan (1974–1991) [Chinese], National Research Institute of Chinese Medicine, Taipei, 1992.

Chen, C.F. (1994) Studies of Chinese medicines and natural products, *National Science Council Monthly*, **22**, 947–950.

Chen, C.F. (1997) Evaluation of central affective neuro-protective Chinese herbal drugs, *Life Sciences Newsletter, NSC*, **11**, 5–7.

Kuo, Y.H. (1986) Review on chemical studies of natural products, *National Science Council Monthly*, **14**, 1223–1252.

Lee, K.H. (1982) Research underway in medicinal chemistry and natural products in Taiwan, *Proceedings of National. Science Council (ROC)*, **6(1)**, 39–59.

Teng, C.M. (1991) Study on vasoactive-antithrombotic principles from Chinese herbal drugs and new drug development, *National Science Council Monthly*, **19**, 200–205.

Teng, C.M. and Liu, H.O. (1993) Report of the team-project research on Chinese herbs, *National Science Council Monthly*, **21**, 741–761.

Way, E.L., Liu, Y.Q. and Chen, C.F. (1996) Perspective and overview of Chinese traditional medicine and contemporary pharmacology, *Progress in Drug Research*, **47**, 131–164.

16 THE PROGRESS OF CHINESE MEDICINE IN THE UNITED KINGDOM

Kelvin Chan
Henry Lee

Development of Complemetary Medicine in the United Kingdom

INTRODUCTION

A survey of complementary or alternative medicine (CAM) conducted in the early 1980s by the British Medical Association (BMA) concluded that it was a mere "fashion" that such alternative therapies were preferred by the public (BMA, 1986). Over the past two decades, the general public in the UK has been more informed of health care matters and increasingly many are turning to natural medicinal products and other alternative therapies. Several studies (Fulder & Munro, 1985; Wharton & Lewith, 1986; Consumers' Association, 1986; Davies, 1987; and Furnham & Smith, 1988) reported an increase of public demand of complementary medicine and therapies outside the National Health Service system in the United Kingdom. For example, the BMA suggested that more rigorous control over the good practice of CAM is required to safeguard the well being of the public (BMA, 1993). Thomas *et al.* (1991) calculated that there could be four million, or five million as suggested by the Research Council for Complementary Medicine (RCCM, 1997), complementary medicine/therapy consultations annually. It works out at a ratio of 1:55 GP consultations on the National Health service (NHS). In their study, Vincent & Furnham (1996) found that the respondents who were attracted to complementary medicine/therapies frequently cited "lack of effectiveness of orthodox medicine" as the main reason. The Foundation for Integrated Medicine (FIM, 1997) suggested that there is "a degree of public dissatisfaction with what people see as the limitations of orthodox medicine and concern over the side effects of ever more potent drugs".

As pointed out in Chapter One, very little is known concerning the reasons for the increase in popularity of CAM in developed countries Untested assumptions include the side-effects of synthetic drugs, general dissatisfaction of orthodox treatment, diseases that cannot be cured by OM, and patients with chronic illnesses demanding more attention from OM practitioners. Research is urgently needed in these areas to improve healthcare planning (Chan, 1996). CAM treatments are recommended for chronic pain affecting spine, joints or muscles, for the control of nausea, eczema, and other skin complaints, asthma, cancer and migraine etc. (Lewith, Kenyon & Lewis, 1996). There are over 100 different therapies available as CAM treatments, but the five discrete clinical disciplines (acupuncture, chiropractic, herbal medicine, homeopathy and osteopathy) are distinguished by having established foundations of training and professional standards (British Medical Association, 1993).

Today, some CAM treatments are being used in National Health Service (NHS) clinics and hospitals. What are the driving forces behind such development in a developed country with advanced medical care and services? There has been a general trend of growing demand for complementary medicine in the UK when compared with other developed countries. A number of factors have stimulated this:

- Some prime professional organisations from the complementary and alternative medicine sector (see Table 1.1 in Chapter One), e.g. those representing osteopaths and chiropractors have recently sought and obtained statutory regulation.
- The British Medical Association (1993) published the report of a survey "Complementary Medicine: New approaches to good practice" indicating that such therapies were demanded by patients and might be beneficial. It emphasised those standards for education, training, regulation; professional practice code and research activities are essential to give credibility for patient care.
- The University of Exeter appointed the first Professor of Complementary Medicine at the Post-graduate Medical Centre to improve standard of education, practice and research activities.
- Several universities are establishing and offering first degree courses, masters and research degrees in complementary medicine,
- Increasing numbers of private institutes are offering part-time, full-time or "distant *learning*" courses,
- Some complementary treatments including acupuncture and Chinese medicinal herbal treatment can be obtained from the NHS

Table 16.1 Early development of acupuncture in the UK

Date	Notable events	Reference
16th century	Early knowledge of acupuncture was brought into Europe via connection with Dutch and English East India Co. 1st European text was compiled by Wiliem ten Rhyne	Rhyne, T., 1683
17th century	A comprehensive account of acupuncture moxibustion was written that had great influence on German acupuncture development	Kaempfer, E 1712
	A French Jesuit Du Halde wrote the text book "Description de l'Empire de la Chine" in 1735	Hsu, 1989
1825	A textbook on "A description of Surgical Operation Peculiar to Japanese and Chinese" in 1825 was published by JM Church	BMA, 1986
Early 19th century	Colonisation of Far East countries allowed more acupuncture knowledge reaching the West.	BMA, 1986
1960s	Influence of JR Worsley: Setting up of the first college of acupuncture in the UK— The British College of Traditional Chinese Acupuncture	Hsu & Peacher, 1977
1970s to present	Many private colleges of acupuncture were set up. Private Clinics have increased in numbers from 600 in early 1990s to 3000 in 1998.	Jin, Berry & Chan, 1995 Pharmaceutical Journal, 1998

- Patients are becoming better informed on healthcare related knowledge; they have the right to choose treatment.

HEALTH SERVICES IN THE UK

To understand the impact of the CAM in the UK, it is useful to give a brief description of the British welfare system. In 1948, the government of the day established the present National Health Service (NHS) as part of its welfare expansion programme. The aim was and still is to provide a comprehensive health care service to be available to all, free of charge at the point of delivery and to be financed mainly via taxation. Since its inception, the original aim of the NHS has not changed despite several major reorganisations. In the UK, every person is registered with a general practitioner (GP) to whom they will go for medical treatment. The consultation is free but the prescribed medications attract a fee, which is a proportion of the true cost of the medicine.

The general practitioner also acts as a gatekeeper to filter entry into the hospital system. The general practice, if equipped, can offer services such as minor surgical procedures. Patients are referred to the hospital only if their conditions warrant it as judged by their GPs. This hospitalisation will be free to the patients including treatment and food during their stay. The same principle applies to an individual who reports him/herself to a hospital's accident & emergency department and is later admitted for treatment or investigation.

Within the welfare programme, a person has free access and treatment for all of his or her health needs. This will include health counselling. As highlighted above, these complementary medicine/therapies can be offered on the NHS. But their availability within the NHS, is however, still very limited. Much is at the GPs' discretion. Increasing numbers of GPs wish to make use of CAM for their patients. In the referral model as suggested in the 1993 BMA Report the GP refers care of the patient to a specialist for the duration of a particular episode of treatment, but will retain clinical responsibility for the overall care of the patient. Therefore the professional standard and competence of the CAM therapists and treatment methods will be of importance when delegating care is given to the CAM therapists whose clinical disciplines for treating the patient may be outside the scope of the GP's skill and experience.

Nevertheless most CAM consultations and treatments are private and fee paying. However, patients who have private health insurance can, in most cases, receive a full refund for the cost of treatment. These practising CAM therapists will exercise their own professionalism and self-regulation for the interest of the patients if there is no statutory regulation governing the profession.

SOME OBSERVATIONS ON THE GROWTH OF CAM IN THE UK

Over the past decade we have witnessed the explosion and availability of information and expansion of knowledge in the public domain, and changing patterns of health and disease. One of the members of the Royalty (1997) called this change in the personal value placed on one's own health as "A very real social phenomenon." He, being a believer of both CAM and OM, has done much to raise the status of the CAM. He is also the Patron of the Foundation for Integrated Medicine, which has recently published a discussion paper, *Integrated Healthcare—A way forward for the next five years?* (1997). During the launch of this discussion document, he acknowledged that tremendous advances have been made in scientific and biological research, to the extent that conditions once thought untreatable could now be cured (1997). However, he argued that "Clearly this alone is not fulfilling all our health care needs as large numbers of people are paying to seek help from CAM practitioners. We simply cannot ignore what is a very real social phenomenon." He urged that practitioners of CAM and OM should collaborate with each other for the creation of "more patient centred health care".

The previous Conservative government accepted this phenomenon when it announced that "It is open to any family doctor to employ a complementary therapist to offer NHS treatment within their practice" (Dorrell 1991)

A survey by the National Association of Health Authorities and Trust, now the National Health Services Confederation (1993) found that: "The vast majority of purchasers have a positive attitude to funding complementary therapies."

The British Medical Association (BMA), which in its 1986 report dismissed Complementary Therapies as "passing fashion", has had a change of policy. In 1993, amidst increasing interest in complementary therapies among medical and health care professionals, the BMA produced a positive report calling for improved training and education within complementary medicine.

SOME KEY RECOMMENDATIONS FROM THE 1993 BMA REPORT INCLUDED:

- Priority should be given to research in acupuncture, chiropractic, herbalism, homoeopathy, and osteopathy as the therapies most commonly used in this country,
- The Council of Europe Co-operation in Science and Technology project on non-conventional therapies be approved by the UK Government, and

- Accredited postgraduate sessions be set up to inform clinicians on the techniques used by different therapists and the possible benefits for patients; consideration should be given to the inclusion of a familiarisation course on non-conventional therapies within the medical undergraduate curriculum.

In 1994, the current government wrote "In principle, complementary therapies that have value in health care should be available to NHS patients". It is a necessary part of good practice that general practitioners should have access to a wide choice of therapeutic approaches." (Primarolo, 1994)

Thomas *et al.* (1995) "Estimated 39.5% of GP partnerships in England now provide access to some form of complementary therapy for their NHS patients."

Goldbeck-Wood S (1996) reported in the BMJ that "Complementary medicine is gaining in popularity world-wide, with increases in the number of practitioners and the number of patients consulting them."

The recommendation of the Foundation for Integrated Medicine (1997) that students of the orthodox medicine, Complementary and Alternative Medicine and other healthcare professions should share a common core curriculum, followed by their specialist discipline is most welcome.

THE GROWING INTEREST IN CHINESE MEDICINE IN THE UK

The practice of Chinese medicine (CM) involves acupuncture and related physical techniques and the use of Chinese herbal medicines (CHM). These practices have continued in traditional manner by CM practitioners and pharmacists serving Chinese communities all over the world in Chinese towns of major cities in the west other than those in China. However a few years ago it was virtually impossible to buy CHM crude herbs and ready made-products in the UK. One could, at one's own risk, have ventured into China Towns in Soho London or in other big cities in UK and emerged with a bag of dried herbs if one knew what one was looking for. Or one could, in a desperate attempt, have received acupuncture treatment, in some private clinics or premises, for ailments that were "incurable" by conventional orthodox medicine.

Among western practitioners CHM is one of the most rapidly growing in popularity of the CAM disciplines in the English speaking western world. (Mills, 1996). It is particularly utilised as the second tier of CM treatment by western acupuncturists who have learned how closely CHM and acupuncture are integrated into clinical practice itself in China. It is interesting to observe that in the 1993 BMA Report that more vigorous professionalism and regulation would be placed upon acupuncture and herbalism (being among the top 5 disciplines singled out from the report) in order to safe-guard patients' interests.

Therefore it will be both interesting and important as reference for future progress and development to find out the historical background of the practice of Chinese medicine in the UK. Such information and understanding of the background will be extremely useful for the future development of integrating the practice of CAM, in particular Chinese medicine, with that of orthodox medicine for the benefit of the public at large.

Development of Chinese Medicine in the United Kingdom (UK)

THE EARLY HISTORICAL DEVELOPMENT OF CHINESE MEDICINE IN THE UK

The history of practising Chinese medicine in Europe, particularly acupuncture, dates from the middle of the 16th century. (Peacher, 1975). The early development of CM in UK is quite similar to that in most European countries, that is the practice of acupuncture. The first reports about acupuncture appearing in Europe were those from Wilhelm Ten Rhyne (1647 to 1700) and Engelbert Kaempfer (1651 to 1716). They spent two years in the enclave of Nagasaki in Japan, where the Dutch-East-Indian Trade Company had a registered office, and became interested in the practice of acupuncture. Their publications formed the foundation for European acupuncture. Ten Rhyne, a Dutch surgeon, published his experiences and observations in 1683 in London, while Kaempfer followed with the article on "Curatio colicae per acupuncturam japonicus unitata". Some French Jesuit Priests also brought back with them their knowledge to Europe; for example; Du Halde in 1735 wrote the "Description de l'Empire de la Chine" that included a detailed discussion of CM (Hsu, 1989). Later the publication in 1939 of L'acupunctyre Chinoise' by Soulie de Morant was an extensive discussion of the practice of acupuncture based on direct translation, observation, and actual practice in France. Later on in the mid-1900s with the European influence in the Far East, China, and

Indo-China much more knowledge of acupuncture percolated through into Europe.

The driving force behind the acupuncture development in the UK under the environment of orthodox medical practice has been mainly due to interest groups. The first extensive British text of acupuncture written by Church, a member of the Royal College of Surgeons in the UK, in 1825 (A description of Surgical Operations peculiar to Japanese and Chinese) marked the beginning of acupuncture practice in the UK. Later on, notable English acupuncturists (Dr. Felix Mann and Dr. Sidney Rose-Neil) began their explorations of acupuncture in the late 1950s and had influenced its development substantially in English speaking countries. In the 1960s the interest in acupuncture was extended further by JR Worsley who was a physical therapist and began his study of the subject in 1962 with subsequent impact on the perceptions of many practitioners in the UK and USA. He studied under the Rose-Neil group who set up the British Acupuncture Association & Register (Hsu & Peacher, 1977). Worsley made observations in Hong Kong and Taiwan and later founded the British College of Traditional Chinese Acupuncture and two schools in the USA. Table 16.1 summarises key periods involved in the early development of acupuncture in the UK.

The practice of traditional CM acupuncture by other CM trained practitioners and the adaptation of acupuncture technique by OM practitioners have nowadays led to the development of two main forms of acupuncture practice. These developments have created confusion among the public into believing that acupuncture is separate from Traditional Chinese medicine. For accuracy, TCM or Chinese medicine is a general concept embracing a host of preventive and treatment methods. Figure 16.1 below shows the most commonly used methods in the UK and Europe. Thus after individual diagnosis according to CM principles the patient will be given physical treatment such as acupuncture, Tuina/massage and or medicinal herbs or herbal products depending on the need of the patient. Some of the CM herbs can be utilised as functional food (See Chapter 17 for details) for prevention of disease or maintenance of health purposes during recuperation period.

The first group of acupuncturist practitioners use traditional methods of needle insertion and selection of acupuncture points, based on traditional Chinese principles of diagnosis and disease classification. These acupuncturists practise mainly in China and southeast Asia, though there are a few in Europe. The second group belongs to some

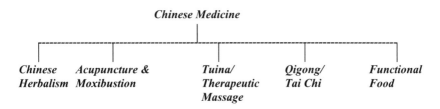

Figure 16.1 The most common methods of Chinese medicine used in the UK and Europe

doctors trained in OM who use a modified form of acupuncture, which places greater emphasis on analgesic effects. The selection of points is based mainly, but not exclusively, on the dermatomical distribution of pain rather than the traditional distribution of points along the meridians. Acupuncturists insert stainless steel needles perpendicularly or obliquely to various depths, depending on prescription. Usually the point is stimulated by rotating the needle or applying a periodic electric current, for about 10–20 minutes at a time.

Both traditional and modern acupuncture procedures may have variants on this technique. A "moxa" prepared from *Artemisia vulgaris* (common mugwort) may be burnt in conjunction with needling (Moxibustion) in the practice of traditional acupuncture. In modern procedure acupuncture points may be stimulated electrically or by laser beams. An instrument called a Dermatron may be used to measure electrical activity at acupuncture points for diagnosis as well as in treatment (EAV or Electro-acupuncture According to Voll). New acupuncture points are also being introduced, particularly on the face, scalp, ear and hand. However, the needle may be broken and may remain in the patient's body for life if good practice is not followed.

RECENT DEVELOPMENT OF TRAINING IN CHINESE MEDICINE IN THE UK

Education and Training Issues: Like those in most other European countries the interest groups of acupuncture and CM herbalism started more formal training of CM on the initial running of and updating of seminars. The earliest group seminars were run during the late 1950s and early 1960s. In recent years, many of the established acupuncture colleges in the UK (also in Australia, see Chapter 10; the USA, see Chapter 17) have introduced courses in CM herbalism. Most of these institutes run part-time courses, mainly in the evenings and weekends, of varying years of duration with certificates and diplomas on graduation (Jin *et al.*, 1995). In at least some cases these courses are rather brief, despite the fact that their graduates face different legislative and professional responsibilities as prescribers of active medications (Mills, 1996). One of the first colleges of acupuncture, the British College of Acupuncture, was founded in 1961. It initially offered only training in acupuncture, but in recent years CM herbalism was also included. In general most of these colleges mainly concentrate on tuition of substantial knowledge of the European interpretation of acupuncture and traditional CM (i.e. acupuncture, CM herbs, Qigong, and Tuina), with some small influence of Japanese variation, Vietnam oriental therapy, and Korean variation. Table 16.2 summarises some of the schools and colleges offering acupuncture and related CM courses in the UK.

In our survey (Jin *et al.*, 1995) we observed from the return of nearly 40% responders of 1248 that the predominant country or region of origin of CM practitioners was British (74.6%), Chinese (8.1%), and Indian (2.7%). The remaining 14.6% consisted of African (2%), the American (12%), Australasian (12%), Asian (20%) and European (23%). Most did not hold qualification in OM practice; 69% had received training in acupuncture, CM herbalism, or acu-pressure (4.9%); eleven (1.7%) were CM pharmacists. Training was mainly on a part-time basis (78.9%) of up to 5 years duration; 21.3% received full-time training of similar duration. Of these 71.9% trained, in some of those schools or colleges mentioned in Table 16.2, in Britain; 19.4% in China, 3.2% in Hong Kong and 2.3% in the USA.

In the past few years, several new universities have expanded their academic courses to cope with the increasing demand of training professionals and practitioners in complementary and alternative medicine (CAM). The main aim has been to formalise courses for CAM and to raise the standard of training for professionals in these areas. A 5-year degree course has been developed for Chinese medicine (both acupuncture and herbalism) at the Middlesex University taught in conjunction with the Beijing University of Traditional Chinese Medicine in China (see details in Chapter 18). Westminster University offers a degree course in Acupuncture in partnership with the British College of Acupuncture. The Northern College of Acupuncture has joined partnership with Bangor University to offer a Master course in acupuncture.

Table 16.2 Some societies and colleges of acupuncture & related Chinese medicine in the UK (Information collected from survey by Jin, *et al.*, 1995, and from journals of CAM available)

Society/register	Associated school/college	Year established
British Acupuncture Council, (formerly Directory of British Acupuncturists) CFA	5 major acupuncture schools/colleges: BAC, CSAC, BAAR	1982/1995
The Register of Chinese Herbal Medicine, RCHM	no affiliated colleges	Recent
The Register of Traditional Chinese Medicine, RTCM	no affiliated colleges	Recent
Association of Traditional Chinese Medicine	no affiliated colleges	1992
British Acupuncture Association and Register (BAAR)	British College of Acupuncture (BAC)	1961/1964
International Register of Oriental Medicine, IROM	The International College of Oriental Medicine	1975/1972
The Traditional Acupuncture Society, TAC	College of Traditional Acupuncture	1976
Chung San Acupuncture Society member of International Federation of Acupuncture	Chung San Acupuncture School (CSAC)	1984
Eligible for CFA membership	Northern College of Acupuncture	1988
Associated Register?	The London School of Acupuncture & TCM	1988?
Associated Register?	College of Integrated Chinese Medicine	1988?
Associated Register?	The London College of Traditional Acupuncture	recent
Associated Register?	The London Academy of Oriental Medicine	1991

THE PRACTICE OF CHINESE MEDICINE (CM) AND THE USE OF CM HERBS AND HERBAL PRODUCTS IN THE UK

The practice of CM

The popularity CM practitioners of consulting (with the public) in the UK, on a largely private basis, has grown since the late 1980s. The number of acupuncture/CM practitioners had increased from 708 in 1981 to 1248 in 1991 (Jin *et al.*, 1995). Consultations with CM practitioners average around an hour in the first instance. Treatment with acupuncture may be combined with CM herbs and advice on diet and exercises (based on Tuina, *Qigong* routine or *Tai Chi*). The consultation fees varied from £30 to £50 and the cost of herbal prescription (to make the decoction) about £5 to £10. Today, many consultation fees include the first course of treatment starting from £35. The herbs are traditionally provided as mixtures of individual dried herbs (plant parts) that the patients have to cook according to instructions at home. Such a procedure can be very trying for patients who are not used to the taste and smell. The alternative is the use of ready made (proprietary) CM herbal products of standard formulations (Fu Fang) that are recorded in the Chinese Pharmacopoeia. These may be in the conventional oral dosage forms such as capsules, pills, tablets and external preparations such as ointments and creams. Very few herbal manufacturers can be identified in the UK for the production of these CM herbal products. In a nation-wide survey of the practice of CM and use of CM herbs and herbal products we observed that several major herbal importers are responsible for import and exports of CM crude herbs and herbal ready-made or proprietary products. In this survey we enquired about the types of CM treatment patients prescribed by the CM practitioners. About 45.5% of the responding practitioners used CM herbs, 54.4% offered some physical therapies other than treatment with CM herbs. Most practitioners treated patients solely with acupuncture (72%), some used acupuncture with CM herbs (12%), or herbal treatment alone (5.3%). Of those who prescribed herbal medications 47.7% used ready-made CM herbal products, 23.8% dried crude herbs, 15% powders, and 13% tinctures.

In a recent seminar organised in Beijing, China under the Sino-British Co-operation theme, it was reported by some British delegates that there were some 3000 "CM clinics" in the UK and these were popular not only with Chinese residents, but also with the population as a whole in UK (Sino-British Co-operation, 1998). These clinics are run privately in most cases. However, there are also few NHS funded centres. One can observe the rapid growth in the numbers of clinics providing CM treatment (from 1248 to 3000 since 1991)

The use of CM herbs and herbal products

We found that nearly all of the locally available CM herbs and herbal products have been imported from abroad. Two importers, East West Herbs and Mayway, out of nine provided 86.5% herbs obtained locally (Jin *et al.*, 1995). Of the 13.5% purchased abroad 44%·came from China, 26% Hong Kong and 11% USA. Tables 16.3 and 16.4 summarise these surveys on the use of CM crude herbs and proprietary (ready-made) CM products in the UK. Importers of CM herbal materials based mainly in the UK supply these.

Majority (62.4%) of users considered herbs supplied to be of good quality, 35.4% of satisfactory and 2.2% of poor quality. All crude herbs suffer the complication of being natural products grown or collected from different sources. With the rapidly increasing demand of CM herbs and herbal products in the West there is greater temptation for suppliers to supply fake substitutes, inferior herbs or even adulterated finished ready made herbal products. Problems are more likely when buying from unfamiliar or small suppliers, especially those providing ready-made formulation or products. (Mills, 1996).

Table 16.3 The top fifteen most widely prescribed CM crude herbs in the UK

No	TCM herbs	English description	Percent of total
1	Dang Gui	Chinese Angelica Root	80
2	Gan Cao	Liquorice Root	64
3	Bai Shao Yao	White Paeony Root	61
4	Fu Ling	Indian Bread	60
5	Huang Qi	Astragalus Root	57
6	Shu Di	Cooked Rehmannia	56
7	Bai Zhu	White Atractylodes Tuber	47
8	Sheng Di	Raw Rehmannia Root	45
9	Dang Shen	Codonopsis Root	37
10	Mu Dan Pi	Tree Poeony Root	29
11	Chai Hu	Chinese Thorowax Root	29
12	Chuan Xiong	Lovage Tuber	26
13	Dan Shen	Red Sage Root	23
14	Ban Xia	Processed Pinellis Tuber	22
15	Fang Feng	Divaricate Saposhnikovia Root	21

(Adopted from Jin *et al.*, 1995).

Table 16.4 The top ten most widely prescribed patent TCM products in the UK

No	Patent TCM products	Percent of total
1	Xiao Yao Wan	73
2	Ba Zhen Wan	45
3	Bu Zhong Yi Qi Wan	39
4	Yin Chiao Chieh Tu Pian	30
5	Liu Wei Di Huang Wan	30
6	Er Chen Wan	24
7	Gui Pi Wan	24
8	Qing Qi Hua Tan Wan	18
9	Bi Yan Pian	18
10	Gan Mao Lin	15

(Adopted from Jin *et al.*, 1995).

From our survey we also found that the practitioners would like to see a guarantee of no fake herbs or adulterants (37%), better quality (15.2%), greater rangers of products (12.8%) and reduced cost (34.5%). In general herbs continued to reach the UK and other European countries without proper quality control. Fortunately there are a number of responsible importers in the market, some of whom use Chinese Pharmacopoeia as reference and pharmacognostic techniques and expertise through their production process, and who favour dealing with the State Administration of TCM in China for good quality control.

The success of a double-blind clinical study in the early 1990s, using a CHM composite prescription of 10 different herbs in the form of an aqueous decoction, for the cure of atopic eczema (Sheehan & Atherton 1992) that has been resistant to orthodox treatment, has created greater interest and attention in the use of CM herbs and ready-made products. Increasing concern and fear, observed from incidents of kidney and liver failures consequential to consumption of CM herbs, has also been expressed over the unsupervised use, efficacy, toxicity and quality of these natural products as well as the legal responsibilities of practitioners. Inclusion of orthodox medications such as antibiotics, non-steroidal drugs and steroids in CM ready-made products was not considered as a positive attribute of CM in the West. The use of fake or wrong herbs has contributed a negative opinion about the safety and efficacy of CM products. Many popular and expensive CM herbs are in short supply and inferior substitutes or fake crude herbs have been found in the UK market (Yu, Zhong, Chan & Berry, 1995; Yu, Berry, Zhong & Berry, 1997). Thus the safety, quality, and effectiveness of CM natural products are jeopardised. The leading professional group of practitioners of CM Herbalism, the Registrar of Traditional Chinese Medicine recommended some guidelines and precautions in the use of CM herbs and herbal products (Table 16.5)

Chinese Medicinal Herbs and Herbal Products in the UK Legislation

GENERAL INFORMATION ON THE LEGISLATION OF HERBAL PRODUCTS IN THE UK

Legislation on herbal medicines is a global problem. A survey conducted by the World Health Organisation (WHO, 1998) pointed out that most developing and few developed countries do not consider herbal products as medicines that require control similar to pharmaceuticals used in orthodox medicine for treatment of diseases. However in some countries herbal medicinal products or remedies are considered as medicines that require the same controls as those for synthetic pharmaceuticals in the form of product licenses.

In the UK almost all the licensed herbal remedies on the market have been available for some time and most held old *Product Licenses of Right (PLR)* that may gradually expire and may be subjected to further

Table 16.5 Recommendations from the register of Chinese herbal medicine in the use of CM herbs

---

- Use reputable supplies, enquire quality control measures to prevent fraudulent substitution of herbs
- Avoid using obscure herbs (About 200 taught by the schools and colleges i.e. London School of Acupuncture & Traditional Chinese Medicine, have been thoroughly investigated for toxicity)
- Confine to dosages recommended in Official Pharmacopoeia
- Monitor patients monthly
- Never prescribe a patent TCM Product unless ingredients are known. Some may contain synthetic drugs
- Set up own effective reporting system for TCM induced adverse reactions with RCHM council

---

reviewed before registration or renewal is approved. Many products of these PLR's were granted as far back as 1971 (about 39,000 PLR's) without scientific assessment. The European Community (EC) legislation required that review of these PLR products be completed by 1990. Therefore with effects from January 1991 all manufactured herbal products herbal products should comply with the new Directive of the EU. The Directive (65/65/EEC) requires herbal medicinal products to possess marketing authorisation if they are "industrially produced" in a similar standard of pharmaceuticals for orthodox medicine. However this term is not defined in the UK or EC law. The UK Government has adopted the view that herbal medicines currently exempted under the Medicines Act are prepared or supplied on a small scale or by traditional processes that take them outside the implication of "industrially produced".

Thus, this exemption has given herbal practitioners the flexibility they need to prepare their own remedies for individual patients without the burden of licensing and to allow simple dried herbs to be readily available to the public. This situation will be changed as EU legislation on herbal medicines has progressed on towards harmonisation among EU members. However this may take some times.

SOME KEY PLAYERS INVOLVED IN REGULATING HERBAL REMEDIES IN THE EUROPEAN UNION (EU) AND THE UK

At present there is little harmonisation in European legislation for the registration of herbal or natural products for medicinal purposes. The legal status of herbal remedies within Europe and the problems involved in harmonising their assessment have been indicated (Deboyer, 1991; Cranz, 1994 and Keller, 1994). In the UK herbal products are available through various retail outlets such as pharmacies, health food shops, supermarkets, departmental stores and even mail order companies. Some are loosen dried plant materials; others are in ready-made pharmaceutical forms (capsules, tablets liquids, creams and ointments). Some of these may contain mixtures of several herbal ingredients. The legal status of these products is complicated by the fact that in most EU countries they could be imported as herbal remedies, "foods" or "dietary supplements" (Cranz, 1994). National procedures implemented by EU member states to comply with the 65/65/EC Directives for reviewing all licensed herbal remedies differ due to different interpretation of medicinal or otherwise use of the same product. An important initiative in the harmonisation process on quality efficacy and safety of herbal materials and products for medicinal uses has been the establishment of the European Scientific Co-operative for Phytotherapy (ESCOP) in 1989 as an umbrella organisation representing national associations for phytotherapy.

It will be important to make a brief review on the roles of some key agencies in the UK and EU that are involved in regulating the import and export of herbal and natural products for medicinal or other uses.

The Ministry of Agriculture, Fishery and Foods (MAFF): The majority of herbal products in the UK are marketed as food supplements without medicinal claims are controlled by food legislation sets out by the **MAF**. It is because of difficulties in defining the status of products occupying the borderline between medicines and foods. Such legislation control is considered not appropriate as some herbal or natural products are with potent medicinal properties though marketed as food supplements without medicinal claims.

The Medicine Control Agency (MCA): MCA, the body responsible for regulating all medicinal products, recently reviewed such situation. It will soon be amended according to the definition of a medicinal product set out by the MCA (MAL 8, 1995) in accordance with the Article 1 of Directive 65/65EEC (EC 1965):

- "A medicinal product is any substance or combination of substances presented for treating, or preventing disease in human beings or animal". An interpretation of the product by presentation.
- "Any substance or combination of substances which may be administered to human beings or animals with a view to making diagnosis or to restoring, correcting or modifying physiological functions in human beings or animals is likewise considered a medicinal product". An interpretation of the product by function.

Guidelines are available from the MCA for manufacturers of herbal products the definition of medicinal products. In the near future such guidelines may be reviewed in consultation with the **European Agency for Evaluation of Medicinal Products (EMEA)**

European Scientific Co-operative on Phytotherapy (ESCOP) is an organisation representing 14 national phytotherapy associations across Europe. *ESCOP* was set up in January 1989. The ESCOP's views on phytomedicines have been:

- "Phytomedicines, or herbal medicinal products are medicinal products containing as active ingredients only plant, parts of plants or plant materials, or combinations thereof, whether in the crude or processed states.

- "Plant materials include juices, gums, resins, essential oils and other directly derived crude plant products. They do not include chemically defined isolated constituents either alone or in combination with plant materials. However phytomedicines may contain excipients of plant or non-plant derivation".

The objectives of ESCOP are:

- Developing a co-ordinated scientific framework to assess phytomedicines
- Promoting the acceptance of phytomedicines especially within general medical practice.
- Supporting and initiating clinical and experimental research in phytotherapy
- Supporting all appropriate measures that would secure optimum protection for those who use phytomedicines.
- Producing reference monographs on the therapeutic use of plant drugs.

In its centenary anniversary meeting in January 1999 ESCOP together with the MCA, EMEA and the WHO Organisation Collaborating Centre for International Drug Monitoring have set targets for promoting the assessment and assurance of the quality, efficacy and safety aspects of herbal medicines:

- To start mutual recognition procedure to bring HMPs (Herbal Medicinal Products) to European Market
- To identify major problems involved: They are listed as follows:
  - Differences in assessment of quality, safety and efficacy of HMPs
  - Complexity of HMPs
  - Interpretation of bibliographic data
  - Better guidance towards mutual recognition of HMPs
- To form an EMEA and hoc working group on Herbal Medicine Products (HMPWG)

The Medicines Control Agency (MCA), UK—Initiatives on control of HMPs.

- Extension of the yellow card scheme to unlicensed HMPs
- Review of toxic herbal substances (in progress)
- Withdrawal of some HMPs making unsubstantiated claims.

The WHO Organization Collaborating Centre for International Drug Monitoring have set targets to monitor reports on adverse drug reactions (ADRs) due to HMPs. The causes of ADRs could be classified as follows:

- A single-ingredient herbal product as the sole cause
- A multiple ingredient ("Combination") herbal products as the sole suspected cause
- A product containing both herbal and non-herbal ingredients as the sole suspected cause
- Simultaneous use of herbal products and non-herbal products as the suspected cause

LICENSING OF CHINESE HERBAL MEDICINAL MATERIALS AND PRODUCTS.

The licensing of CHM products may be more complicated than those herbal products that are produced locally in the UK used in European herbalism. Chinese herbal medicinal (CHM) products used in the UK are mainly imported from abroad (see previous sections of this Chapter). They will be classified unlicensed herbal products. In a recent symposium (Sino-British co-operation, 1998), the group manager for policy on unlicensed medicines of the MCA pointed out that under the present law in the UK some CHM products might be classified as medicines, others as foods or cosmetics. The MCA will be responsible for deciding if or not a product is a medicine according to the general definition. Products classified as medicines will require a product license. Some potent herbal remedies can only be sold through pharmacies. It was observed that there were responsible CHM manufacturers exporting crude herbs and herbal products into the UK; however there were concerns over the imports from some scrupulous manufacturers. For instances, some skin creams contained undeclared steroids, some toxic herbs, such as *Aristochia* species, were sold as substitutes for *Stephania tetrandra* and come products contained unacceptably high concentration of toxic heavy metals such as arsenic and mercury.

Importers and exporters of CHM to the UK should make clear the legal status of a product (whether as food, cosmetic, or medicine) and identify the regulations that applied to that category of products. They should also make sure that products imported came from manufacturers with high quality of practice accompanying with good documentation and clear labelling of products for the category claimed. The present legislation on imported herbal products will be changed in line with those from the EU and in response to public pressure over concern for public health.

RESTRICTED USE OF CHINESE MEDICINAL MATERIALS (CMM FROM NATURAL SOURCES) IN THE UK AND EU

The recent episodes of poisoning or damage of kidneys and livers due to ingestion of Chinese herbal products containing potent CM herbs have urged the Regulators to tighten control over imported CMM. In order to fulfil the demands from EU and U.K government, the Medicine Control Agency (MCA) is planning to regulate the use of imported CMM products and to control the quality, safety and efficacy of these products in the British markets, after consultation with the herbal practitioners. Imports and manufacturers of CMM will be required to get products licenses if they are sold in the British market. This means that CMM can be approved and accepted by British government and get the legal status on U.K., perhaps it is a good chance and also a good future for CMM to enter the British market. But the problem is the fees for registration in the U.K. will be very expensive.

The Royal Botanical Garden in Kew has now set up an authentication centre on CMM in the U.K. to cope under this condition. It is said that the centre may become an official legal administration in the U.K., and later an international centre for authentication and identifying CMM. In the very near future the centre will start working with importers of Chinese medicinal products and their Association, the Chinese Medicine Association of Suppliers on this burning issue.

In the Netherlands because there is higher level of heavy metals in 6 CMM decoctions, Liu Shen Wan, Tian Wang Bu Xing Wan, Niu Huang Jie Du Pian, Niu Huang Jian Ya Wan and Zuei Feng Tu Gu Wan are prohibited from use by Dutch police.

Some CMM are also banned in Europe. They are: Mu Xiang (*Radix Aucklandiae*), Xi Yang Seng (American *Ginseng*), Gan Sui (*Radix Euphorbiae*), Lu Uh (*Aloe*), Lu Shen (Deer Kidney), Lin Yang Jiao (Antelope's horn), Ye Ming Sha (Bat's faeces), Lu Jiao (Deer horn), Lu Jiao Shang (Deglued antler powder), Lu Rong (Pilose deer horn), Shui Niu Jiao (Bufalo horn), Du Pie Zhong (Ground beetle), Ku Lian Pi (*Cortex meliae*), Wu Lin Zhi (Trogopterus dung), Xiong Dian Fen (Bear gall), Yue Ji Hua (Chinese rose), Me Kui Hua (*Flos rose Rugoae*), Mu gua (*Fructus chaenomelis*), Shuang Zha (*Fructus crataegi*), Wu Me (*Fructus mume*), Jin Ying Zhi (*Fructus rosae laevi-*

gatae), Pi Pa Ye (*Folium eriobotrae*), E Jiao (Donkey hide gelatin), Shi Hu (*Herba dendrobii*), Ying Su Ke (Poppy capsule), Dang Gui (*Radix Angelicae Sinensis*), Huang Qi (*Radix Astragali sen Hedysari*), Chai Hu (*Radix Bupleuri*), Long Dan Cao (*Radix Gentianae*), Xue Jie (*Resina Draconis*), Ku Xing Ren (*Bitter apricot kornel*), She Xiang (Musk), Bai Hua She (*Agkistrodon acutus*), Bai Ji li (*Fructus Tribuli*), Zhe Bei Mu (*Bulbus Frieillariae Thanbegii*), Niu Huang (*Calculus bovis*), Xian He Can (*Herba Agrimoniae*), Ye shan shen (*Radix Genseng*), Da Fu Pi (*Pericarpium Arecae*), Lu Jiao Jiao (*Colla cornus cervi*), Jiang Xiang (*Lignum Dalbergiae odoriferae*), Cao wu (*Radix Aconiti Kusnezoffii*), Qu Mai (*Herba Dianthi*), Quan Xie (*Buthus martensi*), etc.

THE ESTABLISHMENT OF CHINESE MEDICINE ASSOCIATION OF SUPPLIERS (CMAS)

As intimated above, in UK, Chinese medicine is neither recognised nor licensed by MCA as medicine despite the fact that CM has been around for more than two thousand years. Instead, most of these medicinal herbs and ready-made products are being sold as herbal teas and food supplements, which do not require a licence. The current clinical trial methodologies and processes used for orthodox medicine (OM) are ill equipped to assess the treatment effectiveness of Chinese herbs. A treatment of Chinese herbal medicine consists of a blend of several sometimes up to ten or more different herbs. This has so far confounded western scientists to bring Chinese medicine within the parameters of existing clinical trial regimes. However such approach has also proved unsatisfactory according to the orthodox pharmaceutical requirement for licensing because these herbs invariably comprise unknown and unidentified chemical components and their overall effect cannot be simply assumed by reference to the perceived single active constituents as in synthetic-based drugs.

In an unregulated environment disgruntle comments from CM practitioners and importers and sellers of CM herbs and products in the UK are inevitable. Many small importers complain that they simply make a living and some accuse the motives of bigger organisations for agreeing to the future legislation of CM herbs and herbal products. Such accusations will continue so long there is no properly and professionally organised group to speak with one voice in the same manner as that for the British Medical Association who speaks with authority on behalf of all OM practitioners.

In April 1999, the CMAS was launched with the following mission statement, aims and objectives and code of practice:

The Mission Statement of the CMAS: The registered members will be guided by the Association's code of practice to uphold both quality and safety in the supply of Chinese medicines.

Aims and Objectives: The Chinese Medicine Association of Suppliers is a professional organisation for the suppliers of CM products. The Association will act as a self-regulatory body, which will lobby in the interest of its members within the bounds of the public safety. The aims and objectives of CMAS are to:

- Create a self-regulated association that will assure safety and quality of Chinese herbs in the UK, through regulation of its members.
- Work closely with regulatory authorities, in particular the MCA, to secure a safe and successful future for Chinese herbal medicines in the UK.
- Lobby for a new regulatory category for herbal medicines that will help to ensure that Chinese herbs are safe and properly regulated.
- Represent suppliers and importers of Chinese herbal medicines and to act on their behalf.
- Develop a recognised kite-mark which will act as assurance of safety for both the public and members.
- Enforce a code of practice.
- Oversee the supply of good quality Chinese medicine to practitioners.
- Preserve the pharmacopoeia and promote the benefits of Chinese medicine outside China

Code of practice of the CMAS: Each member shall act, at all times, in such a manner as to:

- Supply authenticated individual herbs and herbal products.
- Safeguard the biodiversity in the use of Chinese medicine.
- Act with due regard to laws, customs and practices of the land
- Promote good working relationships with other members, manufacturers, practitioners and consumers

- Maintain and improve his/her professional knowledge and competence
- Use appropriate designatory letters on letterheads and in advertisements and publicity providing that the placement and content of such advertising materials always conform to the high standards of professional practice.

A detailed paper on the Code of Practice will be available to all members

Discipline: All members are subject to the CMAS's Code of Practice. CMAS reserves the right to investigate any reported incident of misconduct or breach of its Code of Practice and to take whatever action it deems to be appropriate in the interest of CMAS, the public at large and Chinese medicine.

Progress of Practice and Research in Chinese Medicine in the UK

ASSURANCE OF QUALITY, EFFICACY, AND SAFETY OF CHINESE HERBAL MEDICINAL PRODUCTS

Research of Chinese medicine in the UK, as a whole has been very limited until the early 1990s. Previously studies on the application of acupuncture in anaesthesia within orthodox medical practice had created some interests. Moreover the negative survey in 1986 carried out by the British Medical Association (BMA Report, 1986) did not encourage research in complementary medicine in general. However the more positive approaches to "Good Practice" of complementary medicine suggested in the 1993 report (BMA, 1993) has made some improvement. The formation of the Research Council for Complementary Medicine has created an opportunity for all professionals engaging in various aspects of complementary medicines to meet up and air their difficulties in carrying out practice research. Very little literature in English language is available for basic research on both acupuncture and Chinese herbalism in the UK. There is, however, a considerable and growing literature of basic research and clinical evidence published in Chinese language (see Chapter 6). Much of the evidence cited from studies from China are uncontrolled clinical trials and the regulatory agencies in the Australasia, N. America, and Europe will not accept Chinese data in support of their application for licensing as medicinal products.

According to the UK Medicines Act Leaflet (MAL) 8 and MAL 39 (1986) for products containing herbal ingredients, illustrating the making of Zemaphyte as an example, the whole GMP production is not unsimilar to those stipulated for manufacturing of orthodox pharmaceuticals. The major difference can be identified in the contents of ingredients. One of the difficulties of quality assurance for natural products is their inconsistent composition of many constituents with unknown chemical structures. Research in methodology in these areas is urgently needed.

THE CALL FOR EVIDENCE ON COMPLEMENTARY AND ALTERNATIVE MEDICINE BY THE HOUSE OF LORDS

At the time of writing this chapter in October 1999, the House of Lords Science and Technology Committee has established a sub-committee III chaired by Lord Walton of Detchant. This Committee has to prepare a report on complementary and alternative medicine. To help focus attention from the public, the Committee is inviting submissions by mid December1999, in the forms of answers to the following key questions:

Evidence—What is the role of patient satisfaction in evaluating the effectiveness of complementary and alternative treatments and in determining availability? Do all medical and health care interventions have to be backed by the evidence of controlled clinical trials and the orthodox scientific thinking?

Information—What are the best sources of information for patients and doctors on complementary and alternative medicine? Is it desirable or possible to control the quality of public information available on such treatments?

Research—Should research funding for evaluations of complementary and alternative medicine be increased? If so, where should the extra money come from? What types of additional research would be most useful?

Training—Should the increased interest in complementary and alternative medicine be reflected in medical training and training of other healthcare professionals?

Regulation and risk—Are there areas of complementary and alternative medicine where lack of regulation causes unacceptable risk to the public? Are there practicable forms of regulation that would provide protection without unduly restricting patient choice?

NHS provision—Should public healthcare attempt to integrate elements of complementary and alternative medicine into the mainstream of healthcare? How might this be done? Should access to complementary and alternative treatment through the NHS be limited to those areas that (a) an established evidence base and (b) formal regulatory systems, can minimum required standards of evidence and regulation be defined?

It is apparent these enquiry topics will be applicable for the practice of Chinese medicine in the U.K.

Conclusion

It is obvious that regulatory approaches towards both practitioners and treatments methods and products have been the priority in all complementary medicine in the UK. Chinese medicine has been practised in China for thousands of years and its integration into OM practice in China has been unique. The use of CM in a hospital in Germany (See Chapter 15) and the health service in Taiwan (See Chapter 11) have also pointed towards similar integration and direction. Until the quality of the CM practitioners and the treatment methods and CM herbal products in the UK and EU and other developed countries in the west has been sorted out and regulated one can see there is a definite place in the health service in these countries.

References

BMA (1986) Alternative Therapy: Report of the Board of Science & Education, London: British Medical Association, United Kingdom.

BMA (1993) Complementary Medicine, new approaches to good practice, Oxford; Oxford University Press.

Cameron-Blackie, G. and Mouncer, Y. (1993) Complementary therapies in the NHS (research paper No. 10) London: National Association of Health Authorities and Trusts.

"China to open 30 TCM clinics around the world" reported in the BBC World Service 27.11.97

Consumers Association (1986) Magic or medicine? *Which?*, October, 443–447.

Coward, R. (1986) The whole truth: the myth of alternative medicine, London, Faber & Faber.

Cranz, H. (1994) Medicinal plants and phytomedicines within the European Community. *Herbalgram*, **30**, 50–53.

Davies, P. (1987) Report on trends in complementary medicine, Institute for Complementary Medicine.

de Wit (1981) Quoted in BMA (1986), Alternative Therapy: Report of the Board of Education, London: British Medical Association.

Deboyser, P. (1991) Traditional herbal medicines around the globe: modern perspectives. *Swiss Pharmacy*, **13**, 86–89.

EC (1965) Council Directive 65/65/EEC. *Official Journal of European Community*, **22**, 369.

Foundation for Integrated Medicine (1997) Integrated Healthcare—A way forward for the nest five years? London.

Fulder, S. and Monro, R. (1985) Complementary medicine in the UK—patients, practitioners and consultants, *Lancet*, 7 September, 40–47

Furnham, A. and Smith, C. (1988): Choosing alternative medicine—a comparison of the beliefs of patients visiting a GP and homoeopath, *Social Science Medicine*, **26**, 685–687

Goldbeck-Wood, S. (1996) Complementary medicine is booming worldwide; *British Medical Journal*, **313**, 131.

HRH Prince Charles (1997) Quoted in *The Times*, 22.10.97

Johnson K *et al.* (1993): Can sensory stimulation improve the functional outcome in stroke patients? *Neurology*, **43**, 2189–2192

Hsu, E. (1989) Outline of the history of acupuncture in Europe. *Journal Chinese Medicine*, 28–32.

Hsu, H. and Peacher, W. (1977) Chen's History of Chinese Medical Science. Modern Publishers. Taipei.

Jin, Y., Berry, M.I. and Chan, K. (1995) Chinese herbal medicine in the United Kingdom. *Pharmaceutical Journal*, **255** (**suppl**), R37.

Keller, K. (1994) Phytotherapy on the European level. *European Phytotelegram*, **6**, 40–49.

Lewith, G. *et al.* (1996) Complementary Medicine: an integrated approach. Oxford University Press, Oxford.

MAL (1995) Medicines Act Leaflet: A Guide to what is a Medicinal Product. Medicine Control Agency, December 1995.

Morgan, D. (1997) HIV/AIDS and complementary medicine: seeking information on alternative treatments. *The AIDS Letter*, No 63 Oct/Nov 1997, The Royal Society of Medicine Press.

The NHS Confederation (1997) Complementary medicine in the NHS—managing the issues. *Research paper* No. 4

Primarolo, D. (1994) Complementary Therapies within the NHS, Public Information Unit, The Labour Party, London

The Quality Assurance Agency for Higher Education (1997) Subject Review Handbook—October 1998 to September 2000.

Research Council for Complementary Medicine (RCCM:1997) Public usage of complementary medicine: an overview.

Sino-British Co-operation (1998) Traditional Chinese Medicine in Britain: Report of a Seminar. *Pharmaceutical Journal*, **261**, 641.

Scottish Home Office Department of Health (1996), Complementary Medicine and the NHS—an examination of Acupuncture, Homeopathy, Chiropractic and Osteopathy, The Stationery Office.

Sheehan, M.P. and Atherton, D.J. (1992) A controlled trial of traditional Chinese medicinal plants in widespread non-exudative atopic eczema. *British Journal of Dermatology*, **126**, 179–184.

Thomas, K.J. *et al.* (1991) Use of non-orthodox and conventional health care in Great Britain, *British Medical Journal*, **302**, 207–210

Thomas, K.J. *et al.* (1995) National survey of access to complementary health care via general practice, University of Sheffield.

Tomlinson R (1996), China tightens up TCM courses; *British Medical Journal*, **312**, 20 April 1996.

Vincent, C. and Furnham, A. (1996) Why do patients turn to complementary medicine?—an empirical study, *British Journal Clinical Psychology*, **35**, 37–48.

West, R. (1992) Alternative medicine: prospects and speculations. In Saks M (Ed): Alternative Medicine in Britain, Oxford: Clarendon Press

Wharton, R. and Lewith, G. (1987) Complementary medicine and the general practitioner, *British Medical Journal*, **292**, 1498–1500.

Worth, C. (1997) Guidelines for selecting practitioners of complementary and alternative medicine within the health service 1997/1998

Yu, H., Berry, M., Zhong, S. and Chan, K. (1997) Pharmacognostical investigations on traditional Chinese medicinal herbs: Identification of six herbs from the UK market. *Journal of Pharmacy & Phrmacology*. **49** (**supp 4**), 114.

17 THE PROGRESS OF CHINESE MEDICINE IN THE UNITED STATES OF AMERICA

Ka Kit Hui
Jun Liang Yu
Lidia Zylowska

Introduction

In the United States, the progress of Chinese Medicine (CM) is an integral part of the growing field of complementary and alternative medicine (CAM). Although often used together or interchangeably, the term *complementary* refers to therapies used *in addition* to standard medical treatments while the term *alternative* describes medical practices used *instead* of the standard medicine. Also known under such headings as holistic, natural, mind-body or Oriental medicine, the field of CAM to a great extent incorporates and draws from the CM tradition. Elements and principles of four major disciplines of CM—acupuncture, herbal medicine, massage and Tai-Chi/Qi-Gong exercises—can be frequently found throughout the field of CAM. As a result, any comprehensive discussion of CM progress in America has to acknowledge progress of its elements within the context of other CAM techniques. Over the last three decades, the trend toward complementary and alternative medicine has become a significant area of exploration by the public, health care industry and the academia. Most of the interest has been driven by a growing consumer demand for "natural medicine," forcing western medical practitioners to rethink their attitudes about alternative medicine.

KEY EVENTS INFLUENCING THE PROGRESS OF CM IN THE U.S.

1972—President Nixon's visit to China promoted interest in Chinese culture and opened new avenues of exchange. Traveling with Nixon, a *New York Times* columnist, James Reston, reported benefits of an acupuncture treatment he received while in China. After an emergency appendectomy, Reston had acupuncture, which successfully relieved his post-operative gastrointestinal discomfort. His praising account of the experience and the featured TV shows about surgical operations with acupuncture anesthesia in China were widely publicized and prompted a great interest both among the public and the medical establishment.

1992—NIH (National Institute of Health) established the Office of Alternative Medicine (OAM). The establishment greatly promoted the research and regulation of alternative medicine.

1993—Dr. David Eisenberg *et al.* at Harvard University conducted a study that was published in *The New England Journal of Medicine* (Eisenberg *et al.*, 1993). The article showed that approximately one third of Americans used alternative medicine in 1990. The study sparked further interest and research activities.

1994—FDA (Food and Drug Administration) passed the Dietary Supplement and Health Education Act (DSHEA), (FDA 1995) in order to regulate herbs as dietary supplements. Like vitamins, herbs only need to meet the standards of dietary supplements to be sold on the market and are not subject to the rigorous regulations applied to standard drugs. This act greatly promoted the development of herbal medicine in the U.S.

1996—FDA reclassified acupuncture needles, upgrading the supplies from Class III (experimental use) to Class II (general medical use) (Moffet 1996a, Villaire 1998).

1997—NIH successfully sponsored an Acupuncture Consensus on Acupuncture Efficacy. The meeting confirmed the efficacy, application and safety of acupuncture (NIH 1998, Villaire 1998) for selected conditions.

1998—In October, OAM was renamed as the National Center for Complementary and Alternative Medicine (NCCAM) with substantial increase in its budget.

1998—In November, several major American medical journals (*Journal of the American Medical Association, Arch. Intern Med. et al.*) joined focused on CAM and about 90 articles on alternative medicine were published. That event elevated alternative medicine to a new level of development and identified it as an area in need of further research. The journals acknowledged the significance of complementary medicine, described some of its potential uses, and called for further exploration. Attention was called to regulation and safety of complementary medical treatments.

1999—Government-sponsored Botanical/Dietary Supplements Research Centers are proposed (NIH 1999).

Evolution of the CAM/CM Field

TRENDS IN CAM AND THE STATUS OF CM IN THE U.S.

In the past several years, numerous survey studies have examined the practice of CAM in the United States. Most often quoted is the pioneering study done by David Eisenberg *et al.*, (1993, 1998) at Harvard University published in 1993 and updated in 1998. The comparative results from surveys taken in the U.S. in 1990 versus 1997 indicated a significant increase in the proportion of the population seeking alternative therapies. Specifically, the use of alternative therapies in the general population leaped from 33.8% in 1990 to 42.1% in 1997. The types of alternative medicine most used included relaxation exercise, herbal medicine, massage chiropractic and acupuncture. In both the 1990 and 1997 surveys, alternative therapies were used most often for chronic medical problems such as pain related conditions (headaches, neck and back problems, arthritis); stress related conditions (depression, anxiety, and insomnia), fatigue, allergies, lung problems, digestive problems and high blood pressure. There were more alternative medicine users among women than men, and more among people aged 35–49 than other age groups. The studies found that the largest group of consumers consists of white, well-educated, comparatively affluent individuals who are more likely to live in the West than elsewhere in the United States. When accounting for the U.S. population growth, comparison of out-of-pocket expense for alternative medicine services between 1990 and 1997 suggests a substantial increase in total visits to alternative medicine practitioners, surpassing the number of total visits to all U.S. primary care physicians. The total estimated amount of $27.0 billion spent on alternative medicine in 1997 represents an amount comparable to the projected 1997 out-of pocket expenditures for all U.S. physician services (Figure 17.1).

Focusing on CM only, a study surveyed 575 Chinese medicine users in the United States from six clinics in five states (Cassidy 1998a, 1998b). The study demonstrated that demographics of the patients and conditions for which help was sought were similar to the CAM study by Eisenberg *et al.* The majority of CM users reported "disappearance" or "improvement" of symptoms, improved quality of life, and reduced use of selected measures, including prescription drugs and surgery. Respondents reported utilizing a wide array of practices in addition to Chinese medicine, and expressed extremely high satisfaction with CM care. Ninety-nine percent of respondents had received acupuncture,

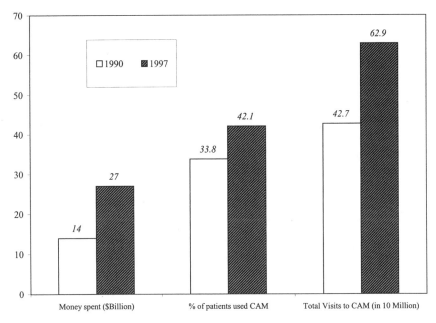

Figure 17.1 CAM use in the US (Data from Eisenberg *et al*, 1998)

59.7% had received moxibustion, and 35.5% had received Chinese herbs. No respondent reported experiencing important adverse events from acupuncture treatments.

Acupuncture

Among alternative medicine practices in the U.S., acupuncture is the most recognized branch of CM. This component of TCM is practiced by a large group of licensed acupuncturists, significant number of physicians and being the area of CM most commonly covered by medical insurance companies. It is estimated that 10 million treatments are performed each year to more than 1 million American patients. Currently, there are more than 10,000 non-physician acupuncturists and close to 3,000 physicians who incorporate acupuncture in their practice (Ulett *et al.*, 1998). More than 53 acupuncture and oriental medicine schools have been founded in the U.S., about 36 states have established acupuncture committees or government agencies to control and regulate the practice of acupuncture, and several national acupuncture associations for acupuncturists and physicians have been organized nationwide (NIH 1997, 1998). Since most non-physicians, licensed acupuncturists incorporate other CM techniques in their practice; the profession largely represents the general CM practitioners in the U.S.

Among the plethora of styles seen in the U.S.—including traditional Chinese acupuncture, French energetic acupuncture, auricular acupuncture, Korean and Japanese acupuncture five element theory and myofascial or tender point-based acupuncture—CM acupuncture is often considered the classic form from which other styles originate and borrow from.

REGULATION OF ACUPUNCTURE

The practice of acupuncture has been regulated on two basic levels: 1) acupuncture needles and 2) training and licensing requirements. Some of the regulations apply nationwide but many exist only at the state level contributing to wide discrepancies between amount of training required of the practitioners.

Regulation of acupuncture needles

When acupuncture was first becoming popular in 1972, after recommendations of an advisory committee, the FDA cautiously labeled acupuncture needles as "investigational devices". By 1980, the FDA recognized the low risk use of acupuncture needles by qualified practitioners and modified its regulations to allow increased availability of acupuncture needles. In 1994, a petition by scientists, acupuncturists, and M.D.s practicing acupuncture urged NIH and FDA to review the investigational designation of acupuncture needles. Finally, in 1996 the FDA formally recognized acupuncture needles as a legitimate medical device and approved it for "general acupuncture use" by licensed, registered, or certified practitioners (Feely 1999, Lytle 1996, Moffet 1996a, Wu 1996). Reclassification of the needles improved the image of acupuncture as a medically approved treatment, increased its accessibility, allowed medical insurance coverage, and expanded research funding for acupuncture.

Regulation of the acupuncture practitioners

In the U.S., those who want to treat patients with acupuncture have to have some kind of medical privilege such as license in medicine, osteopathy, dentistry, and acupuncture. The certification and licence standards of acupuncturists have grown steadily since 1970s. Since the first laws were passed in California in 1972, 35 other states and the District of Columbia have approved the practice of acupuncture and identified licensing requirements. Although efforts are underway to standardize the field of acupuncture, regulations vary from stringent to nonexistent, and many states support a double standard: medical doctors, dentists, and osteopaths can practice the procedure without formal training, but acupuncturists must complete a specified number of training hours and pass a licensing examination (Mitchell 1995, 1996, 1997; Moffet 1996b; Acupuncture Committee 1997). A compendium of laws and practice requirements in every state, published by the National Acupuncture Foundation, may be obtained from the National Acupuncture and Oriental Medicine Alliance (Bailey and Leef, 1999).

NON-PHYSICIAN ACUPUNCTURE

Over two-thirds of all acupuncture in the U.S. is done by non-physician graduates of acupuncture/Oriental medicine colleges, many of which were created in the last two decades. Several years after acupuncture practice started to take root in the U.S., a need for quality assurance was recognized. In 1981, three organizations—ACAOM (Accreditation Commission for Acupuncture and Oriental Medicine), CCAOM (Council of Colleges of Acupuncture and Oriental Medicine) and NCCAOM (National Certification Commission for Acupuncture and Oriental Medicine)—were established to set standards of practice and regulate the field of acupuncture (Bailey and Leef, 1999). The practice of acupuncture covers a wide range of modalities and tools and the title of acupuncturist is the starting point to practice other CM techniques such as herbal medicine, Oriental massage (Tui-Na), acupressure, breathing techniques, exercise, or nutrition. At this time there is no uniform licensing required to practice other CM techniques and the state-specific acupuncture regulations often determine the scope of CM practice. In some states, acupuncturists can order medical tests and prescribe herbal treatments and nutritional supplements. In 24 states, acupuncturists can practice independently. In 10 other states, they must have patients referred to them before they can get paid from insurance or be supervised by a practicing physician, however, three of the ten states have introduced legislation to remove the restriction (Acupuncture.com 1999).

Training standards
Generally, the current standard for training is the master's degree level acupuncture program, with three to four academic years of profes-

sional study in an accredited acupuncture school. Students need to have a minimum of two years of undergraduate courses before attending a program. A clinical doctoral program in Oriental medicine is being proposed by ACAOM as the post-graduate degree; and if approved, it may eventually replace the master's degree as the entry-level degree (ACAOM 1998).

CM and acupuncture schools

According to the National Acupuncture and Oriental Medicine Alliance and the National Acupuncture Foundation, there are presently over fifty acupuncture colleges in the U.S., with a total enrollment of over 6,500 students in 1999 (Bailey and Leef 1999). Most schools are private, each with its own history and philosophy. The majority of schools are members of the Council of Colleges of Acupuncture and Oriental Medicine (CCAOM) and, of those that are members of the council, most but not all are accredited by ACAOM. In addition to insuring quality of education and future competency of the practitioners, the accreditation of a college allows its students to obtain financial assistance from the Federal government and makes them eligible to take the national examination (Moffet 1996b).

According to *The Guide to Accredited and Candidate Colleges* published by the CCAOM, most of the acupuncture and Oriental medical schools tend to cluster around the east or west coast regions, with a few schools scattered in between. Reflecting general acceptance of acupuncture, many of the colleges on the east coast are located in New York, Massachusetts and Florida. On the west coast, colleges are prevalent in California, Washington and Oregon. The schools can vary widely in size, from ten or twenty students in smaller schools to over four hundred in larger ones. The student body is ethnically diverse, with Caucasians and Asian students being the predominant populations.

There are different traditions among the acupuncture/Oriental medicine schools, and their curriculums are far from uniform. While the CM tradition is the most prevalent one, other philosophies taught include Japanese, Five Element, and French Energetics acupuncture. Some schools may require that students acquire the knowledge of Chinese herbal medicine and take western medicine courses as a part of their training but other colleges may offer such courses only as an elective or not have them at all.

Licensure

Licensure laws for non-physician acupuncturists vary from state to state, with differences in exam processes, titles, and scope of practice (Mitchell 1995, 1996, 1997). The acupuncture examination for non-physician acupuncturists accepted by most licensing agencies throughout the country is given either by the National Certification Commission for Acupuncture and Oriental Medicine (NCCAOM) or by state certification. Some states, such as California, only accept state certification examination and not the NCCAOM exam (Acupuncture Committee 1997). Most examinations include a written exam and a practical part, such as the Practical Examination of Point Locations Skills (PEPLS) and the Clean Needle Technique Examination (CNTE). Some states may have additional competency examinations, such as a practical portion on diagnosis and herb recognition (California). In order to be eligible for the NCCAOM or state acupuncture examinations, applicants must complete a three to four-year master's-level course. Additionally, those enrolled after July 1, 1999, must be graduates of accredited schools to be eligible for the national exam.

PHYSICIAN ACUPUNCTURE

While the public interest continues to grow, fueling creation of numerous CM and acupuncture schools in the last three decades, the medical establishment has been slow to warm up. For a long time, many physicians treated acupuncture as a curious but unproved technique and only a minority incorporated it into their practice. The establishment of the Office of Alternative Medicine (OAM) at National Institutes of Health (NIH) in 1992 significantly revitalized physician interest in acupuncture. It now appears that many mainstream physicians believe in the effectiveness of acupuncture and refer their patients for such treatments.

Professional societies and academies

- 1973—First physician and surgeon organization in the U.S. dedicated to acupuncture: The New York Society of Acupuncture for Physicians and Dentists.
- 1982—A Continuing Medical Education (CME) acupuncture course was established at the University of California, Los Angeles, where many U.S. physicians continue to receive their training in the principles of acupuncture.
- 1987—First *national* physician and surgeon organization dedicated to acupuncture: The American Academy of Medical Acupuncture.

Although it is not mandatory for physicians to be affiliated with or certified by external societies or academies in order to practice acupuncture, several of these organizations have set up guidelines for physician acupuncturists. For example, the American Academy of Medical Acupuncture has more than 1,200 members and is the sole professional acupuncture society for physicians in North America. The Academy publishes materials on acupuncture, sponsors continuing education programs and maintains a patient referral service for its practicing members. Its members provide consultation to physicians on how to incorporate acupuncture into their practices and apply for hospital privileges.

Certification by the American Academy of Medical Acupuncture (AAMA) requires an active M.D., dentist, or D.O. license; a minimum of 220 hours of university approved Category 1 Continuing Medical Education (CME) credits; completion of a one-year distance learning program of video training; and two years of experience practicing medical acupuncture (AAMA 1999). The members are also required to complete 50 additional hours of CME in courses on acupuncture or related topics every three years. Some states, such as New York, may require a total of 300 hours of Category 1 CME credits. In Hawaii and Montana, all health-care practitioners, including medical doctors, have the same three-year training requirements and must pass the same national examination as licensed acupuncturists. In contrast, other states do not have any requirement of training credit for M.D.s, dentists or D.O.s who can practice acupuncture without additional certification or a license.

NIH CONSENSUS CONFERENCE ON ACUPUNCTURE

In 1997, a landmark event demonstrated formal recognition of acupuncture by the biomedical establishment. The NIH sponsored a Consensus Meeting on Acupuncture during which high quality research data was reviewed by a panel of scientists and clinical investigators (NIH 1997, 1998). The NIH consensus listed several conditions for which acupuncture can be clinically useful. The panel also acknowledged the need for further research to uncover additional areas where acupuncture can be applied.

According to the NIH statement, conditions for which efficacy of acupuncture is adequately established:

• post-operative and chemotherapy nausea and vomiting
• post-operative dental pain.

Conditions for which acupuncture is recommended as an adjunct treatment or an acceptable alternative:

- addiction
- stroke rehabilitation
- headaches
- pain syndromes such as menstrual cramps, tennis elbow, fibromyalgia, myofascial pain, osteoarthritis, low back pain, carpal tunnel syndrome
- asthma

Herbal Medicine

HISTORICAL BACKGROUND

Throughout most of the twentieth century, the practice of botanical healing has been largely excluded in the development of modern medicine in America. This contrasts with European countries, especially Germany, where herbs were systematically incorporated into the general medical practice and are now prescribed and regulated in ways similar to standard drugs. In the U.S., this division between mainstream drugs and herbal therapies can be attributed to the following key historical factors: 1) low acceptance of herbal medicine by the medical establishment, 2) the development of pharmaceutical industry based on research and mass-production of purified chemicals, and 3) federal regulatory policies, mainly FDA divergent policies on standard drug versus medicinal herb use.

REGULATION OF HERBS AND RELATED PRODUCTS

Since its inception in 1906, the Food and Drug Administration has been involved in several legislative acts that affected herbal sales (O'Hara *et al.*, 1998). The most important legislation—one which has greatly contributed to the current boom in the herbal market—is the 1994 Dietary Supplement Health and Education Act (DSHEA) (FDA 1995, Henney 1999). The act was passed with the goal of regulating the growing herbal industry without limiting the availability of herbal products. Specifically, the DSHEA classified herbal and other botanical products as dietary (i.e. food) supplements and allowed herbal products to be freely marketed as long as they do not claim to treat, diagnose, cure or prevent a disease. However, they may claim to have effect on the structure or function of the body. As dietary supplements, herbs and herbal products are thus excluded from the rigorous approval process required of the standard drugs. In order to take an herbal product off the market, FDA would have to demonstrate its potential health risks.

To protect consumers and provide regulation of the herbal industry, the 1994 DSHEA has: 1) set rules for the distribution of third party literature, 2) described the standards and procedures for setting health claims concerning supplements, 3) specified the supplement ingredient and nutrition labeling information (Baker 1997, FDA 1999), and 4) authorized the FDA to describe mandatory conditions in which dietary supplements must be "prepared, packed or held" (so called good manufacturing practices, or GMP).

Effective March 1999, the FDA has a new regulation on the labeling of dietary supplements. All dietary supplements must bear a nutrition information label entitled "Supplement Facts" (Baker 1997, Friedman and Shalala 1998, Hubbard 1997, Kurtzweil 1999, Schultz 1997a, 1997b). The label must state the name and the quantity of each ingredient in the product, must identify the product as a "dietary supplement" and in the case of herbs, the part of the plant from which the product is derived must be stated. If known, the standard recommendation for daily consumption of each ingredient must be included.

Recognizing the need for further exploration in the area of herbal and nutritional products, the DSHEA also created the Office of Dietary Supplements within the National Institutes of Health (NIH). The office's function is to oversee research and to serve as a source of information about nutritional supplements to other federal agencies.

DIETARY SUPPLEMENT AND HERBAL MARKET

Since the passage of DSHEA, the dietary supplements industry, including herbals, has blossomed. Most surveys show that more than half of the U.S. adult population uses dietary supplement products and spend approximately $3.5 billion annually on herbs (O'Hara et al., 1998). In January 1999, National Public Radio, Kaiser Family Foundation and Harvard's Kennedy School of Government surveyed 1,200 adults 18 years and older nationwide and found that 52% of all surveyed believed that dietary supplements were good for people's health and well-being and 18% identified themselves as regular users (NPR 1999). The results showed that regular users come from all demographic groups, including lower-income and less-educated Americans. There

appeared to be no particular socio-demographic group over represented in regular users.

Currently, numerous herbal products are easily available in most
mainstream stores such as pharmacies, grocery stores, health food stores,
etc. These mainstream herbs are sold in consumer-appealing packaging
with FDA regulated standard labeling. Many have brand names suggesting their therapeutic use such Mense-Ease TM (menstrual discomfort
aid) or Dissolve TM (gall stone aid) and are priced higher than generic or
wholesale products. The herbs chosen for marketing come from many
traditions, mainly European, Asian, or Native American. Among all
herbs, the few selected CM herbs are very popular; however, many other
Chinese herbal preparations are still unfamiliar to the average herbal
consumer. This situation will likely change in the future as the methods
by which Chinese herbs are sold and used are transformed to fit the
growing interest in botanicals. For example, before herbs became
popular in today's worldwide markets, most of CM herbs were displayed
and sold in their original form as raw, dry plants. The original stores
selling herbs were often located exclusively in Chinese-American shop-
ping districts and most of the customers were of Asian descent. Regions
with high Asian American populations still have stores where herbs are
sold in a way reminiscent of ancient CM practice but most herbal
products have been modernized. Many CM herbs are now processed
to achieve powder or extract forms which are then packed in the form
of liquid, tablets, gel, and capsules (Antoniak 1994). Preparations can
be made from a single herb or from a combination of herbs, vitamins, or
minerals. An increasing number of herbal products is made by domestic
companies, but many processed and raw herbs are imported from
abroad (China, Taiwan, Japan, Korea, and Germany). In addition to
the over-the-counter herbs, herbs can be purchased by health care
practitioners directly from the suppliers or can be ordered by consumers
individually via the Internet.

Herbal consumers

Most consumers buy herbs without the need for a prescription; they are
either self-educated about the products they buy, follow someone else's
advice, or an anecdotal account. Most of the available information about
herbs come from advertisements, Internet, magazine articles, books on
herbs, herb bottle labels, and store clerks. Typical buyers of herbs are
characterized as generally healthy and taking the supplements usually for
a single specific problem such as pain, constipation, insomnia,
depression, low energy, aging, and memory impairment. If the herbs

appear to help, most consumers will continue to use it. In the NPR study (1999), 72% of respondents stated that they would continue using a dietary supplement that works for them, even if a government agency said that the supplement is often ineffective. Most consumers are self-diagnosing and self-medicating. Some may consult with health care practitioners on their use of herbs while others may not.

Herbal sales

A 1997 *Prevention* magazine poll by International Communications Research found that 33% of American adults spent an average $54 a year on herbs for an estimated national herbal market of $3.24 *billion* (MacDonald 1998). The ranking of top-selling herbs can vary geographically and depends on the herbal sellers surveyed. According to a recent report published in HerbalGram (Brevoort 1998), the top selling herbs in the U.S. are listed as follows:

Top selling herbs in 1998

Name of herbs	InUS $—millions	% of growth in one year
Gingko	138	140
St. John's wort	121	2801
Ginseng	98	26
Garlic	84	27
Echinacea	33	151
Saw palmetto	27	138
Grapessed	11	38
Kava	8	473
Evening primrose	8	104
Echinacea/Goldenseal	8	80
Cranberry	8	75
Valerian	8	35
All Others	31	
Total:	663.4	

HERBAL MEDICINE PROFESSION

Although most users of herbal remedies are self-diagnosing and self-treating, many patients still seek advice from herbal medicine practitioners. In the U.S., patients can choose from a variety of professionals such as acupuncturists, naturopathic physicians, lay herbalists, chiropractors, nutritionists, as well as a subset of medical doctors, nurses and pharmacists interested in herbal medicine. Since herbs have been classified as dietary supplements, generally there is no licensing requirement for those who practice botanical medicine (Wicke 1995, Silverglade 1995). Texas is the first state establishing the Chinese herbology licensure separate from the acupuncture licensure (Bailey and Leef 1999). The profession of herbalists therefore varies greatly in the amount of training, scope of herbal knowledge and range of herbs used. Most formal training is given in acupuncture schools (CM herbal medicine) and naturopathic schools (Western herbal medicine predominately). Herbal courses are also slowly incorporated into medical school curricula and the number of botanical medicine seminars and articles for physicians is increasing. Other health care and lay herbal practitioners are self-taught or learn through an apprenticeship, through variable non-licensing training programs, or through family and community education (ethnic communities or families with strong multigenerational histories of herbal use). Many herbalists in the U.S. use combinations of herbs in their practice (Chinese herbs and herbs from other traditions). CM concepts of herbal medicine are not always utilized even when traditional Chinese herbs are used. Rather, most practitioners in the U.S. pay more attention to the knowledge of pharmacological effects and clinical application of herbs in terms of Western diagnoses than the CM paradigm (Jensen 1998, Winslow and Kroll 1998). Many alternative medicine practitioners in the U.S. use single herbs or standard herbal formulas rather than prescribing individualized herbal mixtures for each patient.

CM herbalists

Majority of CM/acupuncture schools require courses in Chinese herbology and therefore acupuncturists are by far the major providers of CM herbal medicine. In 1994, of the 25 accredited schools of acupuncture in America, 15 have required training in Chinese herbology and 5 others offered elective courses on the subject. Hours of training varied among schools from 22 to 364. Starting in 1994, NCCA established a certification in Chinese herbology that can be acquired by interested candidates (NAF 1999). The certification bestows the title of "Diplomate of Chinese Herbology" on those who pass a national examination and provide a verification of experience. So far, herbal certification is the only—yet not required—proof of herbal competency and no nationwide licensing procedure is currently in place. Several states have specific legislation allowing acupuncturists to practice Chinese herbology, while other states tolerate acupuncturists' herbal practice even though there is no legislation addressing the subject of botanical medicine. Only one state, Virginia, prohibits acupuncturists without proof of herbal training from using herbal medicine and the general leniency is attributed to the overall low incidence of herbal side effects and complaints.

Among the different regions in the U.S., the quality of CM herbal training is probably the highest and most consistent in the states of New York and California where the acupuncture/CM schools have the longest tradition. Historically, these two states have had large populations of Chinese immigrants and many teachers of their acupuncture schools were originally trained in China.

PROBLEMATIC ISSUES IN BOTANICAL MEDICINE

As described earlier, the 1994 DSHEA classified herbs as dietary supplements and enabled a rapid expansion of all available herbal products. Although attempts to regulate the booming market are currently undertaken, assurance of safety, efficacy and quality control of herbal products continue to be sub-optimal. Reports of side effect, drug-herb interactions, inadequacy or contamination of herbal products have appeared and posed questions about the future of the botanical market (Angell and Kassirer 1998, Bachorik 1997, D'Arcy 1991, D'Arcy 1993, De Smet 1991, Koff 1995, Kupec 1998, Whitemore 1997, Yarnell and Meserole 1997).

Example of Ephedra

Ephedra (Ma Huang in Chinese) has long been used in CM to treat patient with asthma and upper respiratory discomfort. When monitored closely by an herbal medicine practitioner, short-term use of a small dosage of Ephedra in combination with other herbs have been used safely and effectively. Out of the context of Chinese medicine and without medical monitoring, Ephedra-containing products may cause serious side effects as shown by the problems associated with its mainstream marketing. Having alpha and beta adrenergic receptor agonists as active ingredients, products derived from Ephedra are sold as weight loss pills, energy increasing (or pep pills), and sexual stimulating supplements. Some of such products have contained high dosages of Ephedra in combination with caffeine and without proper labeling and warning. Consequently, over the period of 3 years (between 1994 and 1997) the FDA has received more than 800 reports of side effects caused by products made from Ephedra, including irregular heartbeat, sleeplessness, anxiety, tremors and headaches. Extreme reactions have included seizures, heart attacks, strokes and two deaths (Segal 1997). In June 1997, the FDA proposed a regulation to limit the amount of ephedrine, one of the active ingredients from Ephedra, in herbal products and to require proper informational and warning labels. Some experts fear such measure may not be enough and want Ephedra banned from the market.

Contamination of herbs and related products

Many CM herbs used in the U.S. consist of imported Asian patent medicines. Such medicines are mixtures of several different components including herbs, plants, animal parts, and minerals, which are then formulated for sale into tablets, pills, or liquids. Being manufactured outside of the U.S., some of the Asian patent medicines have been identified to contain unauthorized or toxic ingredients, such as heavy metals, prescription drugs or other adulterants that may or may not be listed on the label. In fact, additives such as steroids, non-steroidal anti-inflammatory agents, prescription antibiotics, sedatives, and narcotics have been found in some Asian patent medicines and domestic herbal preparations (Ko 1998).

Manufacturing differences and mislabeling

Unlike standard medicines, herbal preparations (either single herb or mixtures of herbs) can vary between manufacturers and from batch to batch. The variability presents a quality and safety dilemma since an herb may be either toxic or therapeutic depending on its dose and/or the other components it is mixed with. The medicinal value of botanical preparations is affected by multiple factors, such as growing conditions, storage, handling, and preparation methods. In fact, potency of various products from the same plant can vary up to multifold. While some manufacturers may process a particular herb by simply grounding up the plant and putting it into pill form, other manufacturers may use pharmaceutical methods to extract and assay the desired compounds thus making tablets of consistent strength.

In 1995, *Consumer Reports* magazine looked at the composition of 10 different ginseng products available on the market (Herbal Roulette 1995). Although the amount of ginseng per tablet was listed on the labels, the amount of ginsenosides, thought to be the active component, was not always listed. The magazine found striking differences between different brands of ginseng products—a fact that many herbal consumers may not be aware of.

Herbal labels may be incorrect and/or incomplete either accidentally or intentionally. The same common name may be applied to related plant species that may have different therapeutic effects and toxicity. Botanical products can be misidentified, the wrong part of the plant may be collected, or contamination by other herbs can occur. In two publicized cases, an outbreak of belladonna poisoning was attributed to an herbal tea in New York City, and a life-threatening heart arrhythmia in a young woman was traced to a digitalis-contaminated plantain extract (Slifman *et al.*, 1998, Waxman 1996, Winslow and Kroll 1998).

RESOURCES OF HERBAL MEDICINE INFORMATION/RESEARCH

Multiple pamphlets, books, advocacy publications (magazines, newsletters, etc.) and Internet sites attempt to disseminate herbal information as part of herbal marketing directed to consumers. The information in these sources are not subject to labeling guidelines and may claim anecdotal, untested or erroneous information. In order to promote safe use, several companies and organizations try to provide the public and health care professionals with unbiased, accurate information about botanical products. Examples include American Botanical Council (ABC), United States Pharmacopoeia monographs on selected medicinal herbs, the 1999 Physicians Desk Reference (PDR) for Herbal Medicines, and Internet/web sites such as the FDA access to "MEDWATCH". Another valuable source describing the state of herbal field in the U.S. is *Botanical Medicine*. It is a comprehensive compendium of U.S. botanical trends, policies and issues of botanical research discussed during the 1994 historical "Symposium on Botanicals: A Role in U.S. Health Care?" organized by the NIH Office of Alternative Medicine and the FDA.

Therapeutic Massage

Among alternative medical techniques, therapeutic massage has been very popular in the US and its profession has been growing exponentially. Eisenberg's study (1993) showed that 7% of the U.S. population used massage in 1990 and identified massage therapy as the third most popular alternative therapy after chiropractic and relaxation therapies. A comparison of 1997 and 1998 surveys commissioned by the American Massage Therapy Association (AMTA) showed the number of Americans that used massage in one year increased from 8% to

13% between 1997 and 1998 (Opinion Research Corporation 1998). The study also showed that 30% of people surveyed stated they would see a massage therapist for a specific healthcare reason and 52% thought of massage as therapeutic. A look at trends in massage therapy shows that: 1) consumers visit massage therapists about 75 million times annually; 2) the therapy is equally popular among men and women and sought out by all age brackets; 3) the therapy is especially popular among well-educated, well-off consumers (similar to demographics of other CAM therapies consumers) (AMTA 1999a). The therapy is also gaining acceptance among the medical establishment. Over two-thirds of patients who discussed massage with their medical doctor reported a favorable attitude by the physician (Opinion Research Corporation 1998). One national survey showed that more than half of primary care physicians would find massage therapy useful and of those; two-thirds would refer their patients for massage therapy (Grant *et al.*, 1995).

PROFESSION OF MASSAGE THERAPY

Examples of popular massage techniques available in this country are Sweden's massage, Shiatsu, the traditional Chinese massage of Tui-Na, rolfing, and reflexology. Massage is provided in many settings, such as therapeutic massage clinics, physical therapy facilities, acupuncture clinics, health and athletic clubs, spas, chiropractor's offices, and even the workplace. The number of massage therapists is estimated to be between 120,000 and 160,000, including students, and the number is expected to rise along with the mainstream acceptance of massage therapy (AMTA 1999b). In the last 10 years, the profession has undergone a transformation and massage therapy has been increasingly perceived as a type of medical treatment. In 1993, AMTA was founded to promote and upgrade the massage therapy profession by encouraging high educational and practice standards, funding research, and establishing national certification procedures (AMTA 1999c, Precht 1997). During the last decade, the membership of AMTA has tripled and the organization currently has over 35,000 members (AMTA 1999b). Since its first examination 6 years ago, the National Certification Board for Therapeutic Massage and Bodywork has certified over 33,000 practitioners (NCBTMB 1999). As of 1998, 25 states and the District of Columbia have laws requiring massage therapists to be licensed, registered, or certified, and 11 others are considering such legislation. Although licensing laws vary from state to state, most require completion of at least 500 hours of classroom instruction (including courses in anatomy, physiology, ethics, and massage and bodywork theory and application) and passing some type of proficiency exam (state or national) (AMTA 1999d). Much of the movement towards professionalism in massage therapy appears to be driven by medical insurance plans, some of which are interested in including massage therapy in their CAM benefits packages but want a proof of competency from massage therapists.

TRADITIONAL ORIENTAL MASSAGE

The full medical potential of oriental massage is yet to be discovered by physicians. Well-designed research investigating oriental massage therapy is needed in order to alert health care professionals about the value of this type of massage, promote its integration into standard medical therapies, and encourage learning among physicians. Recent studies (AMTA 1999e) on massage therapy have shown benefits for a spectrum of conditions such as chronic pain syndromes, chronic fatigue syndrome (Field *et al* 1997a), asthma in children (Field *et al.*, 1997b), fibromyalgia (Sunshine *et al.*, 1996), PMS (Oleson and Flocco 1993), depression, anxiety (Field *et al.*, 1992), post-mastectomy lymphedema treatment (Zanolla *et al.*, 1984), and inflammatory bowel disease (Yoachim 1983). Hopefully, more research will appear in scientific publications, leading to a better overall acceptance of medical massage, further upgrading of its profession, and discovering the therapeutic value of oriental massage.

Tai-Chi and Qi-Gong

In association with the rapid development of acupuncture and herbal medicine, the Chinese style of body-mind regulated technique, Tai-Chi and Qi-Gong, are also gradually accepted by many Americans. Tai-Chi and Qi-Gong exercises are offered by a variety of CM practitioners as well as the specialists, so-called Tai-Chi Masters. To teach Tai-Chi and Qi-Gong, no proof of knowledge such as a medical certificate or license is needed and many Tai-Chi and Qi-Gong exercise studios have been opened in areas where people seek CM. In California, almost every college or university has an extension of Tai-Chi and/or Qi-Gong class and there are daily morning TV programs with Tai-Chi exercises.

Together with Yoga, Tai-Chi comprises the most popular non-conventional exercise techniques in America.

TAI-CHI

Though this style of exercise is different from the traditional western fast, high impact exercise, Americans have been gradually recognizing the value of Tai-Chi. The slow movement of Tai-Chi helps relax, tones muscles, improves balance and regulates the flow of Qi. The technique promotes wellness, and alleviates stress and many chronic illnesses. Tai-Chi has been shown to be of benefit in the treatment of chronic illness and aging related conditions. In the U.S., the exercises have been especially advocated for older people who, due to age-related physical deterioration, are at risk of falling. A 1995 analysis of seven studies showed that, while any regular exercise lowers the risk of falling in people over the age of 60, Tai-Chi students had by far the best results. In comparison to regular conventional exercise, which lowered the risk by 13%, and to workouts including balance drills, which decreased the risk by 25%, Tai-Chi exercise provided an impressive 48% improvement (Atlanta FICSIT Group et al., 1997, China et al., 1996, Judge et al., 1993, Al et al., 1993, Lan et al., 1996, Lan et al., 1998, Province et al., 1995, Scholer 1996, Wolf et al., 1996, Wolfson et al., 1996, Young et al., 1999).

QI-GONG

Associated with Tai-Chi, Qi-Gong is slowly being recognized in the U.S. Efforts are underway to promote scientific exploration of Qi-Gong and to spread the practice in the mainstream America (Reading 1997, Sandier 1996). In November 1997, the East West Academy of Healing Arts (EWAHA) sponsored the Second World Congress on Qi-Gong in San Francisco, California, which was attended by over 600 people from 15 countries (Stone 1998). The goal of the meeting was to increase awareness of Qi-Gong as a self-help method with documented beneficial health effects. Attendees ranged from medical researchers to those seeking medical knowledge for their own health; from experienced Qi-Gong masters to newcomers to the discipline.

During the meeting, the research on the effect of Qi-Gong practice on asthma, diabetes and the effect of emitted Qi on cancer cells were presented. Other sessions dealt with explorations of connections between Qi-Gong and related disciplines such as acupuncture, craniasacral therapy, naturopathy, and homeopathy. It is further encouraging that articles exploring effects of Qi-Gong in areas such as hypertension, brain activity, kidney function, enzyme and immune function and sex hormone levels started to appear in the American literature (Sancier 1996).

Adverse Effects of CAM

With increased use of CAM in the U.S., it is expected that some of the services will be of substandard quality, misused, done inadequately, or produce side effects alone or in combination with other standard medical treatments. In addition to adverse effects of herbal products (as discussed earlier in the chapter), reports of problems due to acupuncture, massage, and chiropractic treatment have been found.

David Student *et al.* (1998) recently reported on the medical malpractice implications of alternative medicine. The data collected from malpractice insurers was used to analyze the claims experience of chiropractors, massage therapists, and acupuncturists for 1990 through 1996. Analysis of malpractice suits against massage therapist shows that most complaints relate to minor injuries (61%), although a significant proportion (14%) relate to sexual misconduct. Top three claims against chiropractors include disk problems, fracture, and failure to diagnose. Side effects associated with acupuncture are rather minor, such as failure to remove needles (usually no injury post removal), infections, and minor tissue trauma; however, more serious, often isolated cases have been described: irreversible nerve damage, burns, pneumothorax, and hepatitis B infection. In general, the study shows that claims against alternative medicine practitioners occurred much less frequently and typically involved injury that was less severe than claims against physicians during the same period.

Medical Insurance

Unlike most of the other developed countries, United States has no universal medical coverage and instead has established a complex medical insurance industry. In the U.S. system, numerous medical insurance companies offer medical benefits plans that specify which medical services the insurance will pay for (often labeled "the standard medical care"). Any services outside these specifications have to be paid for by the patient. Ignored, even ridiculed by the mainstream physician, alternative medicine (by definition, not a part of the *standard* care) had to suffer such status of "an outsider" for a long time. Medical coverage for CM or other CAM treatments was non-existent and any interested patients had to pay out-of-pocket for alternative medical care. Such extra expense can present a barrier for those with limited resources and selects for either well-off patients able to afford the cost or those who turn to alternative medicine as a treatment of last resort.

This bleak situation has been changing in the last few years, mainly as a response to continuous patient interest in alternative care. Series of surveys demonstrating wide consumer demand for CAM therapies have sparked the interest of the medical insurance industry. One survey done by an insurance company (a managed care company) Oxford Health Plans, Norwalk, CN shows that 33% of its 1.5 million members have sought alternative treatment in the last 2 years (Chowka 1998a, 1998b). Responding to the growing market for CAM, a number of health care insurers decided to start offering medical coverage on complementary medical procedures. The interest of medical insurance companies has been instrumental in the regulation of the CAM field since to be included in a package of benefits, an alternative medicine practitioner must present proof of proficiency such as a professional license.

Most of the major private insurance companies in the U.S. have developed insurance programs to provide benefits for alternative medicine (mainly chiropractic, acupuncture, and therapeutic massage). For the government-sponsored medical insurance, legislation addressing CAM benefits is also being developed. In fact, insurance coverage of chiropractic treatment is mandated by law in at least 42 states, acupuncture—in 7 states, and naturopathy—in 2 states (Studdert *et al.*, 1998). As a mark of the growing legal acceptance of CAM, a bill passed in 1997 in California included acupuncturists as treating physicians in the workers' compensation system (CAAOM 1998).

American Specialty Health Plan (ASHP)—a quickly expanding managed care insurance company in the western part of the U.S. for chiropractors and acupuncturists—has a benefit package, which includes acupuncture and traditional Chinese herbal medicine. As of 1998, patients are allowed 20–40 annual visits to network acupuncture providers and $500 per year is allotted for the traditional Chinese herbal supplement benefit.

CM and Conventional Medicine

After a long period of getting the cold shoulder from mainstream physicians, CAM therapies are starting to be acknowledged by the American medical establishment. The inter-phase between conventional and alternative medicine is created in several areas, which include 1) research, 2) medical education, and 3) clinical practice.

RESEARCH

In response to the high prevalence of alternative therapies in the U.S., the American Congress initiated the creation of a central agency coordinating and sponsoring research into complementary and alternative medicine. In 1992, the Office of Alternative Medicine or OAM was founded within the National Institutes of Health in Beheads, Maryland, with the goal to 1) facilitate the evaluation of alternative medical treatment modalities, 2) gather and disseminate information about CAM, and 3) promote the integration of effective therapies into the mainstream medical practice. Initially awarded a modest $2 million budget, the Office has since undergone an exponential growth reflecting the extent of government investment into studying CAM practices. In October of 1998, the OAM was expanded and renamed as the National Center for Complementary and Alternative Medicine (NCCAM) with an increased budget of $20 million in 1998 and $50 million in the 1999 fiscal year.

The OAM and NCCAM fiscal year budget

1992	1993	1994	1995	1996	1997	1998	1999
$2M	$3.5M	$3.5M	$5.4M	$7.4M	$12M	$20M	$50M

Since its conception, the OAM and now the NCCAM, have been instrumental in promoting research in the field of alternative and complementary medicine. The office has established research links with multiple institutes within NIH, the U.S. Food and Drug Administration (FDA), the Agency for Health Care Policy and Research (AHCPR), and other federal agencies. It has launched several large clinical trials, provided "seed grants" for the development of novel projects, and by 1999 appointed thirteen CAM Research Centers. The Research Centers are expected to act as long-standing sources of high-quality CAM research and serve as the research training and career development sites. In 1998, an intramural training program was begun which currently supports four research fellows. The investigations sponsored by the NCCAM focus mostly on common chronic illnesses, women's health, and addictions (see list below). Grant proposals for other conditions that may benefit from CAM are encouraged and reviewed by the NCCAM.

CAM research center grants
- Stroke and Neurological Conditions (Kestrel Institute for rehabilitation, West Orange, NJ)
- HIV/AIDS (Boaster University, Kenmore, WA)
- General Medicine Condition (Beth Israel Hospital, Harvard Medical School, Boston, MA)
- Women's Health Issues (Columbia University College of Physicians and Surgeons, New York, NY Dentistry, Newark, NJ)
- Addictions (Hangmen County Medical Center/ University of Minnesota Medical School, Minneapolis, MN)
- Aging (Stanford University, Palo Alto, CA)
- Asthma, Allergy, and Immunology (University of California at Davis, Davis, CA)
- Pain (University of Maryland School of Medicine, Baltimore, MD)
- Cancer (University of Texas Health Science Center, Houston, TX)
- Pain (University of Virginia School of Nursing, Charlottesville, VA)
- Pediatrics (University of Arizona, Tucson, AZ)
- Cardiovascular Diseases (University of Michigan at Ann Arbor, MI)
- Chiropractic (Palmer Center for Chiropractic Research, Davenport, IA)

Apart from research funding, the NCCAM is expected to continue the OAM's function in providing technical support in the form of grant-writing workshops, clinical research workshops and consultations on clinical investigations. Since their creation, the OAM and now the NCCAM have organized a number of conferences for medical professionals on CAM-related topics such as wellness, acupuncture, cancer treatment, botanicals, research methodology, and insurance reimbursement. In addition to educating health professionals, the NCCAM also serves the public by disseminating reliable information about CAM.

MEDICAL EDUCATION

In the last few years, several studies confirmed increasing tendency to teach CAM courses at U.S. medical schools. A study in 1995 by the Alternative Medicine Interest Group of the Society of Teachers of Family Medicine showed that about one-third of the family medicine departments at medical schools and one-third of family practice residency programs offered CAM teaching (Carleton 1998). Only 3 years later, a study by Wetzel *et al.* demonstrated that almost two-thirds of all U.S. medical schools offered courses in complementary or alternative medicine (Wetzel *et al.*, 1998). Of the 123 courses reported, 68% were stand-alone electives, 31% were part of required courses, and 1% were part of an elective. Departments most active in teaching such courses were family practice and internal medicine; however, most courses did not have a single department responsible for its teaching. Some courses were offered in affiliation with outside CAM institutes or centers, some were initiated by an individual school's office of medical education, and others were interdepartmental. The format and content of instruction varied greatly between institutions, from short electives to month long clerkships; from lectures only (majority) to diverse, hands on experience (selected few schools). In general the CAM education at medical schools is widely supported by such organizations as the OAM and the AMA and many schools are now establishing separate departments of complementary and alternative medicine. Much of the investment in teaching CAM is student driven and multiple student interest groups have extended their exposure to CAM beyond what their medical school offers (organizing "brown bag" lunches with different CAM practitioners or visiting CAM practice sites) (Daly 1996, Milan *et al.*, 1998, Shaw 1999).

CLINICAL PRACTICE

Prompted by the high demand for CAM and its promise of business or academic opportunity, many conventional medicine practices and universities have attempted to establish integrative treatment sites. After the initial excitement wore off, such task has proven to be a challenging endeavor requiring in-depth knowledge of western as well as eastern medicine (Astin *et al.*, 1998, Berman *et al.*, 1998). Some clinics have experienced difficulties since their establishments (few had to close down), some are successfully thriving, and others are being formed. Many western medicine health systems are opening the so called "center of complementary medicine" in response to patients' interest. Among examples of clinics/programs that aim to integrate conventional and CAM medicine are: the UCLA Center for East-West Medicine, the Center for Spirituality and Healing at the University of Minnesota School of Medicine, the Center for Integrative Medicine at Jefferson Medical College, and the California Pacific Medical Center's (CPMC) Health and Healing Clinic (Shaw 1999).

UCLA Center for East-West Medicine

A clinical, educational and research center, UCLA Center for East-West Medicine was formally established in 1993 and is devoted to full integration of western and traditional Chinese medicine. The center has a successful East-West medicine clinic run by experienced western medical doctors familiar with CM and licensed acupuncturists trained in western medicine and modern sciences. These clinicians work in unison throughout the diagnostic and therapeutic process. An individualized management plan is designed for each patient using western medical drugs, therapeutic massage, acupuncture, and education on dietary and herbal supplements, physical therapy, and Tai-Chi/Qi-Gong exercise.

As a part of a major university in the U.S., the center also serves as an active educational and research base. Since 1996, the Center sponsored several international conferences on integrative East-West medicine for physicians and other health care professionals. The meetings covered broad range of topics from chronic pain management to successful aging. The center also has selective courses on integrative medicine for first year, fourth year medical students and medical residents. The center explores effective ways of integrating eastern and western medicine in medical practice and uses creative ways in teaching integrative medicine to students (for example, use more clinical cases and hands-on experience in teaching). The clinic also serves as an innovative laboratory where the efficacy of various CM techniques is evaluated.

Conclusion

The field of alternative medicine in the U.S. including TCM has undergone a tremendous growth in the last decade. Individual branches of CM have entered the mainstream at different rates with acupuncture leading the progress. Despite making some strides, the field continues to be in a state of flux. The merger of CAM and conventional biomedicine is ongoing in diverse ways and in different settings. New data about popularity and efficacy of alternative therapies compete with reports of side effects, failed expectations and warnings of quackery. As such, the field of alternative medicine is seen by some as an area of great promise and opportunity and by others as untested waters, murky and deceiving. Despite contradictory information, those believing in the great potential of CAM hope that this transitory state will lead to a better, more integrated medicine and an overall improvement in people's health. We feel that the principles of CM paradigm can provide the guiding framework for the transformation.

Acknowledgements

The authors would like to thank the following people for contributing their time and effort in facilitating the completion of this chapter: George Hsu; Jie-Jia Li, LAc; Steve Liao, BS; Jennifer Mankowski; Elaine C. Pang, MA, MPH, CHES; Angela Tan, BS; and Anna Wang, BS. Special thanks to Agnieszka Goeller for critiquing the chapter. The Balm and the Gerald and Virginia Oppenheimer Foundations provided financial support for this research work for which the authors are deeply grateful.

References

ACAOM (1998) Up-date on the doctorate program. *National Acupuncture and Oriental Medicine Alliance Newsletter*, **Winter 1998–1999**, 28, 30.

Acupuncture Committee. (1997) *Laws and regulations relating to the practice of acupuncture*, State of California, Department of Consumer Affairs, Sacramento, California.

Acupuncture.com (1999) States seek to remove medical intervention [Internet] Available from: <http://www.acupuncture.com/News/3.99News/state-news3.99.html> [Accessed April 9, 1999].

American Academy of Medical Acupuncture. (1999) American academy of medical acupuncture [Internet] Available from: <http://www.med-icalacupuncture.org/> [Accessed April 13, 1999].

American Massage Therapy Association (1999a) Trends in Massage Therapy & Complementary Healthcare [Internet] Available from: <http://www.amta-massage.org/publications/marketresearch.htm> [accessed April 26, 1999].

American Massage Therapy Association (1999b) Massage therapy in the United States: Meeting the growing demand among consumers [Internet]

Available from: <http://www.amtamassage.org/publications/ market-trends.htm> [Accessed April 26, 1999].

American Massage Therapy Association (1999c) Research shows massage therapy works [Internet] Available from: <http://www.amtamassage.org/publications/mat-research.htm> [Accessed April 26, 1999].

American Massage Therapy Association (1999d) States continue to pass massage therapist licensing laws [Internet] Available from: <http://www.amtamassage.org/ publications/mat-states.htm> [Accessed April 26, 1999].

American Massage Therapy Association (1999e) Massage therapy in the United States: Scientific studies on the effects of massage therapy [Internet] Available from: <http://www.amtamassage.org/publications/sciencere-search.htm> [Accessed April 26, 1999].

Angell, M. and Kassirer, J.P. (1998) Alternative medicine—the risks of untested and unregulated remedies. *The New England Journal of Medicine*, **339**, 839–841.

Antoniak, M. (1994) New awareness for ancient Chinese herbs. *Vitamin Retailer*, **April**, 18ff.

Astin, J.A., Marie, A., Pelletier, K.R., Hansen, E. and Haskell, W.L. (1998) A review of the incorporation of complementary and alternative medicine by mainstream physicians. *Archives of Internal Medicine*, **158(21)**, 2303–2310.

Atlanta FICSIT Group, Barnhart, H.X., Coogler, C.E., Ellison, G.L. and Wolf, S.L. (1997) The effect of Tai chi Quan and computerized balance training on postural stability in older subjects. *Physical Therapy*, **77(4)**, 371–381.

Bachorik, L. (1997) FDA warns against consuming the arise & shine product "chomper" [Internet] Available from: <http://vm.cfsan.fda.gov/~lrd/hhschomp.html> [Accessed May 18, 1999].

Bailey, A. and Leef, L. (1999) Acupuncture Alliance Forum. *National Acupuncture and Oriental Medicine Alliance Newsletter*, **Spring 1999**, 20.

Baker, D. (1997) The commission on dietary supplement labels [Internet] Available from <http://web.health.gov/dietsupp/> [Accessed May 7, 1999].

Berman, B.M., Singh, B.B., Hartnoll, S.M., Singh, B.K. and Reilly, D. (1998) Primary care physicians and complementary-alternative medicine: training, attitudes, and practice patterns. *Journal of the American Board of Family Practice*, **11(4)**, 272–281.

Brevoort, P. (1998) The booming U.S. Botanical Market: a new overview. *HerbalGram*, **44**, 33–48.

CAAOM (1998) 1997–1998 Legislative activities [Internet] Available from: <http://caaom.org/legislat/9798/199798.htm> [Accessed May 10, 1999].

Carlston, M. (1998) The revolution in medical education: complementary medicine joins the curriculum. *Healthcare Forum Journal*, **November/December**, 25–31.

Cassidy, C.M. (1998a) Chinese medicine users in the United States part I: utilization, satisfaction, and medical plurality. *The Journal of Alternative and Complementary Medicine*, **4(1)**, 17–27.

Cassidy, C.M. (1998b) Chinese medicine users in the United States part II: preferred aspects of care. *The Journal of Alternative and Complementary Medicine*, **4(2)**, 189–202.

Chowka, P.B. (1998a) Major U.S. Health Insurers Turn to Complementary Alternative Medicine. *Natural Healthline* [Internet] Available from: <http://www.acupuncture.com/News/Insurance2.htm> [Accessed August 31, 1998].

Chowka, P.B. (1998b) Majority of HMOs plan to offer alternative medicine in near future [Internet] Available from: <http://acupuncture.com/News/HMO.htm> [Accessed August 31, 1998].

Daly, D. (1996) Alternative medicine courses at U.S. medical schools: an ongoing listings. *The Journal of Alternative and Complementary Medicine*, **2(2)**, 315–317.

Dalzell, M.D., ed. (1999) Health plans and alternative medicine—where do physicians fit in? *Managed Care*, **April**, 14–23.

D'Arcy, P.F. (1991) Adverse reactions and interactions with herbal medicines. Part 1—Adverse reactions. *Journal of Alternative and Complementary Medicine*, **10(4)**, 189–208.

D'Arcy, P.F. (1993) Adverse reactions and interactions with herbal medicines. Part 2—Drug interactions. *Adverse Drug React. Toxicol. Rev.*, **12(3)**, 147–162.

De Smet, P.A.G.M. (1991) Is there any danger in using traditional remedies? *Journal of Ethnopharmacology*, **32**, 43–50.

Eisenberg, D.M., Davis, R.B., Ettner, S.L., Appel, S., Wilkey, S., Van Rompay, M. and Kessler, R.C. (1998) Trends in alternative medicine use in the United States, 1990–1997: results of a follow-up national survey. *The Journal of American Medical Association*, **280(18)**, 1569–1575.

Eisenberg, D.M., Foster, C., Kessler, R.C., *et al.* (1993) Unconventional medicine in the United States. *N Engl J Med.*, **328**, 246–252.

Feely, R. (1999) Acupuncture history [Internet] Available from: <http://www.americanwholehealth.com/library/acupuncture/acuhis.htm> [Accessed April 9, 1999].

Field, T., Henteleff, T., Hernandez-Reif, M., Marting, E., Mavunda, K., Kuhn, C. and Schanberg, S. (1997b) Children with asthma have improved pulmonary functions after massage therapy. *Journal of Pediatrics*, **132**, 854–858.

Field, T., Morrow, C., Valdeon, C., *et al.* (1992) Massage reduces anxiety in child and adolescent psychiatric patients. *Journal of the American Academy of Child and Adolescent Psychiatry*, **31(1)**, 125–131.

Field, T., Sunshine, W., Hernandez-Reif, M., Quintino, O., Schanberg, S., Kuhn, C. and Burman, I. (1997a) Chronic fatigue syndrome: massage therapy effects on depression and somatic symptoms in chronic fatigue syndrome. *Journal of Chronic Fatigue Syndrome*, 3, 43–51.

Food and Drug Administration (1999) Dietary supplements now labeled with more information [Internet] Available from: <http://vm.cfsan.fda.gov/~~lrd/hhssupp2.html> [Accessed April 10, 1999].

Food and Drug Administration Center for Food Safety and Applied Nutrition. (1995) Dietary supplement health and education act of 1994 [Internet] Available from: <http://vm.cfsan.fda.gov/~dms/dietsupp.html> [Accessed September 3, 1998].

Friedman, M.A. and Shalala, D.E. (1998) FDA proposes rules to make claims for dietary supplements more informative, reliable and uniform. HHS News [Internet] Available from: <http://vm.cfsan.fda.gov/~lrd/hhssupp.html> [Accessed September 3, 1998].

Grant, W., Kams, C., Blumberg, D., Hendricks, S. and Dewan, M. (1995) The physician and unconventional medicine. *Alternative Therapies in Health and Medicine*, 1, 31–35.

Herbal roulette (1995) *Consumer Reports*, **November**, 698–705.

Hubbard, W.K. (1997) Food labeling; nutrient content claims: definition for "high potency" and definition of "antioxidant" for use in nutrient content claims for dietary supplements and conventional foods [Internet] Available from: <http://vm.cfsan.fda.gov/~~lrd/fr97923c.html> [Accessed May 17, 1999].

Jensen, C.B. (1998) Clinical trials of herbal and pharmaceutical products: a comparison. *Alternative & Complementary Therapies*, **February 1998**, 30–35.

Judge, J.O., Lindsey, C., Underwood, M. and Winsemius, D. (1993) Balance improvements in older women: Effects of exercise training. *Physical Therapy*, 73(4), 254–262.

Ko, R. (1998) Adulterants in Asian patent medicines. *New England Journal of Medicine*, 339(12), 847.

Koff, R.S. (1995) Herbal Hepatotoxicity: revisiting a dangerous alternative. *JAMA*, 273(6), 502.

Kupec, I. (1998) FDA warns consumers against taking dietary supplement "Sleeping Buddha" [Internet] Available from: <http://vm.cfsan.fda.gov/~~lrd/hhbuddha.html> [Accessed May 18, 1999].

Kurtzweil, P. (1999) An FDA guide to dietary supplements [Internet] Available from: <http://vm.cfsan.fda.gov/~~dms/fdsupp.html> [Accessed May 17, 1999].

Lan, C., Lai, J.S., Chen, S.Y. and Wong, M.K. (1998) 12-month Tai Chi training in the elderly: its effect on health fitness. *Medicine and Science in Sports and Exercise*, 30(3), 345–351.

Lytle, D. (1996) History of the Food and Drug Administration's regulation of acupuncture devices. *The Journal of Alternative and Complementary Medicine*, 2(1), 253–256.

MacDonald, S. (1998) Herbal alternatives. *The Cincinnati Enquirer*, February 11, 1998, pp. E1, E5.

Milan, F.B., Landau, C., Murphy, D.R., Balletto, J.J., Sztykowski, T., Hart, J.A., Rybeck, C.H. and Cyr, M.G. (1998) Teaching residents about complementary and alternative medicine in the United States. *JGIM*, **13**(8), 562–567.

Mitchell, B.B. (1996) Educational and licensing requirements for acupuncturists. *The Journal of Alternative and Complementary Medicine*, **2**(1), 33–35.

Mitchell, B.B. (1995) *Legislative handbook for the practice of acupuncture & oriental medicine*, National Acupuncture Foundation, Washington DC.

Mitchell, B.B. (1997) *Acupuncture and oriental medicine laws*, National Acupuncture Foundation, Washington DC.

Moffet, H. (1996a) Acupuncture and oriental medicine update, special report: FDA ruling on acupuncture needles and their use. *Alternative and Complementary Therapies*, **January/February**, 32–34.

Moffet, H. (1996b) Acupuncture and oriental medicine update, special report: acupuncture education: focus on the profession. *Alternative and Complementary Therapies*, **July/August**, 266–269.

National Acupuncture Foundation (1999) *Acupuncture and Oriental Medicine Laws*, 1999.

National Certification Board for Therapeutic Massage and Bodywork (1999) Emerging standards [Internet] Available from: <http://www.ncbtmb.com/Publicat/emerging/winter99.htm> [Accessed April 26, 1999].

National Public Radio, the Henry J. Kaiser Family Foundation, and Harvard University's Kennedy School of Government (1999) Survey of Americans and Dietary Supplements [Internet] Available from: <http://www.npr.org/programs/specials/survey/front.html> [Accessed March 26, 1999].

NIH Consensus Statement (1997) Acupuncture [Internet] November 3–5, 15(5): in press. Available from: <http://odp.od.nih.gov/consensus/cons/107/107_statement.htm> [Accessed February 9, 1998].

NIH Consensus Conference (1998) Acupuncture. *JAMA*, **280**(17), 1518–1524.

NIH (1999) Centers for dietary supplements research: botanicals [Internet] Available from: <http://www.nih.gov/grants/guide/rfa-files/RFA-OD-99-007.html> [Accessed March 23, 1999].

O'Hara, M., Keifer, D., Farrell, K., Kemper, K. (1998) A review of 12 commonly used medicinal herbs. *Arch. Fam. Med.*, **7**, 523–535.

Oleson, T. and Flocco, W. (1993) Randomized controlled study of premenstrual symptoms treated with ear, hand, and foot reflexology. *Obstetrics and Gynecology*, **82**(6), 906–910.

Opinion Research Corporation (1998) 1998 Massage therapy consumer fact sheet [Internet] Available from: <http://wwwamtamassage.org/news/survey-fact.htm> [Accessed April 26, 1999].

Precht, R. (1997) American massage therapy association encourages more research on how therapeutic massage works [Internet] Available from:

<http://www.amtamassage.org/news/moreresearch.htm> [Accessed April 26, 1999].

Province, M.A., *et al.* (1995) The effects of exercise on falls in elderly patients. A pre-planned meta-analysis of the FICSIT Trials. Frailty and Injuries: Cooperative studies of intervention techniques. *JAMA*, **273**(17), 1341–1347.

Reading, M.M. (1998) Qi-Gong shows promise: needs controlled research studies. *The Journal of Alternative and Complementary Medicine*, **4**(1), 117–118.

Sancier, K. (1996) Medical applications of Qi-Gong. *Alternative Therapies*, **2**(1), 40–46.

Schultz, W.B. (1997a) Food labeling; notification procedures for statements on dietary supplements [Internet] Available from: <http://vm.cfsan.fda.gov/~lrd/fr97923d.html> [Accessed May 17, 1999].

Schultz, W.B. (1997b) Food labeling; requirements for nutrient content claims, health claims, and statements of nutritional support for dietary supplements [Internet] Available from: <http://vm.cfsan.fda.gov/~lrd/fr97923b.html> [Accessed May 17, 1999].

Segal, M. (1997) FDA warns against drug promotion of "herbal fen-phen". *FDA Talk Paper* [Internet] Available from: <http://vm.cfsan.fda.gov/~lrd/tpfenphn.html> [Accessed September 3, 1998].

Shaw, G. (1999) Taking an integrative approach to complementary medicine, *Association of American Medical Colleges*, **March 1999**, 10–11.

Silverglade, B. (1995) The state role in dietary supplement regulation. *Journal of the Association of Food and Drug Officials*, **59**(3), 24–29.

Slifman, N.R., *et al.* (1998) Contamination of botanical dietary supplements by *Digitalis lanata*, *NEJM*, **339**(12), 806–811.

Stone, A. (1998) The second world congress on Qi Gong and the first American Qi Gong association conference [Internet] Available from: <http://www.acupuncture.com/News/qgconf.htm> [Accessed May 20, 1999].

Studdert, D.M., *et al.* (1998) Medical malpractice implications of alternative medicine. *JAMA*, **280**(18), 1610–1615.

Sunshine, W., Field, T., Schanberg, S., Quintino, O., Kilmer, T., Fierro, K., Burman, I., Hashimoto, M., McBride, C. and Henteleff, T. (1996) Massage therapy and transcutaneous electrical stimulation effects on fibromyalgia. *Journal of Clinical Rheumatology*, **2**, 18–22.

Ulett, G.A., Han, J. and Han, S. (1998) Traditional and evidence-based acupuncture: history, mechanisms, and present status. *Southern Medical Journal*, **91**(12), 1115–1120.

Villaire, M. (1998) NIH consensus conference confirms acupuncture's efficacy. *Alternative Therapies*, **4**(1), 21–25.

Waxman, S. (1996) Lawsuits blame women's death on unregulated herbal products. *The Washington Post*, **March 24**, A1ff.

Weeks, J. (1999) *The Integrator for the Business of Alternative Medicine*, Integration Strategies for Natural Healthcare, Seattle, Washington.

Wetzel, M.S., Eisenberg, D.M. and Kaptchuk, T.J. (1998) Courses involving complementary and alternative medicine at US medical schools. *JAMA*, **280**, 784–787.

Whitemore, A. (1997) FDA Warns Consumers against dietary supplement products that may contain digitalis mislabeled as "plantain" [Internet] Available from: <http://www.fda.gov/bbs/topics/NEWS/NEW00570.html> [Accessed May 18, 1999].

Wicke, R.W. (1995) The right to practice herbology, legal history and basis. Rocky Mountain Herbal Institute [Internet] Available from: <http://www.rmhiherbal.org/a/f.ahr3.rights.html> [Accessed September 3, 1998].

Winslow, L.C. and Kroll, D.J. (1998) Herbs as medicines. *Arch Intern Med*, **158(9)**, 2192–2199.

Wolf, S.L., Barnhart, H.X., Kutner, N.G., McNeely, E., Coogler, C. and Xu, T. (1996) Reducing frailty and falls in older persons: An investigation of Tai Chi and computerized balance training. *Journal of the American Geriatrics Society*, **44(5)**, 489–497.

Wolfson, L., Whipple, R., Derby, C., Judge, J., King, M., Amerman, P., Schmidt, J. and Smyers, D. (1996) Balance and strength training in older adults: Intervention gains and Tai Chi maintenance. *Journal of the American Geriatrics Society*, **44(5)**, 498–506.

Wu, J. (1996) A short history of acupuncture. *The Journal of Alternative and Complementary Medicine*, **2(1)**, 19–21.

Yarnell, E. and Meserole, L. (1997) Toxic botanicals: Is the poison in the plant or its regulation? *Alternative & Complementary Therapies*, **February**, 13–19.

Yoachim, G. (1983) The effects of two stress management techniques on feeling of well-being in patients with inflammatory bowel disease. *Nursing Papers*, **15(47)**, 5–18.

Young, D.R., Appel, L.J., Jee, S. and Miller, E.R. 3rd. (1999) The effects of aerobic exercise and Tai Chi on blood pressure in older people: results of a randomized trial. *Journal of the American Geriatrics Society*, **47(3)**, 277–284.

Zanolla, R., Mazeglio, C. and Balzarini, A. (1984) Evaluation of the results of three different methods of postmastectomy lymphedema treatment. *Journal of Surgical Oncology*, **26**, 210–213.

SECTION FOUR
CONCLUDING ISSUE

18 A CURRICULUM MODEL FOR TEACHING AND TRAINING CHINESE MEDICINE IN ENGLISH

Henry Lee
Kelvin Chan

Introduction

During recent years many reports (Goldbeck-Wood, 1996; NAHAT 1993) have repeatedly emphasised the increasing popularity of traditional Chinese medicine (TCM). Some of the reasons offered are; there are fewer side effects compared with orthodox medicine (OM), and it is also proving especially effective in the treatment of chronic conditions such as eczema, for which OM has yet to offer long term help or solution. Other medical conditions popularly treated include serious and chronic conditions such as arthritis, HIV/AIDS, malaria, cancer, chronic pain affecting spine, joints, muscles, control of nausea, hepatitis C and skin conditions (Lewith G *et al.*, 1996, Morgan D. 1997). However, there is still a paucity of information on TCM to enable the public to make informed choice and more importantly for the OM practitioners to be confident to make informed referral to TCM practitioners.

The popularity of TCM is also reflected in the UK, the demand for education and training in Chinese medicine has also increased. There are at least 11 known private schools offering part-time pro-grammes of variable length of time in either herbs or acupuncture which are the two major branches of TCM (See Table 18.1 in Appendix 1). There is no available evidence by which to judge either the depth or rigour of these programmes or to compare them with those offered in China, the birthplace of the TCM. This Chapter describes a five-year full-time programme operative in China that is taken as the benchmark for development within the Middlesex University in the UK.

The Middlesex-Beijing Model

SETTING THE ACADEMIC STANDARD

The popularity of the complementary medicine/therapies (CMT) gathered pace since they first captured the public imagination in the 1980s. In 1993, the British Medical Association acknowledged that CMT's rise in popularity was not due to a passing fashion. For traditional Chinese medicine education and training, 1997 must be viewed as the final breach in the cultural frontier when Middlesex University (MU) and Beijing University of Traditional Chinese Medicine (BUTCM) designed and validated a joint five year full-time BSc (Hons) TCM programme (Lee, 1998). This programme also claimed to be the world's first undergraduate programme of this kind. The Middlesex-Beijing model is based on the principles of BUTCM's own five-year full-time programme, which is devised and devolved down by the State Administration of Traditional Chinese Medicine (SATCM). In China, the SATCM controls and regulates the curricular content and practice of the TCM programmes. It is then delegated for delivery in the nominated TCM universities and colleges of whom BUTCM is one. In other words, other eight selected universities offer similar programmes. They are also highly prized universities by the TCM students. Of course, there are now many other universities and colleges which offer degree programmes in TCM (see Chapter 11).

When Middlesex University undertook the development of this programme as part of its portfolio of academic programmes in complementary medicine/therapies, it was already offering a degree in western herbal medicine, and post-healthcare professional registration programmes in reflexology and aromatherapy. At the time both the public and professional healthcarers were increasingly concerned that the TCM education and training programmes available in China were being misused. This led to the then Deputy Minister of Public Health and Director of SATCM, making a public statement in 1996 that "non-doctors who acquire some knowledge from short courses should not practise (Chinese) medicine". Tomlinson (1996) also reported in the British Medical Journal that "China is tightening supervision of Chinese medicine and pharmacology courses for foreigners and will stop institutions from granting advanced training certificates to non-medically trained students."

During the validation of the MU-BUTCM programme, one of the members of the External Validating Panel hailed the programme as

"The gold standard for TCM education" (Lee, 1998). This notable success was due to the considerable work and effort invested into the programme by all concerned, so that it can:

- Satisfy the rules and regulations of both universities and the State Administration of TCM(SATCM) in China;
- Meet funding criteria of the Higher Education Funding Council for England (HEFCE);
- Meet the programme quality criteria set by the Quality Assurance Agency for Higher Education;
- Reassure the then Confederation of National Association of Health Authorities and Trusts (now Confederation of NHS Trust), the Scottish Office Department of Health and the British Medical Association that TCM is safe and can complement OM to enhance the quality of patients' life;
- Address and reconcile with both universities' philosophy and vision;
- Include both universities' mission and objectives;
- Facilitate the future growth of the collaboration;
- Meet the public expectations both in the quality of the programme and of professional practice;
- Nurture safe, competent and reflective practitioners.

Quality Assurance Agency for Higher Education

In meeting the funding criteria of the HEFCE, the programme had benefited from the criteria, which were published just in time by the Quality Assurance Agency. These criteria guide the institutes of higher education to develop and manage quality education experiences for their students. They are also the subject review guidelines, "to establish a graded profile and an overall judgement on the quality of *the education* provision" (QAA, 1997) for the institutes of higher education to assess their own quality assurance. These six aspects of provision are:

a) Curriculum Design, Content and Organisation—*examines* the structure and content of the curricula, the intended outcomes of the curricula and currency and innovative features.
b) Teaching, Learning and Assessment—*examines* the strategy and methods for teaching, learning and assessment, observations of teaching and learning activities and assessment.

c) Student Progression and Achievement—*examines* the student profile, progression and completion rate and student achievement.

d) Student Support and Guidance—*examines* Admission and induction arrangements; Academic guidance and tutorial support; pastoral and welfare support and Careers information and guidance.

e) Learning Resources—*examines* learning resources strategy; library resources; equipment and information technology; Teaching and social accommodation and Technical and administrative support.

f) Quality Management—*examines* the internal quality assurance for the subject; quality enhancement."

Whilst the programme is first and foremost an academic programme, it is so developed to enable the graduates to practise as Chinese medicine practitioners. Their status and standing will be equal to those practitioners who were trained in the eight SATCM designated TCM universities. Apart from the QAA guidelines, Middlesex University was able to tap on several publications, which have major impacts upon the practice of complementary medicine/therapies guidelines for the professional side of the course development.

— *The National Health Services Confederation (1997)*, represents all NHS hospitals and health authorities, produced a set of guidelines on purchasing complementary therapies and medicine in three specific areas such as: "professional registration (*which is presently not regulated*), insurance; and qualification".

— *The Scottish Office Department of Health* (1996) which recommended that when purchasing CMT services the purchasers should consider the aspects of safety and competence. With safety, the practitioners should demonstrate that they operate within "a code of practice which provides guidance on ethics and conduct. The practitioners should be bound by the Code of Practice on confidentiality which applies to all staff working in the NHS". The practitioners should also be able to offer a level of care, which reflects their level of competence in their practice, which does not yet have statutory recognition in terms of training and continuing professional education.

— *The British Medical Association (BMA)* (1986 and 1993) also provided important pointers for the members of the programme development group. Their recommendations included:

— Priority should be given to research in acupuncture, chiropractic, herbalism, homoeopathy, and osteopathy as the therapies most commonly used in the UK,

— The Council of Europe Co-operation in science and Technology project on non-conventional therapies be approved by the UK government

— Accredited postgraduate sessions will be set up to inform clinicians on the techniques used by different therapies and the possible benefits for patients' consideration should be given to the inclusion of a familiarisation course on non-conventional therapies within the medical undergraduate curriculum.

For more details of these reports please refer to chapter 16.

PROGRAMME DEVELOPMENT OF THE BSC (HONS) IN TRADITIONAL CHINESE MEDICINE

During the course development, the Programme Development Committee (June 1996–July 1997, see Appendix 2 of the Chapter) and the Curriculum Planning Group (June 1996 to present see Appendix 2 of the Chapter) recognised that a common misconception existed among the public that traditional Chinese medicine only deals with Chinese herbs and herbal products. The traditional Chinese medicine is a generic term. It embraces Chinese herbal medicine, Tuna, Medicinal food, Qigong, Acupuncture, Cupping and Moxibustion. They are all methods of treatment underpinned by the Chinese medicine philosophy and principles. This concept is diagrammatically presented in chapter 16. Whilst there was no apparent difficulty in developing the programme based on the traditional philosophy, the implications, the advantages and the disadvantages of basing the curriculum solely on the traditional philosophy, were nevertheless debated and examined. The Programme Development Committee decided that the programme should be a bridge between tradition and modernisation. This is clearly represented in the structure and contents of the programme. The following sections illustrate aspects of the traditional Chinese medicine philosophy, the programme philosophy and the aims and objectives of the programme.

The traditional Chinese medicine philosophy

It is important to understand that traditional Chinese medicine is a medical practice of both an art and a science of healing based on the harmonious coexistence of yin and yang. Despite many scientific developments and innovations, the traditional Chinese medicine philosophy and principles are still deeply rooted in the yin and yang theory, handed down through many generations of experiences and practice.

Traditional Chinese medicine is inherently holistic and focuses on the unity of man with its environment. It identifies the nature and location causing the diseases through the understanding of the individual's environment, emotional state and life style. The aim is to restore the yin and yang harmony in the individual.

Diagnosis is achieved by triangulating three sets of data derived from yin and yang, the Five Elements and the Qi. Their influences and effects can be observed through close examination of patient's tongue; pulse, auscultation; olfaction; palpation and careful questioning to explore the signs and symptoms of the diseases. Treatments are based on the evaluation of the diagnosis to rebalance the yin or yang deficiencies or excess in the body and environment.

For a detailed illustration of these theories and philosophy readers are referred to Chapter 2.

The programme philosophy

The programme rests on a set of explicit values and beliefs about the client, the nature and context of clinical practice and the possession of a body of knowledge based on the traditional Chinese medicine philosophy and principles. This body of knowledge is the tool for the professional TCM practitioner. The Programme believes that;

1   The human body houses a biological, psychological and social being who is in constant interaction with a changing environment. Each person possesses individual needs which are determined by his/her innate characteristics, environment and culture.

2   In a multi-cultural society, this individual's responses to critical incidents in his/her life cycle are influenced by sociocultural factors.

3   TCM practitioners must apply the principles of care and promote the optimum quality of life for the individual, his/her family, and the community within the politico, socio-economic environment in which they work and live.

4   TCM practitioners must accept responsibility to commit themselves to lifelong learning and to seek out opportunities for their own professional development and advancement to enable them to operate in this dynamic changing world, both inside and outside the British NHS.

5   The concept of care is fundamental to the quality of service provided to the individual, groups and society as a whole. This concept involves activity and affective components, which are, linked by the concern society expresses for its members and the service provided. This concept acknowledges the right of the individual to be actively involved in the care given.

6   Learning is a growth process involving changes where individuals and groups actively participate. This process is chiefly self-initiating and includes both planned and unplanned life experiences.

7   Knowledge is a collection of facts, values and information gained through study, research, intuition and experience. Education is a life-long process whereby individuals and groups attempt to achieve self-actualisation.

The Programme reflects the Vision and Mission of both MU and BUTCM. It aims to prepare the individuals within these beliefs, to treat patients competently and safely in a wide variety of clinical and social settings.

The programme is organised so that students' learning and praxis are incremental from being an "observer/assistant" during the first five semesters. Throughout semester 2 of year 3 and semester 1 of year 4, the students will develop their clinical skills further to become "assistant practitioners" progressing to "safe practitioners" in semester 2 of year 4. Finally, after they successfully complete the programme they will become "competent practitioners".

The programme aims

The aims of the programme are to:-

1. Provide a programme of comparable quality and content to that taught in BUTCM, for those wishing to become competent, safe and caring practitioners in either A & M or CHM outside China. They are now combined as one outcome.

2. Provide the students with a thorough preparation in the principles and applications of TCM underpinned by sufficient knowledge and understanding (over 1000 hours) of orthodox medical anatomy, physiology, pharmacology, pathology and diagnostic processes and procedures to enhance their clinical competence.

3. Develop reflective and autonomous lifelong learners with the professional curiosity to want to seek up-to-date knowledge, understanding and skills and to conduct research to underpin their practices.
4. Include the principles of evidence-based practice but still underpinned by the traditional philosophy.
5. Broaden and enrich the students' clinical experiences by undertaking a six month hospital internship in China.

The programme objectives
At the end of the programme the graduates will be able to:

1 Apply and transfer knowledge into practice within the dynamic context of changing health care services.
2 Practise TCM in their own right in a safe, competent and caring way within the ethical and legal framework of the time in a wide range of rapidly changing general health expectations.
3 Critically evaluate patient problems with relevant information taken from history and assessment, and where appropriate, propose a differential diagnosis.
4 Demonstrate logical reasoning and decision making on options for managing the treatment programme.
5 Distinguish the significance of recognising unusual and complex conditions and know when to seek help or to refer.
6 Conduct assessment, diagnostic sessions having regard to patients' confidentiality, the medico-legal implications of his/her actions and accept responsibility thereafter
7 Make an accurate diagnostic interpretation of signs and symptoms elicited in the clinical examination.
8 Manage a clinic as a successful business in a safe and legal manner.
9 Recognise effects of ill-health on patients and take appropriate corrective actions to deal with the psychological stress.
10 Communicate and work appropriately and effectively with other professional colleagues to advance patients' welfare.

THE SCOPE OF TCM PRACTICE

Whilst the programme is based on the traditional philosophy, the programme also attempted to bring this healing art into the modern era, particularly in the developed or post industrialised societies whose predominant health care modality is underpinned by the orthodox medicine (OM). This programme acknowledges that OM is very advanced with well defined specialisation. This acknowledgement made obvious that clear and well defined parameters need to be set and these are reflected in the programme contents. For example, Chinese medicine is taught as a practice, which complements and supports OM. It does not claim to be better or an alternative, rather a complementary medicine, which can enhance the quality of life for those patients, suffering from chronic conditions. In response to various official publications and guidelines already mentioned, and in the absence of a Statutory Regulatory Body for TCM, MU has also set up its own TCM Ethics Committee and holds a live register of its graduate practitioners to "police" their professional practice until such time as a regulatory body is set up. The final outcomes of the programme therefore, expect that the graduates will be competent to practise in gynaecology, dermatology, paediatric, psychosomatic, neuropathology, chronic conditions, anaesthesia and palliative care. In cases of special and acute medical/surgical, accident and emergency conditions the practitioners will be competent to recognise them and refer such patients immediately to their GPs or hospital as appropriate, thus explaining why the programme offers over one thousand hours of western biomedical sciences. The students will learn from their OM practitioner colleagues, the skills in interpreting the armoury of investigations involved in OM and acute internal orthodox medicine. They will also spend a specified time in the hospital wards and investigative units to gain greater insight into the diagnostic procedures used in OM. The graduates will practice within the scope of their practice and the code of practice and the ethical framework is to be provided by the University's Chinese Medicine Ethics Committee.

SUPPORTING LIFELONG LEARNING

Despite the programme's academic outcome, the contents reflect more accurately the processes of professionalism. The graduates will be able to:

— Acquire and interpret information about the patients and their influencing factors.
— Decide how to respond to this assessment both immediately and long term treatment strategy.

— Able to implement the actions, including treatment, referral, providing advice etc.
— Manage own professional behaviours and offer on-going monitoring of their patients.

Chinese medicine practitioners like many other Complementary Therapists often operate in isolation and this is unlikely to encourage self development. It will demand greater commitment and personal sacrifices to maintain the "lifelong learner" spirit. To keep this spirit alive, the programme has adopted the student self-assessed learning log book (**SSALLB**), a learning portfolio which instils in the students the concept and culture of self-development. The aims of the programme's approach to lifelong learning are to:

- Achieve integrated learning through and across the modules.
- Include a reflective diary to facilitate the development of reflective skills.
- Record individual learning contracts between the student and teachers to negotiate the teaching and learning to achieve the programme objectives.
- Facilitate records of professional, personal and academic development including feeding from peers, practitioners and patients.
- Help the students to accept responsibility for own life-long development needs.
- Contribute to the students' award.

RESEARCH MODULE IN TRADITIONAL CHINESE MEDICINE

The programme believes that many CM practitioners accept and recognise that their practice must be as evidence-based as that of their colleagues in health care services. This will include "employing consistent; accurate records and reports; accessible publication and willingness to supply further information for research purposes (de Wit 1981).

This programme is also designed to build "bridges" between East and West/the traditional and the progressive. Much has been written as to particular research methods TCM should adopt. The programme's intention is to introduce the students to various research paradigms embracing both psycho-social and orthodox medical models. It is also this programme's intention that Western research methods should be applied to TCM and evaluation be conducted. It is a matter of selecting the best fit approach to a particular investigation. Students will have an opportunity to apply a particular approach when they pursue their end of the programme proposition module. The objective of this approach is to embrace the holistic and analytical principles and provide the graduates with the necessary skills to monitor and evaluate the outcomes of their practices.

THE CHALLENGES FACING TRADITIONAL CHINESE MEDICINE OUTSIDE CHINA

The global popularity of traditional Chinese medicine has significantly influenced and directly induced the progress and modernisation of this traditional philosophy; experience-based medical practice in all aspects in Mainland China (see Chapter 6) and other regions all over the world. In particular, the product-based treatment aspects of the traditional Chinese medicine will be expected to address 3 important issues; quality, safety and efficacy of the medications in a similar manner as for orthodox pharmaceuticals. Graduates when properly trained with this proposed curriculum will be able to appreciate the following key points that can be expected from the public. The future graduates of the traditional Chinese medicine course will have to face the continuing development and modernisation of traditional Chinese medicine.

The Change of Traditional to Science and Technology-based disciplines is the inevitable progress for traditional Chinese medicine to modernise. The future of the traditional Chinese medicine graduates and practitioners will face and lead such development. Some positive actions are needed to:

- use high tech to communicate its knowledge and skills
- Transformation and explosion of interest in TCM to ensure quality, safety and effective health
- provide leadership in the safe practice and treatment of TCM
- Explore its large clinical research data and make them available to the practitioners outside China
- Regulate the quality and safety of herbs and instruments used
- Be more research orientated and research based practice
- Work closely with the importers and the government agencies to assure public safety

- Take a lead in the biodiversity movement to assure the natural products continue to be available for future generations.

The TCM practitioners will be challenged to:

- deliver safe and effective treatment
- collaborate and work inter-professionally to contribute to the World Health Organisation's target to achieve "Health for All by the Year 2000"
- provide concise and essential information to the public to enable them to make informed decision
- practise research-based practice as well as to conduct own research to build up knowledge.

Concluding Remarks

The history of traditional Chinese medicine is as old as the history of the early man searching for food to survive. State Administration of Traditional Chinese Medicine(1995) stated that "In the beginning, primitive people ate wild fruit and dug up roots or plants to appease their hunger. They often ate poisonous plants by mistake, resulting in vomiting, diarrhoea, coma or even death. Out of these experiences, they gradually learned to identify which plants would cause vomiting or diarrhoea and those that were poisonous, those that were harmful and those that were beneficial to the body." This quotation is offered to highlight the difficulties and frustration MU/BUTCM curriculum model had experienced. It was not the mere translation of the curriculum from Chinese into the English language that in itself is a complex task. A good translator should be able to describe and emphasise the original thoughts and ideas therein but also reflect the originality of the text. Translating knowledge and skills from one culture to another is also, therefore, doubly complex. There is immense potential to integrate traditional Chinese medicine into Western healthcare as it is done in China and other regions in the East and this is a very real challenge. This can only be possible if proper training and education can be achieved to deliver quality, safe and efficacious discipline.

The chapter offers a bird's eye view of the complex issues had to be resolved as well as weaved into the programme without lessening the significance of the traditional philosophy evolved over many thousands of years. For example; the programme had to be very carefully constructed to harmonise tradition with modern, the Chinese medical philosophy with the Western medical philosophy which will continue to play the dominant role, and the high tech medicine on one extreme to the minimal technology based practice at the opposite extreme. This programme is now in its third year and much has been learned. One major and several minor changes were made. The students on graduating will now be able to practise both acupuncture and herbal medicine. The minor changes include modifications in the assessment strategy and in the delivery processes. We hope this chapter will assist future programme developers to circumvent the difficulties MU has experienced as described and to be able to improve from it.

References

BMA (1986) Alternative Therapy: Report of the Board of Science & Education, London: British Medical Association, 1986.

BMA (1993) Complementary Medicine: New approaches to good practice, Oxford; Oxford University Press, July 1996.

de Wit, A. (1981) Quoted in British Medical Association (1986), Alternative Therapy: Report of the Board of Education, London: British Medical Association.

Goldbeck-Wood, S. (1996) Complementary medicine is booming world-wide; British Medical Journal 313, 131.

Jin, Y., Berry, M.I. and Chan, K. (1995) Chinese herbal medicine in the United Kingdom. *Pharmaceutical Journal*, 255 (suppl), R37.

Lee, H. (1998) The first Chinese medicine degree programme outside China, Positive Health, September, 1998

Lewith, G., Kenyon, J. and Lewis, P. (1996) Complementary Medicine: An integrated, approach. Oxford University Press, Oxford, 1996.

Morgan, D. (1997) HIV/AIDS and complementary medicine: seeking information on alternative treatments. The AIDS Letter, No 63 Oct/Nov 1997, The Royal Society of Medicine Press.

NAHAT (1993) Complementary therapies in the NHS (research paper No. 10) London: National Association of Health Authorities and Trusts.

Scottish Home Office Department of Health (1996) Complementary Medicine and the NHS—an examination of Acupuncture, Homeopathy, Chiropractic and Osteopathy, The Stationery Office.

Tomlinson, R. (1996) China tightens up TCM courses. British Medical Journal Vol. 312, 20 April 1996

Worth, C. (1997) Guidelines for selecting practitioners of complementary and alternative medicine within the health service 1997/1998

Appendix 1

Table 18.1 Training courses offered by various institutions in acupuncture, Chinese herbal medicine, & other related disciplines in the United Kingdom (Data updated from previous survey, Jin *et al.*, 1995)

No	Institution	Courses	Duration	Contact address
1.	British College of Acupuncture	Acupuncture	3 year	The Registrar, 8 Hunter St, London WCIN 1BN
2.	Chung San Acupuncture School	Acupuncture	part-time	15 Porchester Gardens London W2 4EY
3.	College of Integrated Chinese Medicine	Training in Acupuncture	part-time	40 College Road, reading, RG6 1QB
4.	Institute for Traditional Medicine	Herbs	part-time	5 Waverley Place Finsbury Park, London N4
5.	Japanese Herbal Medicine, Kohoha School	Japanese Herbal Medicine	part-time	C/o 36 Bankhurst Road, London SE6 4XN
6.	London Academy of Oriental Medicine	Acupuncture & Chinese Herbal Medicine	4 Year part-time	7 Newcourt Street, London NW8 7NA
7.	London School of Acupuncture & Traditional Chinese Medicine	B Sc.(Hons.): Acupuncture	3 Year—Full time course	The Registrar, 4th Floor, 60 Bunhill Row, London, EC1Y 8QD
8.	Northern college of Acupuncture	Diploma in Acupuncture	3 year, part time	124 Acomb Road, York YO2 4EY
9.	Northern College Herbs	Part time Training course in Chinese Herbs	2 Year	124 Acomb Road, York YO2 4EY

Table 18.1 Training courses offered by various institutions in acupuncture, Chinese herbal medicine, & other related disciplines in the United Kingdom (Data updated from previous survey, Jin *et al.*, 1995) (*Continued*)

No.	Institution	Courses	Duration	Contact address
10.	Renshu College of Chinese Medicine	Acupuncture & Chinese Medicine	Short courses	629 High Road Leytonstone, London E11
11	School of Chinese Medicine & Clinical Massage	Herbs, Tuina	4 year part-time	253 east end road, London N2 8AY
12.	The Southwest College of Oriental Medicine	short course in Acupuncture & Shiatsu	2 Year part-time	P O Box 795, Bristol, BS 99 5WZ

Appendix 2

We are grateful for those colleagues from various institutes and organisations of Chinese medicine in the UK and China who have helped us to developed this educational module (MU-BUTCM) for the degree course of Chinese medicine at the Middlesex University. Special thanks should go to the then President of the Beijing University of Traditional Chinese Medicine, Professor LONG Zhi Xian and his colleagues who visited Middlesex University in November 1996 and finalised the joint curriculum with the TCM Curriculum Planning Group. Members who were and have been involved in the course development are acknowledged as follows:

MEMBERS OF THE TCM CURRICULUM DEVELOPMENT COMMITTEE BETWEEN JUNE 1996—JULY 1997

Dr J.H. Chen—Practitioner & Representative of the Association of TCM (until November 1996)
Dr B.C. Chan—Private TCM Practitioner
Professor Kelvin Chan—Visiting Professor of Biomedical Sciences, Middlesex University
Dr Lily Cheung—Principal and TCM Practitioner, Chung San School of Acupuncture
Mr. Ming Chee Kwok—Dean, Ming Ai (London) Institute
Mr. Henry Lee—Head of School (Chair), Middlesex University
Dr David St George—Visiting Academic and Orthodox Medical Practitioner
Dr Theresa Shak—Director, Ming Ai (London) Institute
Dr Ellis Snitcher—Senior Lecturer in General medicine, Middlesex University
Mr. Jidong Wu—Senior Lecturer/Practitioner, Middlesex University (since February 1997)
Mr. Wilson Xu—Private TCM Practitioner (until November 1996)

MEMBERS OF THE TCM CURRICULUM PLANNING GROUP BETWEEN JUNE 1996 TO PRESENT

Dr B.C. Chan—Private TCM Practitioner
Dr J.H. Chen—Practitioner & Representative of the Association of TCM (until November 1996)
Professor Kelvin Chan—Visiting Professor of Biomedical Sciences, Middlesex University
Dr Lily Cheung—Principal and TCM Practitioner, Chung San School of Acupuncture

Mr. Henry Lee (Chair)—Head of School (Chair), Middlesex University
Mr. Jidong Wu—Senior Lecturer/Practitioner, Middlesex University (since February 1997)
Mr. Wilson Xu—Private TCM Practitioner (until November 1996)

19 AN ORTHODOX PRACTITIONER'S VIEW OF CHINESE MEDICINE

David J. Atherton

Background

We are told that the plant hunters are out in the forests and mountains of the world looking for new drugs. I have always been puzzled by the focus on medicinal plants used by small-scale communities in the Amazon, for example, when the use of plant medicines in China has achieved such sophistication, and has such a long history of careful study and refinement within a highly cultivated medical framework.

For many hundreds of years, the great civilisation of China evolved largely in isolation from the West. One of the remarkable effects of this seclusion was to allow the development of unique scientific concepts in the absence of any significant exchange of ideas with the cities far to the west in the Near East and in Europe. Whereas some of China's greatest scientific discoveries did make the journey westwards, traditional Chinese medicine (TCM) continued to develop in almost complete isolation right up to the present.

Oddly, this isolation appears to have become greater the closer one gets to modern times. In earlier centuries a number of medicinal herbs was brought from China to Europe and became incorporated in the formularies of orthodox medical practitioners. Well-known examples included liquorice (from *Glycyrrhiza uralensis*) and dittany bark (from *Dictamnus dasycarpus*). However, the rapid decline after the Great War of the prescription of medicinal herbs in orthodox medicine in the West has served to obscure this former link with Chinese medicine. These herbs and others have however continued to be prescribed by herbal practitioners in Europe. Liquorice continues to be popular, though diminishingly so, in confectionery; it also remains the source of a licensed medicine known as carbenoxolone sodium, still occasionally prescribed for the treatment of oesophagitis.

There are remarkable similarities between theories of causation of disease that were current in medieval European medicine, and ones that remain valid in Chinese medicine. A good example is what was known in Europe as the theory of 'element', a concept that was already well established in ancient Greek medicine. The four 'element' are air, earth, fire and water, of which the human body is composed. This is very close indeed to the principle in TCM whereby illness is regarded as the result of an imbalance of the properties of wind, heat, dampness, dryness and cold. Another parallel exists in the concept of 'humours', which also originated in Greek medicine and remained an important influence in orthodox European medicine until the nineteenth century. According to this concept, the body contains four main 'humours',—or fluids—blood, yellow bile, black bile and phlegm. Many diseases reflected imbalances in the content of these fluids within individual organs. These 'humours' had something in common with the Chinese 'organs', such as the liver, spleen, blood and kidneys; their perceived functions have little in common with those of their anatomical counterparts.

There are remarkably similar concepts in Indian medicine, for example, and while all these similarities might be regarded as fortuitous, their existence suggests either that the medical traditions of much of the world arose from a common source, or perhaps more likely, that there was substantial interchange of ideas during their development. This link between Chinese medicine and ancient medical traditions in the West might suggest that TCM is merely of historical interest, and this is certainly the way that it is generally regarded by orthodox Western medical practitioners. However, closer examination shows that Chinese medicine is by no means rigid or unchangeable, that it has changed throughout history, and that the pace of change—as in Western medicine—has progressively accelerated over the last century.

To the practitioner of orthodox Western medicine, the therapies used in TCM comprise 2 principal components, namely herbal therapy and acupuncture. Those unfamiliar with Chinese medicine should be aware that, in present-day China, it is regarded as perfectly normal for TCM practitioners to prescribe Western-type licensed pharmaceutical products alongside acupuncture and herbal therapies. There is no rigid separation of Western-type medicine and TCM as outsiders might imagine, and the training of TCM practitioners has for several decades included substantial amounts of basic Western medical science including anatomy, physiology and pathology. Likewise, those training in China in Western-type medicine are taught the theories of TCM. The result is considerable cross-fertilisation between these 2 disciplines, despite their superficially exclusive natures.

This has been very much to the benefit of patients, who are not infrequently treated simultaneously by both types of practitioner. During my own visits to China I saw this collaboration occurring in many areas of medicine, but perhaps most effectively in the treatment of auto-immune diseases such as systemic lupus erythematosus and dermatomyositis, which are common in China, and in the symptomatic care of patients dying of liver failure, also common in China, and of terminal malignant disease.

The effectiveness of Chinese herbal treatment was first brought to my own attention about 10 years ago, when a child under my care with severe atopic eczema was taken by his parents to see a Chinese doctor, Dr Ding-Hui Luo, in London's Chinatown. He was brought to see me after a few weeks of herbal treatment and I recall today how impressed I was with the resulting improvement. I should add that this was a child with severe and extensive eczema, who had consistently failed to respond to conventional medical measures to treat his distressing skin disease. He had been treated with daily decoctions taken by mouth, made from a mixture of dried herbal ingredients.

Although atopic eczema is generally a mild disease that will respond satisfactorily to simple topical treatments, there is a important minority of children and adults in whom it is severe and disabling. In such patients, the disease may be unresponsive to treatments other than those whose use is associated with substantial toxicity, such as systemic corticosteroids or cyclosporin.

Western dermatologists would all acknowledge the need for more effective and safer treatments for such patients. This was the reason for my own curiosity regarding my patient's remarkable improvement. Of course, anyone who treats patients with atopic eczema knows that from time to time sudden improvements occur which can be hard to explain, and which are often attributed by patients to any type of alternative therapy they happen to be using. For this reason, while I had been impressed by my own patient's experience of Chinese herbal therapy, I remained sceptical in the absence of corroboration. Therefore, over a period of time, I recommended about 30 further children with treatment-resistant eczema to this doctor. They all received similar treatment, though I noted that their prescriptions varied considerably. I recorded that substantial improvements occurred in over half of them. At this point, it occurred to me that decoctions of Chinese medicinal herbs might be generally more effective in the therapy of atopic eczema than the conventional treatments we would otherwise use in Europe and North America. Furthermore, careful observation of patients treated in this way had failed to reveal evidence of any obvious adverse effect other than a little diarrhoea at the beginning of treatment.

Orthodox medical practitioners in the West will generally be sceptical of the theoretical basis for the selection of a Chinese herbal prescription. This is true for myself, despite my acceptance that such prescriptions can be very effective in treating eczema. In practice, what matters is whether a treatment is effective, not whether the hypotheses that profess to explain that effectiveness are convincing. In every medical tradition, therapeutic choices are based on a set of beliefs relating to the causation of disease and the way that treatments work. When a treatment works, the practitioner's confidence in the set of beliefs on which the choice of treatment was based is reinforced. However, the effectiveness of a treatment does not in fact confirm that the rationale for using that treatment is absolute truth, only that it is one that functions. In whatever medical tradition one works, it is wise to reflect upon this.

My own increased awareness of the potentially insecure nature of the theoretical basis for selecting treatments has made me more questioning of the rationales for all the treatments we use in orthodox Western medicine. My choice of treatment is still largely based on the evidence that it actually works. The reliability of that evidence is another source of misgivings between Western and Chinese medicine. In Western medicine we have experienced an ever-increasing emphasis on the importance of having scientifically reliable evidence of the effectiveness of treatments. This has been accompanied by an equal de-emphasis of anecdotal and personal experience as a basis for treatment selection. Doctors in the West find themselves increasingly required to justify the treatments they use according to the scientific evidence for their effectiveness and the value of their own 'clinical judgement' has steadily depreciated. However, there are many treatments whose effectiveness has not been demonstrated scientifically, but which nevertheless appear to be effective. The current trend is to deprecate the use of such treatments, and a doctor who uses them is increasingly at risk of criticism and litigation. Whether rigid adherence to the principle of no treatment without incontrovertible evidence of benefit is always in the best interest of patients is open to question.

The contrast between this trend in Western medicine and the way that treatment selection is undertaken in the practice of Chinese medicine is a stark one. There is virtually no scientific evidence that any Chinese herbal treatment works in any condition. Furthermore, the selection of the elements of an individual patient's prescription, and the doses in which they are prescribed, are highly idiosyncratic, varying to an extraordinary degree between different practitioners. Despite the great variability between prescriptions that might be formulated by different practitioners for a single patient, each practitioner is able to look at a colleague's prescription and understand the basis on which it has been formulated. This flexibility in therapeutic style is inherent in Chinese medicine, and it means that selection of practitioner by patients may have a major effect on outcome. In the West, great efforts are being made to reduce the idiosyncratic element in therapy, in an attempt to increase every patient's chances of receiving the best possible treatment. These two styles could hardly be more different.

The quality of therapeutic materials is regarded as extremely important in the West. By their nature, plant materials vary considerably from batch to batch, both in terms of their content of beneficial therapeutic constituents and of potentially harmful components. While no doubt great care is taken in China to produce medicinal herbs of consistent quality, there will clearly be great variability in quality, which may serve both to reduce therapeutic effectiveness and to increase the risk of toxicity. In addition, there exists a very real danger that plant materials will at least occasionally be wrongly identified. These issues do little to reassure those in Western medicine and undoubtedly serve to increase scepticism.

Paradoxically, plant-derived medicines continue to figure prominently among licensed drugs used in the West. While many single molecules originally derived from plants can now be cheaply synthesised, other compounds continue to be extracted from plants. However, it is a condition of obtaining a product licence for such drugs that both the therapeutic activity and the content of any toxic compounds should be carefully assayed in order to guarantee consistent quality. In contrast, the active compounds in Chinese herbs are largely unknown; thus their activity cannot be measured in the laboratory.

It is possible that Chinese herbal prescriptions generally contain several active compounds that work together to increase benefit to the patient. There is therefore a risk that an obsession with reducing plant medicines to a single molecule will lead to 'the baby being thrown out with the bathwater'. There is nevertheless a great deal that can be done to enhance the quality of herbal medicines, though the benefits that this may bring must be weighed against increased costs and, therefore, the fact that some of those who might benefit might be unable to afford treatment at all.

Batches of herbs can be examined in several ways to increase consistency. They can be examined botanically to verify the identity of the material. Extracts can be examined by chromatographic techniques to provide a 'fingerprint', ie. a profile of constituents which does not require the molecular identity of each constituent to be known, only to be recognised by its position and its normal relative quantity in the chromatogram. Batches can then be discarded if quantitatively important components are present in significantly reduced amounts or if certain components are present in significantly increased amounts. 'Stray' components can also be sought. Contaminants such as insecticides and heavy metals can be measured directly.

Clinical Trials of a Prescription for Atopic Eczema

The strong impression I gained of the therapeutic effectiveness of Chinese herbal medicine in atopic eczema led me to desire both to confirm this effectiveness scientifically, and to go on, if effectiveness could be established, to encourage the development of a quality-controlled product that could benefit large numbers of patients throughout the world.

The next step was to contact Dr Luo, who offered her expertise without hesitation. Although the practice of Chinese medicine normally requires that patients receive individually formulated prescriptions, Dr Luo agreed to devise a limited number of standardised formulae for patients whose eczema fulfilled certain fairly precise criteria. She wrote 4 formulae, and defined the type of patient for which each of these would be most appropriately prescribed. She agreed to dispense these standardised prescriptions to patients that I would identify, and for whom I would prescribe what I believed to be the appropriate formula. These patients would be exclusively ones whose disease had failed to improve adequately on conventional therapy, and the evaluation of response would be on an open basis. This pilot study suggested that these 4 prescriptions could be helpful in as many as 60% of patients selected according to the criteria we had established. Furthermore, blood tests on these patients were reassuring in that they demonstrated no evidence of impairment of renal, hepatic or bone marrow function after 6 months' continuous therapy.

It was my view that a stage had now been reached where it was reasonable to progress to a full-scale clinical trial of one of these 4 prescriptions. The particular prescription selected had been formulated for patients with extensive diffuse atopic eczema, with prominent erythema but without exudation. The main reason for selecting this particular prescription for further study was that it had shown promise for a group of children with a type of eczema that generally proves difficult to treat with conventional topical therapy.

The next task was to find support for the project within the pharmaceutical industry, because we would need quality-controlled materials, which we would have to provide to patients free of cost. I approached Dr Geoffrey Guy, who ran his own small pharmaceutical company and who I knew to be sympathetic to the concept of developing plant-based medicines. Dr Guy offered to help by establishing a small off-shoot of his company to prepare the treatment materials that would be required for our trial; this eventually became Phytopharm Ltd.

The need for the trial to be both placebo-controlled and double-blind provided a challenge. The prescription contained 10 different plant materials, all in common use as medicines in China. Chinese formularies provide a Latin name for each component. With the assistance of experts in the UK and in China, we were able to check these identifications and obtain a species of origin for most of the relevant plant materials.

We were able provisionally to identify the plants in the prescription as: *Ledebouriella seseloides, Potentilla chinensis, Clematis armandii, Rehmannia glutinosa, Paeonia lactiflora, Lophatherum gracile, Dictamnus dasycarpus, Tribulus terrestris, Glycyrrhiza uralensis* and *Schizonepeta tenuifolia.*

Quality controls were run on every batch of herbs purchased, both to verify their identity, and to minimise the possibility of contamination, particularly in respect of heavy metals. Following these quality control procedures, the material was milled to a fine powder, mixed and sealed in porous paper sachets. Two types of sachets were prepared, larger sachets containing the majority of the constituents, and smaller ones containing those which incorporated volatile components that would otherwise be lost during prolonged boiling. The placebo comprised a mixture of inert plant materials of similar appearance, taste and smell, but with no known benefit in eczema. These included bran, hops, barley and small amounts of culinary herbs.

We used a cross-over design, with randomisation of treatment order. Each treatment was given for 8 successive weeks, with an intervening 4 week wash-out period. Forty-seven children of both sexes (age range 1.5–18.1 years) participated, following a blood test to verify normal bone marrow, liver and kidney function. Disease activity was assessed using a simple scoring system. The children attended the clinic every 4 weeks throughout the 5 month trial period. Further blood tests and a 24-hour urine collection were made at the end of each of the two treatment periods.

Parents were instructed to prepare the medication once daily, the number of sachets depending on the child's age:

age 1–7 years: 2 large and 2 small sachets/day
age 8–13 years: 3 large and 3 small sachets/day
age >14 years: 4 large and 4 small sachets/day

The large sachets were placed in 500 ml. of water, which was brought to the boil and simmered for 90 minutes. The small sachets were then added and the liquid simmered for a final 3 minutes. Parents learned to boil the liquid at a rate that would reliably reduce its volume to about 100 ml, which was taken while still warm.

Of the 47 children who started the trial, 37 were able to complete it. Five were unable to take the treatment as instructed on account of its unpalatibility, and 5 others were excluded from the study by protocol, because of the prescription during the study of systemic corticosteroids for asthma, or systemic antibiotics for skin infections. Analysis demonstrated a large and statistically significant superiority of active treatment over placebo [1]. Two-thirds of the children enjoyed greater than 60% reductions in disease activity scores. Most of the improvement was apparent by the end of the 4th week of treatment. The reductions in disease activity scores were mirrored by symptomatic improvements recorded by parents on special diary cards. Some of the children also had asthma, but this was not affected by the treatment.

The children remained well throughout the study, apart from short-lived diarrhoea at the initiation of therapy in a few cases. No child developed any detectable abnormality of bone marrow, kidney or liver function during treatment.

The results of the trial confirmed the effectiveness of Chinese herbs as a treatment for atopic eczema in children. We were subsequently able to show very similar results in a trial in adults [2].

The results of these studies were gratifying for 2 reasons. Firstly, this Chinese herbal formula treatment appeared to offer the most effective new treatment for atopic eczema since the introduction of topical corticosteroids some 40 years ago (apart from a small number of powerful drugs whose use is limited by serious toxicity). Secondly, the benefit was observed in patients for whom orthodox treatment had failed to provide adequate disease control.

Although entry to both these studies had been restricted to patients with a particular subtype of atopic eczema, there appeared to be no reason for similar treatment not to be equally effective in other, commoner types of atopic eczema. Indeed, my own observation of patients treated by Chinese medical practitioners in the UK and in China suggests that it would be. This is an issue that I had hoped to address in further studies.

While we found no evidence of short-term toxicity, either by observation of the patients, or in the limited tests undertaken by way of monitoring, a risk that there might be longer-term toxicity could not be excluded. This was one reason for our wish to extend the trial in any child whose parents wanted to do so. Another reason was to investigate whether treatment could gradually be withdrawn without loss of benefit. We therefore offered a further year's treatment to all 37 children who had completed the initial controlled trial. All of them elected to continue, and were switched to active treatment, whichever limb of the trial had just been completed. The therapeutic aim was to stabilise initial improvement and then to attempt to reduce treatment frequency progressively without deterioration.

At the end of the year, 18 of the 37 children enjoyed at least 90% reductions in eczema activity scores, and 5 showed lesser degrees of improvement. Fourteen children withdrew from the study, 10 due to lack of response, and 4 because of treatment unpalatability or difficulty of preparation. By the end of the year, 7 of the children had been able to discontinue treatment altogether without relapse. The other 16 required continued regular treatment to maintain control of their eczema, but only 4 of these still required daily treatment.

Asymptomatic elevation of serum aspartate aminotransferase to values 7–14 times normal were noted on one occasion in 2 children whose eczema was so well controlled that the therapy was stopped; restarting would not have been clinically indicated. Unfortunately routine clinical chemistry in our hospital did not at that time include a measurement of serum alanine aminotransferase, which is more liver-specific and other measures of liver function were normal. The reason for the abnormality could not be identified and routine clinical chemistry was normal when rechecked 8 weeks later in both cases.

My co-workers and I concluded that our Chinese herbal formula appeared to provide a therapeutic option for children with extensive atopic eczema that had failed to respond to other treatments. Over a period of a year it had continued to prove helpful for approximately half the children who originally took part in our placebo-controlled trial, and withdrawal of treatment without relapse appeared possible in at least a proportion of cases. The possibility had however been raised that it might occasionally provoke hepatic abnormalities.

MODE OF ACTION OF CHINESE HERBAL MEDICINES

The pharmacology and mechanism of action of this formulation of herbs is unknown. This is true for almost all Chinese herbal treatments. Plant medicines of this type contain large numbers of pharmacologically active compounds, and these are certain to possess a wide spectrum of biological effects. We were particularly anxious to be able to rule out any corticosteroid-like activity as a basis for its effectiveness, and we were able to do so by demonstrating that the treatment did not alter patients' patterns of endogenous steroid excretion in the urine [3]. The principle of this test is the fact that giving steroid from outside ('exogenous') will suppress the body's own ('endogenous') steroid production, and therefore the appearance of recognisable compounds in the urine.

A pharmacological basis for the combination of several different plant components in a single prescription, ten in the case of our formula, has not been demonstrated. The Western scientific prejudice would be to believe that the therapeutic activity is likely to reside in one or two of the components and that the others will be more or less superfluous. Personally, I find it hard to accept that that this is the case. The use of plants in Chinese medicine has evolved over an extraordinarily long period of time, and it is probable that 'trial and error' has been the main driving force throughout. I would suspect that the predilection for compound prescriptions genuinely reflects either superior effectiveness or reduced toxicity—or, most probably, both of these. I believe that every component of a compound prescription is included for a reason, either because it increases therapeutic benefit, or because it counteracts some unwanted effect or perhaps improves palatability, but I do not believe that Chinese doctors always, or ever, know the reasons; they have simply inherited the accumulated experience of their predecessors. It is known by Chinese doctors that some plant components should be used in combination with certain others, and there are general rules to help. In China, compound prescriptions are often explained in terms of each constituent having a role like a member of an imperial court: an emperor, an empress, a chief minister, and so on. The scientific Westerner should not expect to gain much pharmacological insight from such rules, whose real purpose and value is to help the Chinese doctor to formulate a prescription that will work as well as possible because it is based on principles that have stood the test of time.

Although the obsession with single molecule therapy in Western medicine is a relatively modern one, it is now firmly entrenched. This is true of the medical profession, the pharmacologist, the pharmaceutical companies and licensing authorities. It will be very difficult to change this, but I believe it will change when all these bodies recognise that there are effective treatments which do not conform to this limited model. It seems paradoxical that we recognise the complex interactions of millions of different molecules within living organisms, yet we can only conceive of treatment with single molecules. In practice, doctors often employ combinations of single molecules. Many over-the-counter headache formulations combine a variety of single molecules to obtain enhanced effectiveness with a reduced risk of unwanted effects. The use of combination therapy is probably most highly developed in oncology, in which therapy will most characteristically comprise combinations of several anti-neoplastic agents. Other agents may be added to reduce adverse effects, for example an anti-emetic. Each individual component will have achieved all the requirements of the licensing authority as a single molecule, but there will have been no prior testing whatsoever of the effectiveness or safety of the combinations in which it will actually be most frequently used. Combination therapy is also commonly employed in the treatment of infectious diseases, but in reality it features to some degree in almost all areas of Western medicine, including my own speciality of dermatology. It is possible that many of the components of a Chinese herbal prescription would have little effect when given alone, and will only provide benefit when given in appropriate combination with others. If Chinese herbal medicines are ever to be licensed in the West, the licensing system will somehow have to take this possibility into account.

Toxicity of Chinese Herbal Medicines

A number of reports in the medical literature have served to heighten anxiety about the toxicity of Chinese plant medicines in general. These have largely been of an anecdotal nature, and it could be argued in nearly every case that the causal relationship between the medicine and the unwanted event has not been proven. In some of the reports the evidence for such a relationship is very weak indeed; in others it is stronger. It is however a reasonable assumption that, like any other form of pharmacological therapy, Chinese herbal medicines will be accompanied by a risk of adverse effects. I have occasionally been reassured by Chinese doctors that Chinese herbal medicine, "is safe". I presume that they are saying that with the proper training, experience and good quality herbs, the risks are likely to be far outweighed by the benefits. I would accept that this is the case.

In relation to the toxicity of Chinese herbal therapy, one needs to consider several sources of risk, which can be listed a follows:

1. inadequate training of the practitioner
2. excessive dose of a single herb
3. failure to prescribe a smaller dose when:
   a) several herbs are given simultaneously
   b) the patient is a child
   c) the patient has a kidney or liver problem that delays breakdown or excretion
4. simultaneous drug treatment which is not admitted to the practitioner
5. idiosyncrasy (an unpredictable liability of a particular patient to react adversely against a particular drug given in the correct dose)
6. variation in quality of herbs, particularly in respect of content of the relevant pharmacological activity
7. contamination of herbs by heavy metals, insecticides, herbicides or other toxins, e.g. fungal toxins due to poor storage conditions, or human faeces (often used as a fertiliser, carrying a risk of transmission of viral hepatitis)
8. dispensing of the wrong herb, as a consequence of:
   a) accidental mislabeling by supplier
   b) substitution of herbs by a supplier
   c) dispensing errors

This article is not the place to elaborate on these, but it will be clear to the reader that proper training of supplier, practitioner and pharmacist will reduce the risks substantially, and quality control of herbs, as discussed earlier in this chapter, would further reduce the risks.

PALATABILITY OF CHINESE HERBAL MEDICINES

As anyone who has ever taken a Chinese herbal decoction will know, palatability is an issue. A high proportion of pre-school children—and even many adults—find them impossible to swallow. It is hard to see how one would ever be able to solve this, if the practitioner is to retain the great flexibility that characterises Chinese medicine and which may be fundamental to its effectiveness. Patent medicines are often prepared in more palatable forms, eg. pills; these can be useful, but are regarded as invariably less effective than freshly-made decoctions.

In our own trials, we were all impressed how few children were unable to take the decoctions, only around 10%, though a greater proportion reported some difficulty. However, I would imagine that the proportion of patients experiencing difficulties with palatability would be far greater in a less motivated group. Because we were using a fixed herbal formula it was possible to develop a more palatable presentation. In fact, Phytopharm succeeded in producing a more or less tasteless presentation. This comprised very small pills, which we called 'mini-tablets', which contained freeze-dried extract, which were then lacquer-coated to make them tasteless. The mini-tablets were packed in small sachets, allowing different doses to be prescribed according to the age of the patient. It has proven simple even for small children to wash down these mini-tablets with a drink. We have now been able to show that these mini-tablets retain effectiveness as a therapy for atopic eczema [4].

Potential for Controlled Clinical Trials

Our studies have demonstrated that it is perfectly feasible to undertake controlled clinical trials of Chinese herbal medicines. The short-cut in our case was to use a standardised formula, so that all patients received the same treatment. However, this goes against the principles of Chinese herbal medicine. It is nevertheless possible to devise ways of undertaking controlled trials of variable herbal formulae prescribed for a single disease, such as psoriasis, and at one time we had planned such a study. A belief in the value of such trials is not a feature of Chinese medicine, and we should never underestimate the genuine ethical issues that arise when it is consciously planned to withhold treatment from some patients. I have no doubt, however, that the acceptance of the scientific basis for Chinese herbal medicine, if not its actual survival, will ultimately depend on more convincing verification of effectiveness and safety.

Having made the case for controlled trials of Chinese herbal medicines, the question arises how such trials could be funded. This is a very real problem. In orthodox Western medicine, we have reached a situation where the great majority of clinical trials of therapies are funded by pharmaceutical companies, in return for exclusive commercial rights through the patent laws. Without the protection of patent, spending by pharmaceutical companies on Chinese herbal medicines will simply not happen.

Practitioners' Qualifications

Before ending this chapter, I am keen to say that while I am personally enthusiastic regarding the therapeutic promise of Chinese herbal medicine and would not hesitate to seek help from a good practitioner myself if it were appropriate, I am very anxious about the variability of the qualifications of practitioners currently treating the general public in the UK. I have a feeling that less than 10% of all practitioners now working in the UK are qualified doctors of TCM with a full training that would be recognised by the best of them. I do not blame the practitioners themselves as their activities lie within the law as it is, and I believe that most of them are very careful not to take risks with their patients' healths. However, many of them have a very limited understanding of the principles of good prescribing of herbal medicines, so that their patients are unlikely to receive the most effective treatment, and may be at increased risk of toxicity for many of the reasons I listed earlier.

I believe that we must establish a minimum requirement for practitioners for the protection and reassurance of patients, and to encourage practitioners to train properly.

My personal preference would be for a standard examination in the principles and practice of Chinese medicine. It could greatly benefit the development of Chinese medicine in this country in a variety of ways. It would enhance the academic status of Chinese medicine, and it would encourage and reward the well-qualified practitioner. Moreover, it would increase the confidence of the public and of the scientific community in Chinese medicine.

Conclusions

For me, it has been exciting to learn of the potential of Chinese herbal medicine, and to undertake controlled trials of a herbal medicine that has proved helpful for atopic eczema. I confess disappointment that others in orthodox medicine have not taken more interest in the potential of Chinese herbal treatments in their own fields of medicine, but there are reasons. The step from seeing apparent benefit in patients treated by a Chinese doctor to embarking on a controlled trial is a big, bold and difficult one. Local ethics committees will want more than anecdotal evidence of effectiveness and safety to permit such trials, and funding is problematic. Furthermore, the motivation of the orthodox practitioner will be limited if the pharmaceutical industry is unlikely to develop a product for wider prescription?

It will be clear to the reader that there are many problems to be faced if Chinese herbal medicine is to be integrated into the front line of modern medicine, but I, for one, would be delighted if this were to happen.

References

Sheehan, M., Atherton, D.J. (1992) A controlled trial of traditional Chinese medicinal plants in widespread non-exudative atopic eczema. *Brit. J. Dermatol.* **126**, 179–184

Sheehan, M.P., Rustin, M.H.A., Atherton, D.J. *et al.* (1992) Efficacy of traditional Chinese herbal therapy in adult atopic dermatitis: results of a double-blind placebo-controlled study. *Lancet* **340**, 13–7

Taylor, N.F., Sheehan, M.P., Dawson, H.A., Atherton, D.J. Lack of glucocorticoid effect of a traditional Chinese herbal decoction used for treatment of atopic eczema (unpublished)

Lomas, D.E., Atherton, D.J. Efficacy of a palatable Chinese herbal medicine for atopic eczema (in preparation)

Acknowledgements

Our research was conducted with the support of grants from the National Eczema Society and the Roger Waters Trust and with the invaluable advice of Dr Luo Ding-Hui.

THE WAY FORWARD FOR CHINESE MEDICINE

Kelvin Chan
Jian-Qian Zou

A Summary of the Present Progress of Chinese Medicine in the West

WORLD-WIDE INTERESTS AND CONCERNS ON THE USE AND PRACTICE OF CHINESE MEDICINE

In the west, the practice of traditional Chinese medicine is comparatively new. As a consequence, substantive clinical practice and
research in the field is fairly limited. Information from Section 2
(Chapters 5 to 13) undoubtedly illustrates the increasing interests and
concerns over the use and practice of Chinese medicine (CM) in the
west among the public of rich developed and developing countries. It
is also obvious that Chinese medicine, in particular the practice of
acupuncture, has been on the top of the list of complementary medicine among those practiced in these countries, but not accepted
officially into the main stream of the healthcare system. On the other
hand in China and Japan as well as some countries and regions in the
east, the use and practice of CM have been included as part of the
healthcare system together with orthodox medicine (OM). Apart from
the difference of tradition, training, regulation as well as culture, there
is also a definite gap in the knowledge of Chinese medicine between
east and west; in particular in the understanding of how CM uses
medicinal plants for treatment.

Both acceptance and skepticism on the usefulness of Chinese medicine (CM) in healthcare exist among orthodox medical practitioners in
the west. In the UK and other developed countries there has been a
rapid growth of interest in complementary and alternative therapies as
a whole and in acupuncture in particular. This interest has lead to
increasing research into acupuncture, but not into Chinese herbal medicine (CHM). Research to date in the UK has been mostly initiated by
practitioners of CM rather than orthodox medical professionals. It is
noteworthy to point out some of the most common concerns shared by

the professionals in the orthodox medical circles in the east and the west (See Chapter 3 and those chapters in Section 2).

THE WESTERN PERSPECTIVE OF CHINESE MEDICINE

Using Chinese medicine (CM) as an example of complementary and alternative therapies, the practice of acupuncture is gaining acceptance in the developed countries while the other equally important part of CM practice, Chinese herbal medicine (CHM) is not widely accepted. Both disciplines are receiving worldwide attention. Since the early 1990s the popularity of CHM products has been increased in the West due mainly to the successful treatment of atopic eczema that was resistant to OM treatment in a double blind controlled clinical trial using the decoction of 10 Chinese herbs (See Chapter 3). Over the last 10 years there has been a steady increase in the number of "clinics" (all private), a recent count of some 3000, of traditional Chinese medicine in the UK (See Chapter 12) and similar increase in numbers in other developed countries. These were not only popular with Chinese residents, but also with the population as a whole. The fact that this number of clinics exists, and that they are paid directly by their patients, bears some witness to the perception of generally beneficial results achieved by patients. Without widespread patient satisfaction, these therapies would not thrive. However it is important to recognise that satisfaction may not reflect safety and efficacy.

Safety and efficacy of acupuncture

Like all complementary and alternative medicine, the absence of a formal system for reporting adverse effects makes it difficult to assess acupuncture's safety in daily treatment of patients. However, it appears to be relatively safe with a low incidence of serious adverse events. An extensive worldwide literature search identified only 193 adverse events (including relatively minor events such as bruising and dizziness) over 15 years. The more serious events were usually related to poor practice. For example, cases of hepatitis B infection typically involved bad hygiene and unregistered practitioners have been reported. A prospective study of over 55,000 acupuncture treatments given in a college for medically trained acupuncturists confirms that acupuncture is probably safe in qualified hands. Only 63, mostly minor, adverse events were identified, and no cases of serious adverse events such as pneumothorax infection, or spinal lesions were reported, although these have been described in the literature (See Part 3 of Chapter 6).

Different concepts of acupuncture among global practising centres

In its original practice for over thousands of years acupuncture has been based on the principles of traditional Chinese medicine. Thus the workings of the human body are controlled by the vital force or energy "*Qi*" that circulates the 12 main meridians that connect the *Zhang Fu* organs. Although some of these organs have the same names (such as *Heart, Liver, Spleen, Lung, Kidney* and *Stomach*), Chinese and orthodox medical concepts of the organs correlate only very loosely. The *Qi* energy must flow in the correct strength and quality through each of the meridians and vital organs to maintain health. The acupuncture points are located along the meridians and provide one means of altering the flow of *Qi*. All traditional acupuncture theory is based on the Daoist concept of balancing *Yin* and *Yang*. Illness is seen in terms of excesses or deficiencies in various exogenous and endogenous pathogenic factors. Treatment is aimed at restoring balance using acupuncture or herbs. Traditional diagnoses often relate to the terms such as "*Kidney-yang deficiency, water overflowing*", "*damp heat in the bladder*", etc.

Since the introduction of acupuncture into the west in the 16th century, the details of practice differ between individual schools that were developed in the west and from those in the east. Many orthodox medical health professionals who practise acupuncture have dispensed or ignored with such concepts, yet results of clinical benefits have also been observed. In the modified western concepts acupuncture points are viewed as those corresponding to physiological and anatomical features such as peripheral nerve junctions, and diagnosis is made in purely orthodox terms. An important concept used by such acupuncturists is that of the "trigger point". It refers to an area of increased sensitivity within a muscle that is said to cause a characteristic pattern of referred pain in a related segment of the body. Even in terms of insurance cover for practising acupuncturists there are a clear and firm distinction between traditional and western acupuncture, but the two categories overlap considerably. Yet the traditional acupuncture originated from ancient China is not a single historically unchangeable therapy as shown by research activities mentioned above (See Part 3 of Chapter 6). Other eastern countries have taken up modifications to form many different schools. For example, Japanese Kampo practitioners differ from Chinese counterparts by using mainly shallow needles. Acupressure, a variant of Chinese medicinal Tuina/massage involving firm pressure on selected traditional CM acupuncture points, is practiced as Shiatsu in Japanese Kampo medicine.

The perceptions on the use of Chinese herbal medicinal (CHM) products in the west

The use of these remedies and medications in the UK, EU and other developed countries poses a number of questions.

- What is known about the quality, safety and efficacy of the CMM used? Recently the Medicines Control Agency has placed a ban on the use, sale and supply of *Aristolochia* species which are used as ingredients of several Chinese herbal prescriptions and medicinal products.
- Do CHM products have to pass through the same strict legislative procedures as pharmaceutical medicines? Nearly all of the Chinese herbal prescriptions and herbs have been "trialed" or used in treating human diseases for thousands of years.
- What is the level of education and training of practitioners of Chinese medicine who diagnose and prescribe CM treatments in the UK and other developed countries? Many of them have been locally trained by private schools whose standard have not been validated officially by any recognised academic or professional body.
- What do UK pharmacists and medical practitioners know about acupuncture and CMM products and are they aware that their patients may be using a dual approach to health-care by indulging in orthodox and Chinese medicine at the same times?
- Why are composite mixtures prescribed in Chinese medicine? The western conventional approach of research and development with clinically effective medicinal plant extracts has been to find out the active principles (chemical compounds) and then isolate, purify and structurally identify the compounds as pure pharmaceutical entities. This approach has not been proven successful to obtain novel compounds from CM herbs and effective according to the Chinese medicine principles (Chan, 1995). Each CM prescription contains the following components: the "Principal" herb (treating the main symptoms of the disease), the "Associate herb" (aiding the principal herb in its action and acting against other symptoms), the "Adjuvant" herb (reinforcing the "Principal" herb and moderating toxicity, and the "Messenger" herb directing activity to a particular site. Not many orthodox medical practitioners or conventionally trained scientists are knowledgeable nor in agreement with this concept.
- How to obtain guaranteed good quality of crude and ready-made CHM products with assured safety and efficacy? A regulatory problem needs solution.

Regulatory viewpoints on Chinese herbal medicinal (CHM) materials and products in the west

CHM products in the UK and other EU countries present a number of problems. Firstly, the exemptions from licensing only apply to products where all the active ingredients are of herbal origin. In other words, products containing for example, inorganic substances or animal parts are not covered by the exemptions and should by law hold product licences. This, however, is not the case in Germany where specific regulations for registration of medications of herbal or natural origins apply under the Commission E guidelines. Other problems arise because some traditionally used CM ingredients are potent plants restricted by existing UK or EU legislation e.g. *Aconitum and Croton species* (see also list of restricted herbs in Chapter 12). In addition, there are concerns about the safety of some CHM products and raw materials and in particular concerns arising from the lack of appropriate quality measures being in place. Lack of adequate authentication coupled with hazardous substitution, use of toxic elements and heavy metals, deliberate addition of synthetic drugs e.g. steroids, and non-steroidal anti-inflammatory drugs (NSAIDs) are well documented in worldwide literature. Specific problems have also occurred in the UK, most notable being the recent two cases of renal failure due to *Aristolochia species* substitution in Mu Tong crude herbs leading to the emergency ban on all *Aristolochia species*. The Regulatory views on quality-related safety concerns may include the followings:

- The lack of adequate authentication (as most control agencies in the west do not have the original crude CHM products for comparison)
- Intentional or accidental inclusion or substitution of orthodox drugs such as antibiotics, NSAIDS and steroids or other herbs
- Use of toxic substances and heavy metals such as arsenic disulphide as in "realgar" and toxic animal materials such as bufo-secretions as in "Chansu" from toads' glands, and
- Inaccurate or inadequate labelling.

In the UK the Medicines Control Agency (MCA) has responsibility to safeguard public health in all areas relating to medicines, licensed and unlicensed. The above particular problems arising with CHM products are under active discussion and MCA is encouraged by the positive response from industry and practitioner groups in the UK. (See chapter 12). One important development has been the extension of the Yellow Card Scheme for report of adverse reactions from orthodox medications to include adverse reactions to unlicensed medicines. Future steps of the MCA will include:

- Reviewing controls of potentially toxic plants
- Considering regulatory options for ensuring that harmful substitutions are avoided
- Consulting importers and practitioners on professional matters relating to CHM products
- Playing an active role in current EU discussions on developing a suitable frame work for herbal medicines
- Deriving schemes to balance consumer choice (unlicensed products) with consumer safety.

Authentication and quality assurance of imported CHM products
The supply of CHM crude substances and manufactured products to the west depends mainly on the integrity of importers and the suppliers in the east. In China, every province has its own authentication centre for herbal materials, which strictly adheres to the Chinese Pharmacopoeia (CP), and hospitals as well as clinics could not use herbs that are not included in the CP. However, in the UK and other developed countries, many species are available that are not included in the CP. There is tremendous variability in the quality of CHM crude materials in the UK; some of them are supplied as adulterated specimens (Yu *et al.*, 1997; Forum, 1999). In response to such difficulties the Royal Botanic Gardens in the UK, is developing an Authentication Centre of Chinese Medicinal Plants for use worldwide. Working with the Institute of Medicinal Plant Development, Beijing, the Centre aims to offer, to a wide audience, an authentication and quality assurance service for all Chinese medicinal herbs on the Western market. In this way the Centre will encourage the use of accurate and high quality herbs only and thereby help improve patient safety. No such quality assurance service is currently available in the west. Working with the recently formed Chinese Medicine Association of Suppliers (CMAS, see Chapter 12), the Centre will ensure the supply of good quality and safe CHM products to the public.

The key role of the Authentication Centre has been to establish facilities for CHM substances and products:

- Herbarium specimens of commonly available CHM crude substances in the western markets
- Catalogues of crude CHM specimens as reference materials

- Anatomical slides
- Chemical profiles
- DNA profiles

The potential users of the service of the Centre include importers/suppliers, manufacturers, regulators, health authorities and the pharmaceutical industry. It is envisaged that other centres of this type may be set up in other developed regions or countries to cope with global demand. The Hong Kong government has suggested the set up as a matter of priority of an International Institute of Chinese Medicine to co-ordinate with expertise existing in China Mainland for the betterment and modernisation in parallel with the proposed actions from the Mainland.

Evidence for patient satisfaction in evaluating the effectiveness and safety of Chinese medicine

As far as many physicians in orthodox medicine in developed countries are concerned, Chinese medicine (CM) has been taken up by the general public without adequate scientific validation to support it. It is imperative that CM is subjected to a much fuller evaluation, which should include primary care studies at clinic level. "Pragmatic" randomised controlled trials (RCTs) using placebo where suitable appear to be essential approaches. Without research, ignorance about the potential benefits of CM will continue. The future development of CM would then remain limited to a small, albeit significant, part of private complementary health care driven purely by public demand rather than sound medical evidence or recommendations. The challenge for those of us engaged in clinical practice in the UK is to encourage clinical research by identifying suitable research partners in mainstream medical research circles and to obtain adequate funds. Primary care studies, which provide pragmatic evidence of efficacy also, have an important role to play. There is an increasing interest within the NHS in directly commissioning CM as part of NHS provision and encouragingly, three quarters of UK doctors think that complementary medicine should be available within the NHS. Public demand is also driving this demand forward and it is very likely that if there is increasing clinical evidence for the use of CM, in particular acupuncture, combined with rigorous cost-benefit analysis, NHS and private purchasing will grow (See Chapters 12 and 20).

Not all complementary therapies can be assessed by randomised controlled trial (RCT) according to orthodox medicinal methodology; such as acupuncture and related disciplines. However good individual case history follow-up with measured outcomes can be used for assessing the efficacy of treatment, provided quality and safety issues are previously considered. It is likely that the general public may not demand objective, scientific evidence of efficacy. Orthodox thinking may not be sufficiently flexible to accept the role of established (but not traditional European) forms of medicine, such as traditional Chinese medicine from outside Europe. Nevertheless the general public should be informed of the importance of the scientific value of the treatment, even for those involving some elements of psychology.

Limited available research funding for Chinese medicine

It has been a problem in the developed countries that there have been insufficient well-controlled clinical studies on complementary medicine, and this should be remedied. The former negative findings of the British Medical Association (BMA, 1986) survey on complementary medicine in 1986 did not help to persuade funding councils to support research in this area. The more recent BMA (1993) report on complementary medicine did identify certain contributions of complementary medicine to healthcare and did encourage the funding of evidence-based complementary medicine practice. In recent years, the Medical Research Council in the UK and the Office of Alternative Medicine under the umbrella of the National Institute of Health in the USA have certainly supported a variety of research programmes in complementary medicine based on good quality design. There should be a trend to increase funding along this direction to investigate the safety and efficacy of complementary medicine treatments.

Training of professionals in Chinese medicine in the west

If there is the desire to use Chinese medicine in the healthcare system in any developed countries there should be training courses that produce practitioners of Chinese medicine of good quality and professionalism to safeguard the public interest and their health. This is to check on those who jump onto the band wagon and to eliminate "cow-boy" practice. In most European countries the interest groups of acupuncture and CM herbalism started more formal training of CM on the initial running of and updating of seminars. The earliest group seminars were run during the late 1950s and early 1960s. In recent years, many of the established acupuncture colleges in the UK (also in Australia and the USA) have introduced courses in CM herbalism. Most of these institutes run part-time courses, mainly in the evenings and weekends, of varying lengths of duration with certificates and diplomas on graduation (Jin, *et al.*, 1995). In at least some cases these courses are rather brief, despite the fact that their graduates face different legislative and professional responsibilities as prescribers of active medications (See Chapters 12 and 16 for details). Such courses may not be of the right level compared to those in the east. In the past few years, several new universities have expanded their academic courses in Australia, Hong Kong and the UK to cope with the increasing demand of training professionals and practitioners in Chinese medicine in conjunction with established universities in China (See Chapters 10, 13 and 16 respectively).

In the west there is also an urgent need of professionals who are trained in plant identification and authentication in order to ensure quality control of the raw materials used in herbal medicines in general and Chinese herbs in particular as these materials are mainly imported. There are very few academic centres that provide this training. However, centres of excellence in pharmacognosy are available within some schools of pharmacy that provide such training and undertake research. In the Kotzting TCM Klinik in Germany university experts are working with hospital for such purposes (See Chapter 5). Collaboration should be initiated between institutes in UK and other developed countries with those in China or Far East where active research in CHM products are focused.

Patients may be at risk from a delay in seeking medical advice for a serious medical condition that is not appropriately treated by complementary therapies. Therefore the practitioner should recognise the need of knowledge in both Chinese medicine and orthodox medical practice. Professionalism and regulations are needed to protect the public.

Demand of Modernisation of Chinese Medicine by the Chinese Government

SOME BACKGROUND INFORMATION ON MODERNISATION OF CHINESE MEDICINE

The practice of Chinese medicine, co-existing with orthodox medicine introduced in the early 1900s, in China has never been stopped throughout the history of the development of healthcare in China. However the improvement of this form of healthcare has not been keeping pace with the advance in science and technology and that of orthodox medicine. The recent increase of interests and concerns of CM practice in the west has indirectly hastened and induced the already planned national decision to implement the "Plan of Modernization of Chinese Medicine". This decision has helped to cope with the increasing demand of good quality crude materials and finished products. The recent "Plan" proposed in general by 15 ministries in China, was led by the Ministry of Science and Technology, jointly with the Ministry of Health, the State Administration of Traditional Chinese Medicine (SATCM), the State Drug Administration (SDA), National Foundation Committee of Nature Science and so on.

The aims of the Plan have mainly been to modernise and internationalise various aspects of Chinese medicine based on inheriting and carrying forward the advantages and distinguishing features of the traditional system of healthcare. The Plan will fully utilise the methodology and measures of modern sciences, draw lessons and experiences from international standards and regulations on materia medica, in order to develop Chinese herbal products that can compete and enter the international medicinal markets. The Plan started in 1995 and aimed to increase the share of the world market from the then 3% to 15% in 10 to 15 years' time. Other areas of modernisation include:

- Provision of training programmes of various CM professionals to strengthening the modernisation programmes
- Linking with overseas universities for the development of training courses and degrees programmes, and research collaboration for Chinese medicine
- Development of the frame work for harmonisation of regulations for control of registration of Chinese herbal medicines, including all aspects of "Good Practices" such as GAP, GLP, GMP and GCTP for Chinese medicines
- Establishing key national institutes and high quality corporations for co-ordinating the national development and modernisation of all aspects of Chinese medicine, including practice and research of acupuncture.

ACTION PLAN FOR THE MODERNISATION OF CHINESE MEDICINE

To implement the modernisation plan nationwide efforts have been called upon. An International Symposium on the Modernisation of Traditional Chinese Medicine was held in Nanjing on 10 to 12 July 1998 Key officials from the 15 ministries gave their viewpoints and plans. Overseas Chinese nationals contributed with positive approaches and ideas. The following points summarise some of the plans for action and implementation.

Policy on research and development of Chinese herbal products to cope with the market-needed (Zou, 1998)

- Screen and evaluate herbal products from good assortments of Chinese herbal prescriptions or formulae in response to disease-directed needs.
- Explore the theory and methodology suitable for developing Fu-Fang (herbal composite prescriptions)
- Concentrate on application of CM theory in developing Fu-Fang formulation products
- Develop Fu-Fang dosage forms following earlier attempts, in order to obtain quality CHM medications with efficacy, stability and good quality. It has been aimed to provide products with "3 Efficiencies" (efficiency in potency, efficiency in rapid onset of actions and efficiency in appropriate duration); "3 Lows" (low in dosage, low in toxicity and low in side-effects), and "3 Eases" (easy to save, easy to take along and easy to use).
- Apply modern technology used for orthodox pharmaceuticals in the R & D of dosage forms development of Chinese herbal products. It should be mentioned that the new dosage forms should be in keeping with the characteristics of Chinese herbal products.

Establishing framework structures for research and development of Chinese herbal products

- Absorb the advantages of modern physical, chemical, and computer sciences and information in order to set up efficient, accurate and rapid methodologies for the isolation of effective components from Chinese crude herbs.
- Establish standardised laboratory models for evaluating methodologies and providing indices suitable for pharmacological screening of Chinese medicinal plants.
- Emphasise the development, protection, and cultivation of Chinese medicinal plants by implementing GAP.
- Explore and strengthen the theoretical and methodological research on Chinese herbal toxicology.
- Strengthen the research on processing of crude Chinese medicinal plants,

- Develop the methodology for quality control on Chinese medicinal plant materials and manufactured products by setting up good practices guidelines such as GAP, GLP, GMP and GCTP that should be adapted for manufacturing of Chinese herbal medicinal products,
- Establish the evolution systems on the overall quality assurance of Chinese herbal medicinal products, which include national screening, standardisation centres, GMP centres and GCTP centres on Chinese herbal products,
- Set up information Internet system on Chinese Medicine, by making use the KDD (Knowledge of Database Discovery), pattern recognition for medicinal plant extracts for identification and quality assurance. etc.

Establishing technology for modern Chinese herbal industries
- Modernise productive technology of Chinese herbal products.
- Apply modern biotechnology in production and cultivation of Chinese herbs.
- Engineer automatic systems for processing of Chinese herbal materials.
- Renew and update equipment and apparatus in processing of Chinese herbal materials and products in accordance with GMP.
- Standardise the procedures for quality assurance of Chinese herbal products. Chinese herbal products contain complex components. It is important to establish the internationally acceptable quality control standards suitable for Chinese herbal products (Zhou, 1998).
- Set up internationally acceptable quality control standards on presence of heavy metals and pesticides in Chinese herbal products

Promoting Chinese herbal products into international markets for medicinal products
- Strengthen the protection of intellectual property of Chinese herbal products.
- Elevate the level of patent on Chinese herbal medicines by protecting the interest of technology and formulation know-how on Chinese herbal products.
- Strengthen international exchange and co-operation by launching international links with various academic institutes and government bodies for information exchange.

- Encourage co-operations in setting up joint research projects on R & D of product development on Chinese herbal products,
- Compile standard CM terminology in various foreign languages for the promotion of knowledge exchange
- Updating analytical information in monographs of herbal materials included the Chinese Pharmacopoeia to cope with new analytical technology such as finger-printings and pattern recognition for herbal extracts (Wang, *et al.*, 1998)
- Promote the formation of Trans-national Corporation on national herbal industries.

Promoting international academic exchange in training professionals of Chinese medicine

In view of the fast development of various schools of Chinese medicine (both acupuncture and Chinese Herbal Medicine) in the west the State Administration of TCM and other appropriate ministries in China have launched joint training and educational programmes. This approach aims to raise the standard and quality of CM practitioners and other related scientists and technicians in Chinese herbal products. Indirectly this helps to build linking bridges between east and west for better understanding of the principles of Chinese medicine.

The Way Forward for Chinese Medicine

There is great potential and scope to make good use of Chinese medicine for primary healthcare within orthodox medical practice in the west. The integration of Chinese medicine with orthodox medicine in China, Japan and other countries in the east has set some positive examples. The uncertainty in the west about usefulness of Chinese herbal medicine has been due mainly to lack of understanding of what Chinese medicine is, the practice by unqualified CM practitioners, the supply of fake herbs and adulterated herbal products. On the other hand when one judges the usefulness of Chinese medicine in terms of orthodox medical approaches there is a lack of randomised controlled trials that are considered acceptable. Acupuncture has been demonstrated to be useful in several clinical situations as practised by orthodox medical practitioners not following Chinese medicine principles. The following suggestions and observations will serve as future guidelines on how to make good use of Chinese medicine for healthcare.

SOME THOUGHTS FOR THE WAY FORWARD OF ACUPUNCTURE

Global therapeutic range of acupuncture

This traditional therapy has puzzled the orthodox medical fields in therapies that conventional medicine has not been successful. Many patients requested acupuncture therapy and related Chinese medicine treatments as their last hope for cure and comfort (See Chapters 5 and 12). Acupuncture has been developed as a relatively global system of medicine. Some western texts refer it to treating diarrhoea, the common cold, and tinnitus. In Europe and North America (See relevant Chapters in Section 3) acupuncture is used to treat benign chronic diseases and musculo-skeletal injury. Other common complaints, found in survey, include anxiety, arthritis, asthma, back pain, digestive disorders, fatigue, hay fever, impotency, menstrual disorders and irritable bowel diseases. It is also used in the treatment of drug and alcohol rehabilitation (particularly in the USA) and HIV (See Chapter 6).

Global research activities in acupuncture

Globally there is also good scientific research evidence that acupuncture has effects greater than placebo. Randomised controlled trials (RCT) have found that true acupuncture is more effective in pain relief than a "sham" point technique (inserting needles away from the true acupuncture points). Numerous studies of acupuncture relieving nausea (a condition often refered to as placebo effect) show that stimulating the true acupuncture points is more effective than that stimulating the false points. Experimental studies showing that acupuncture can affect and anaesthetised animals and give evidence that its positive effects cannot be interpreted as purely psychological influence.

It is less clear whether acupuncture has clinically important benefits in the conditions for which it is typically used. Clinical research evidence comes mainly from hospital-based situations of acute conditions such as post-operative pains rather than those from chronic conditions in primary care. Most trials in these areas have had small numbers of patients and only short-term follow up. Evidence from several RCTs supports the use of acupuncture in some chronic pain conditions such as migraine, headache and postoperative pain. Some RCTs showed acupuncture is effective in treating substance misuse, nausea, and stroke while conflicting results are observed in asthma and hay fever. Acupuncture may not be effective for stopping smoking, tinnitus, and obesity. Very little reliable information is available on the relative effectiveness of various orthodox and traditional forms of acupuncture.

Education, training, professionalism and regulation

There is divergence in the education and training aspects, the professionalism required and the practice of acupuncture in the west and
China. Acupuncture is considered as part of Chinese medicine (CM) in
China. As a whole, CM can be practised as integrated discipline with
OM, while acupuncture can only be practised as a separate medical
tool under the orthodox medical treatment in the west. Plenty of work
will be needed to reach a harmonised agreement in the recognition of
professional standards and treatment safety.

THE REQUIREMENT OF BALANCED REGULATION AND QUALITY IN PRACTICE OF CHINESE MEDICINE

Organisations such as the Foundation for Integrated Health have
clearly stated the need for further research in complementary medicine.
Many patients have benefited from treatment with acupuncture and
Chinese herbal medicine. To maximise these benefits and reduce risks
requires balanced regulation and good practice.

Regulation and risk

In the west the uncertainty of how Chinese herbal medicine works,
whether it is safe and of good quality and the incidents of adverse
effects of substituted herbs has urged the authority in the UK to ban
use of certain Chinese herbal medicinal (CHM) products. Thus there is
a need for regulation on the quality assurance of both practitioners and
products-related treatment involving herbal products for medicinal
uses as those practised in China (See Chapter 11). In the case of
Chinese herbal medicinal products in the UK nearly all of them are
imported. Some are "manufactured" by small herbal firms from
imported dried granules. They are crude herbs and ready-made products of well-used prescription products. Quality assurance and control
of these have been loose and unsatisfactory. They arrive on the UK
market probably as food or nutritional category. There is a lack of
expertise in the professional aspects of checking the identity of them.
Language problem is another aspect (herbal ingredients are supplied
with similarly named substitutes that could be toxic). Appropriate regulations may help to sort out problems on the quality assurance and
control side (See Chapter 16).

One way of giving guidelines for regulation is to spell out monographic
control of herbs and herbal products imported. For some herbs used in
the EU there are monographs issued for all of them in common use. The

Commission E in Germany has produced standard monographs for controlling herbal medicines. The European Scientific Co-operation on Phytotherapy (ESCOP) has commissioned the writing of standards for 50 European herbs. With quality of herbal medicinal products assured the efficacy of them can be assessed by RCT before licenses can be issued. The drawback of such procedures will (certainly single out "cow-boy" practice) discourage manufacturers to register their products as medicines due to the high cost for getting the licences. A suitable approach should be developed without compromising the issue on quality, efficacy and safety of these products (See Chapter 16).

SAFETY ISSUES AND CONTROL ON PRACTICE

Chinese herbal medicinal (CHM) products may be unsafe in a number of ways if they are handled by unqualified practitioners. Products may be unsafe because they are supplied with impure, contaminated, adulterated or non-authentic materials. Concerning purity, over the years a number of herbal products have been found to contain contaminants such as pesticides and heavy metals. CHM preparations for dermatological conditions to which steroids were added may create potential for longer-term toxicity on chronic use. It is noted that substituting one herbal ingredient with another reputedly having similar medicinal properties (even though it may be botanically unrelated), or adulteration of prescribed herbs will cause concerns relating to toxicity (See Chapter 16). Such "cowboy" practice will certainly make assessment of the usefulness of CM rather difficult.

RESEARCH DIRECTIONS USEFUL FOR CHINESE MEDICINE DEVELOPMENT

A new approach for pre-clinical screening of crude CHM extracts

Due to the out-cry over toxicity, poor quality and adulteration of ready made herbal medicinal products in the market the priority of research on products-related treatment, in particular herbal product, is to ensure quality, efficacy, and safety of the end products used by patients. In the majority of the cases, the biologically active chemical compounds of these products are unknown even other known chemical entities are isolated. It has also been shown that single compounds isolated from organic solvents are either too toxic or with no activities. Most traditional medicinal herbs are used as aqueous decoctions. Therefore research projects should be directed towards the development of analytical, bio-activity and toxicological patterns of the herbal extracts (decoctions) for quality assurance and control purposes. These data can be in-put, as characteristic patterns or finger-printings, to the computer program that utilises fuzzy logic, pattern-recognition or neural network computing techniques (Chan 1995). The computer program is trained to recognise the characteristic and specific for each decoction or extract, chemical/analytical (a measure of quality), bio-activity (a measure of efficacy and quality) and toxicological (a measure of safety) patterns or finger-printings of the CHM extract. After a series of "training set" inputs of the authenticated aqueous herbal extract, from single herbs or mixtures of herbs, a "standard" pattern is obtained and can be used as the reference guide for subsequent assessment. This type of approach will generate patterns as standard reference for quality assurance and control purposes. The generated patterns can also be further used for prediction and recognition purposes when searching purer active fractions or single chemical entities from the extract. If the final active CHM product resulting from the crude decoction is submitted for regulatory licensing purposes the finger printings or patterns of the initial extract and that of the final product can be used as the reference standards required by the licensing authority.

Randomised controlled trial for CHM products

To carry out evidence-based research on product-related treatment using orthodox medical research tools will be the logical approach to prove the efficacy of Chinese herbal medicinal (CHM) products. This is because there is no available methodology that is recognised as unbiased measure for assessing the efficacy of medications. However in some of the CM practice, such as that of acupuncture where placebo procedure is not convenient, randomised controlled trials (RCTs) approach may not be applicable. In these cases a well-designed case-study concept is acceptable, provided the trial products have reproducible quality. The preparation of placebo samples for RCTs of (CHM) product is also problematic. Research in this area requires development.

Researching and documenting interactions between CHM products and orthodox drugs

Research on the beneficial and adverse interactions between herbal medicinal products and orthodox drugs should be supported as most patients would be exposed to these treatments either knowingly or unknowingly (accidentally) during their course of illnesses. Knowing the potentiating or adverse effects from the interactions the safety of co-medication of two treatments can be assessed. Proper documentation of these types of clinical data should be encouraged (Chan & Cheung, 2000) The integrated approach in making good use of CM offers potentially useful opportunity to utilise the beneficial interactions between CHM products and orthodox drugs (Chan & Cheung, 2000). The adverse or beneficial effects of combined CM and OM treatments using orthodox therapies and other CM therapies such as acupuncture *qigong, tuina* should also be documented.

REGULATIONS PROVIDING PROTECTION WITHOUT UNDULY RESTRICTING PATIENT CHOICE

All Chinese herbal medicinal (CHM) products when supplied as medications should be licensed for safety, quality and for appropriate evidence of efficacy. It advocates the establishment of a new category of licensed herbal medicines, prepared in accordance with current Good Manufacturing Practice (cGMP), which meet standards for safety and quality, and which are regulated by the Regulators in the countries concerned.

The licensing requirements of this new category with cGMP approval may not be as demanding as those currently apply to licensed pharmaceutical medicines. Specifically, the "level of proof" of activity may not need to be as high as for allopathic medicines. Efficacy may be accepted on the basis of documentation of traditional use over a long period.

Safety may deem to have been demonstrated by virtue of traditional use. However, these products ought to be required to substantiate a history of safe use, as in the EU for the dosage and indications to be approved, and the license should clearly indicate the inappropriate conditions of use (contra-indications). It would be dangerous to agree product safety as the basic, default position. In addition, the "test of time" criterion detects common acute adverse events, but not rare adverse events or those with a long latency. Also, today's users of herbal remedies may differ from those in earlier eras.

The governmental departments in China, such as State Administration of Traditional Medicine and the State Drug Administration, issue regulations and registration guidelines and procedures for herbal medicinal products originated from Chinese medicine R & D. Consultation with these guidelines will help to set up regulations in the UK or other developed countries. Consultation of the Commission E structure from Germany will also help to formulate regulatory guidelines for herbal products as medicines.

It will be most useful and appropriate in the near future to set up an international organisation for the formulation of *international harmonisation* of regulations for registration of Chinese herbal medicinal products and on the qualification of CM practitioners.

THE ADVANTAGE OF INTEGRATION OF CHINESE MEDICINE INTO MAINSTREAM HEALTHCARE

The example of practising integration medicine by combining Chinese medicine (CM) and orthodox medicine (OM) in China (See Chapter 11) and other regions in the Far East can be used to assess the situation developed countries where CM practice exists. Guidelines should be set to ensure adequate quality and availability of practitioners and treatment methods for implementation. Evidence-based assessment should be the minimal requirement for inclusion of CM into the OM main stream practice.

The German experience

The practice of integrated CM and OM in a well-established private TCM hospital in Kotzting, near Munich in Germany, since 1991 has been a success example of integrated practice. Crude CHM materials and products imported from China, are authenticated and quality-controlled by Phytochemists at the Dusseldorf University Department of Pharmacognosy and that of Munich University under the direction of Prof. Bauer and Prof. Wagner respectively. CM practitioners are qualified from Beijing University of TCM. Patients who fail to get cure from orthodox medicine are admitted to the hospital for treatment with CM therapies (such as acupuncture, *Tuina*, *Qigong* and CM herbs) only as a last attempt for medical treatment. All patients are diagnosed by CM method and OM procedure before and after treatment period. Several studies have been carried out on the efficacy and safety of the CM treatment in the hospital. Success rate has been impressive (See Chapter 5 for details).

If there is evidence showing benefits of integrating complementary medicine into orthodox treatment it should be allowed for patient care. Treatment of some diseases such as atopic eczema, strokes, some rheumatic diseases has not been successfully cured by orthodox medicine. These chronic illnesses have been referred to Chinese medicine practitioners legally or illegally for treatment with considerable success. Some aspects of the success have been noted for treatment of skin diseases that are resistant to orthodox medications. Some private proper CM acupuncture clinics with the aid of CM herbal proscriptions show successful cases of treating irritable bowl syndromes that OM has fail to help (See Chapter 7).

The NHS experience in the UK

In an UK National Health Service (NHS) environment at the South Western Hospital in Brixton the use of CM has been successful for treatment of pain, drug dependence and strokes. This Gateway Clinic has been set up since 1983 by a Physiotherapist who became, after subsequent training in the UK and China, a CM practitioner. The Gateway Clinic is a NHS clinic with very little financial support. The Clinic is styled on the "open plan Chinese Medicine Clinic" as seen practised in China; with a large community space where people are all treated as equals together. In this open public forum Chinese medicine is seen for what it is and the results, or failures, or reactions, are in full view. Obviously over the years there have been orthodox medical practitioners, nursing professionals, and physiotherapists and administers who maintain strong opinion and refuse to recognise the evidence of the work being done. As time passes the political climate has had to find new innovations and methods of working, as the allopathic model is too costly and hazardous, incomplete and unpopular. The CM practitioner has commented that there is the need for a Gateway Clinic in every hospital in the U K and it will probably happen in the near future. The general public has welcomed the friendly and sincere attitude and the natural flow of Chinese medicine, particularly as the results have been good. All clients have benefit on some level or another and many have resolved their health issues completely and gone on to learn the Chinese systems of longevity such as *Qi Gong, Tai Chi*, meditation and food therapy etc.

The Hospital Authority is now acknowledging these achievements and is at present developing strategies to utilise these skills to obtain more financial resources to further develop the service. This year the Gateway service has been accepted into the main stream HIV Budget and so its future is more secure than before. Previously the "survival" budget had to be bid on an annual basis (See Chapter 6 for detail).

Training and professionalism in Chinese medicine

The use and practice of CM in China and other regions and countries in the east have been established. However, modernisation and improvement will be needed to make better use of this traditional medical practice for complementing and co-existing with well-advanced orthodox medicine. Implementing and up keeping of existing regulations for both practitioners and product-related treatment is also needed to safeguard the quality of CM for providing and improving healthcare of the population.

In the west in order to be recognised and accepted into practice in healthcare as part of the medical and health professional team, the CM practitioners have to be able to demonstrate their competence of practice and level of their training. The demonstration of profession-alism requires a concerted effort of those who are practising various roles of Chinese medicine. Professional organisations apart from self-regulating their membership (See Chapter 16 for examples from the UK) should be able to demonstrate their working ethics and profes-sionalism in order to obtain national and international recognition by aiming at:

- Maintaining and developing educational standards
- Continuing professional development and modernisation
- Being familiar with oriental affairs (improving linking via transla-tion and culture information)
- Keeping with development of ethics and safety issues
- Being aware of research & development in Chinese medicine as well as those in orthodox practice
- Liaising with government regulation agency for better service
- Helping to develop monographs or formulary of CHM products for local use

BUILDING LINKS BETWEEN EAST AND WEST

The way forward to make better use of Chinese medicine for health-care of the public in a global situation will require tremendous efforts from professionals and health officials in China where Chinese medi-cine originated and those from countries where Chinese medicine is practised. Both east and west have to work closely together to get the right approach for professionalism, regulatory issues for control of quality of practitioners, Chinese herbal medicines and other treatment related therapies. It is not the responsibility of one country to see to the implementation of efficacy, safety and quality of Chinese medicine. The areas for building bridges can be summarised as follows:

- International development for regulation on authentication of Chinese medicinal plants
- Dialogue between regulatory bodies from Chinese regulatory authorities and those from other countries
- Control of quality of import and export of CHM substances
- Co-ordination of Good Agricultural Practice of CHM materials to avoid extinction of endangered species
- Development of methodology for assessment of efficacy of CHM products
- Development of regulatory issues for the international harmonisation of setting monographs for CHM materials and products (Zhang, 1998)

There is great potential for Chinese medicine to make contribution for better healthcare in developed countries where the public is cared for by orthodox medical practice. The integration of CM into OM in China has set positive examples. In order to make better use of CM there is a need to demonstrate the efficacy, quality and safety of the discipline in the west. Modernisation of CM in China can help to make better understanding of the discipline. The development of proper education and training courses for CM in the west and regulatory control over professional qualification and treatment products will be the way forward for Chinese medicine.

References

British Medical Association Report (1986) Alternative Therapy: Report of the Board of Science & Education, London, British Medical Association.

British Medical Association Report (1993) Complementary Medicine: new approaches to good practice. Oxford University Press: Oxford.

Chan, K. (1995) Progress of Traditional Chinese Medicine, *Trends in Pharmacological Sciences*, **16**, 182–187.

Chan, K. and Cheung, L. (2000) Interactions between Chinese Herbal Medicinal Products and Orthodox Drugs, Harwood Academic Publishers, Amsterdam, June 2000, in printing preparation.

Forum (1999) Symposium on Traditional Chinese medicine, organised by the Pharmaceutical Science Group of RPSGB and Middlesex University, 26 to 27 October, 1999, *Pharmaceutical Journal*, **263**, 796–798.

Jin, Y., Berry, M.I. and Chan, K. (1995) Chinese herbal medicine in the United Kingdom. *Pharmaceutical Journal*, **255** (**Suppl**), R37.

Wang, X.M., Xue, Y., Zhou, T.-H. and Takeo, S. (1998) Characterisation of Traditional Chinese Medicine by Liquid Chromatography/Atmospheric Pressure Ionisation Mass Spectrosmetry. *In: Proceedings of the International Symposium on the modernisation of Traditional Chinese Medicine.* 10 to 12 July 1998, Nanjing, China, p. 93–103.

Yu, H., Berry, M.I., Zhong, S. and Chan, K. (1997) Pharmacognostical investigations on traditional Chinese medicinal herbs: Identification of six herbs from the UK market. *Journal of Pharmacy & Pharmacology*, **49** (**Suppl 4**), 114.

Zhang, K. (1998) Some aspects and suggestions of establishing an ICH for Chinese medicinal herbs. *In: Proceedings of the International Symposium on the modernisation of Traditional Chinese Medicine.* 10 to 12 July 1998, Nanjing, China, p. 49–50.

Zhou Hai-Jun (1998) Some Aspects of Standardisation of medicinal plants source materials *In: Proceedings of the International Symposium on the modernisation of Traditional Chinese Medicine.* 10 to 12 July 1998, Nanjing, China, p. 38–39.

Zou Jian-Qian (1998) Research into Pathways for the Modernisation of Chinese Medicine. *In: Proceedings of the International Symposium on the modernisation of Traditional Chinese Medicine.* 10 to 12 July 1998, Nanjing, China, p. 6–24.

Index

Note; page numbers in *italics* refer to figures and tables